Robert Koch and
American Bacteriology

ALSO BY RICHARD ADLER
AND FROM MCFARLAND

*Victor Vaughan: A Biography of the Pioneering
Bacteriologist, 1851–1929* (2015)

Cholera in Detroit: A History (2013)

Mack, McGraw and the 1913 Baseball Season (2008)

BY RICHARD ADLER AND ELISE MARA

Typhoid Fever: A History (2016)

Robert Koch and American Bacteriology

RICHARD ADLER

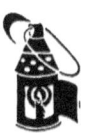

McFarland & Company, Inc., Publishers
Jefferson, North Carolina

LIBRARY OF CONGRESS CATALOGUING-IN-PUBLICATION DATA

Names: Adler, Rich, author.
Title: Robert Koch and American bacteriology / Richard Adler.
Description: Jefferson, North Carolina : McFarland & Company, Inc., Publishers, 2016. | Includes bibliographical references and index.
Identifiers: LCCN 2016041677 | ISBN 9781476662596 (softcover : acid free paper) ∞
Subjects: LCSH: Koch, Robert, 1843–1910. | Microbiologists—Germany—Biography.
Classification: LCC QR31.K6 A35 2016 | DDC 579.092 B—dc23
LC record available at https://lccn.loc.gov/2016041677

BRITISH LIBRARY CATALOGUING DATA ARE AVAILABLE

ISBN (print) 978-1-4766-6259-6
ISBN (ebook) 978-1-4766-2705-2

© 2016 Richard Adler. All rights reserved

No part of this book may be reproduced or transmitted in any form or by any means, electronic or mechanical, including photocopying or recording, or by any information storage and retrieval system, without permission in writing from the publisher.

Front cover illustration of Robert Koch © 2016 iStock

Printed in the United States of America

*McFarland & Company, Inc., Publishers
  Box 611, Jefferson, North Carolina 28640
  www.mcfarlandpub.com*

Table of Contents

Preface 1

Introduction 5

1. Robert Koch: His Life and Role in Bacteriological Research 13
2. Germ Theory of Disease: Origins of Bacteriology 32
3. Bacteriology in 19th Century United States 53
4. The Cartwright Lecture: Belfield vs. Formad 70
5. Training with Koch 91
6. Theophil Mitchell Prudden 105
7. William Henry Welch 126
8. Edward Oram Shakespeare 152
9. Harold Clarence Ernst 168
10. Victor Vaughan and Frederick Novy 174
11. Lydia Rabinowitsch-Kempner 199
12. American Bacteriology After Koch 214

Chapter Notes 221
Bibliography 236
Index 241

Preface

My book *Victor Vaughan: A Biography of the Pioneering Bacteriologist* (2015) told how Vaughan, shortly to be appointed dean of the medical school in Ann Arbor, and a colleague and student, Frederick Novy, traveled to Germany during the 1880s for training under the auspices of Robert Koch in the then nascent field of bacteriology.[1] That Vaughan and Novy went to Germany for developing such expertise, rather than receiving training in laboratories closer to Michigan where they lived and worked, was not unusual for the times. Despite the inconvenience, and cost, numerous physicians and bacteriologists—the two fields, as a rule, being found within the same individual—recognized the training they would receive in German laboratories far exceeded anything they were likely to obtain in the United States. This was certainly the case for bacteriology; this was equally true in nearly all fields of medicine. For that reason, this book can be viewed as a prequel to the Vaughan biography, a description of Koch's research and laboratory and the attraction these had for those American students interested in learning about this newly developing field.

The history of medicine is among my professional interests, and in reading over the years the biographies of many of the American pioneers in that field, I was struck by how common such training in the German school of thought had become by the 1880s. The same tradition of European study had, in fact, developed much earlier in that century, the difference being that prior to the 1850s, Americans largely traveled to France—primarily Paris—for such training. Of course bacteriology as a distinct discipline had not yet appeared during that period.

My own schooling and professional work has been in the field of bacteriology, now termed microbiology in an effort to encompass all fields of microscopic organisms. When dealing with my own students, either in a classroom or laboratory, I expect them not only to understand and apply the common terminology used in this discipline, but to have some knowledge of their origins. A significant proportion of the methodology and terminology produced in that field originated with German researchers, and much of that from the research carried out in the laboratories of Koch, his students and his colleagues. One could make the argument that a "perk" for any writer, about any subject, is that the research carried out on that subject not only provides gist for the publication, but also imparts knowledge to the writer him or herself. In my case, I have been fortunate in learning the origin of many of the medical terms which are now second-nature in the field, as well as the experimentation, and controversies, associated with that early work—historical contexts which are rarely addressed in today's science books.

One could make the argument that much of the most important scientific research, not only in medicine and bacteriology, but science in general between the 1870s and 1914, was carried out in Germany and the German speaking areas of Europe such as portions of Austria.[2] The "Golden Age of Bacteriology," as historians often refer to this period, only ended in Germany with the political and military self-destruction of that country in the years that followed. There were exceptions, of course. France remained a secondary destination for a generation of students, particularly from America, motivated in part by the research carried out at the Pasteur Institute under the guidance of Louis Pasteur.

The question, in part, is how did Germany by the 1870s and 1880s surpass France in becoming the center of research in the new field of bacteriology? And what part did Robert Koch play? Some answers apply even in our own time. Support of the sciences by the German government, both in terms of providing research laboratories and the funding of work in those laboratories, played a key role. The more liberal attitude of the medical establishment, as in the use of cadavers for study, played an important role as well. This was particularly true after the formation of the German Empire following the victory in the Franco-Prussian War in 1871. Beginning in the late 1870s, Koch was the recipient of much of that support, and would remain such nearly until his death. Both of these examples—governmental support and availability of cadavers for medical studies—illustrate key differences with the level of support then found in the United States. A more detailed discussion of this subject is provided in the introduction.

As we attempted to carry out in previous books addressing the broad topic of medical history, I have tried to provide a contemporary feeling to the work which is described. One method of doing so is to utilize direct quotations from the principles, both in their own scientific writing as well as that of their contemporaries; consequently, significant portions of the book include those direct quotations. Robert Koch, whose work represents the underlying theme in this book, was often the target of what today would be considered unprofessional barbs. Occasionally this was the result of nationalism, as was the often the situation with Louis Pasteur of France, and sometimes the result of personal disagreements, as with Henry Formad of the United States, or even Koch's own colleague Max von Pettenkofer. Criticism was sometimes humorous, as seen with some of the comments or discussions included in this book. While much of the book is written for the reader with at least a casual interest in medical history, portions do include more detailed descriptions of contemporary research. I have attempted to include definitions or clarification for those less familiar with the terms or topics being discussed on those pages. Abridged biographies of American physicians or others carrying out research in the field of bacteriology represent much of the second half of the book. Most had at least one aspect of their careers in common: they spent time studying either directly with Koch, or with his students. I have attempted to discuss the impact that was to have on their own respective careers in that field.

Allow me to acknowledge those who helped provide information and expertise for this book: the Office of Research and Sponsored Programs on the University of Michigan–Dearborn campus for providing funds in support of this work. Archivists and personnel at various libraries patiently searched for information and questions which I posed: Margaret Graham from the Legacy Center, College of Medicine at Drexel University, the staff of the Bentley Historical Library at the University of Michigan; the staff of the research library at the University of Pennsylvania; Doug Atkins, National Institutes of Health, National Library of Medicine; Beth Lander, College Librarian, Historical Medical Library, the College of Physicians of Philadelphia; and Elise Mara, a former student, colleague and co-author on the book *Typhoid Fever: A History*.

And of course the members of my family who have provided help when needed: my wife, Sally Adler, and my daughter, Rose Adler.

Introduction

A portion of David McCullough's *The Greater Journey: Americans in Paris* (2011) briefly described the work carried out by aspiring American physicians in Paris during the 1830s, particularly at the École de Médecine, and largely under the tutelage of Pierre-Charles-Alexandre Louis. Louis' more prominent American students included Oliver Wendell Holmes, Sr., an early proponent of proper obstetric hygiene as a means to prevent puerperal fever, Henry Bowditch, known more for his views on abolition but a reformer in the area of public health in Massachusetts, and James Jackson, Jr., one of Louis' most promising students, but a victim of typhoid fever upon his return to Boston. Traveling to France for a proper medical education during this period—the first half of the 19th century—was hardly unusual for those who could afford such "advantages." Medical schools in the United States, and for that matter training in any aspect of the medical field, could be charitably described as abysmal. During this period fewer than twenty-five medical schools existed in the entire United States, with few truly worthy of that designation. Faculty generally consisted of five or six men—no women could yet call themselves a physician—and training was minimal.[1] Faculty were often paid, not by the college, but directly by the students enrolled in their courses. The quality of the teaching was often irrelevant; the more popular and entertaining the instructor, the greater the number of students he might train. Most of those who practiced medicine did not even attend any of these schools; they often earned their title through apprenticing with an older "doctor." France, of course, was not the only destination—England, and institutions in the larger European cities like Vienna and Berlin, were alternative destinations. But it was Paris which had the greatest attraction during these years.

The European destination for American students wishing to train in a medical specialty began to change during the latter third of that century. The quality of French schools began a slow decline, only to be replaced by the rapid development of German teaching and research. Several factors contributed to this transformation, and are briefly outlined in this introduction. A more detailed discussion is presented in the first several chapters. During this same period—the 1870s through the end of the century—an additional revolutionary change was taking place in the medical field: the germ theory of disease, the concept that illness was often the result of infection by a microscopic agent, a bacterium or a virus.[2]

Bacteriology as a discipline barely existed before the 1850s. In retrospect, some of the reasons were obvious. Since microscopes were relatively uncommon, most physicians of the time had no way to observe microscopic agents. Medical "schools" rarely had them. And even if they had studied them, associating these organisms with disease would have been beyond the thinking of most. How could these tiny creatures—even acknowledging they were alive—cause illness in humans and other animals so much larger than they? Theories explaining the basis for disease were abundant, many centering on the idea of miasmas, a form of "bad" or "night air," originating with the putrefaction of sewage in the soil. In a sense, evidence could be found to support this idea: when sewage contaminated soils were treated for the odors, outbreaks of disease often became rare. As James Manley (1781–1851), resident physician of New York City, described the challenge of cholera, then in the midst of an outbreak in Montreal and Quebec: "this disease is not personally communicable; ... that it is an atmospheric disease, whose causes have hitherto eluded the most philosophical [scientific] research: that it is carried on the wings of the wind."[3] If emanations in the air were the cause of diseases such as cholera, the solution was equally obvious: purify the air. Burning of tar, while perhaps lacking in efficaciousness, at least left the authorities feeling they were doing something.[4] It would not be until the 1870s that an understanding of the effects of water purification and proper sanitation on elimination of disease causing organisms was the actual basis for control of outbreaks.

To understand the impact of Robert Koch on the new field of bacteriology, it is helpful to briefly review the state of medical education which existed in the United States, Germany, and to some extent, France, in the decades before Koch entered the field. Koch was trained as a physician, and ultimately much of his research on disease was an outcome of this training. He would have received no equivalent education had he attended school in the United States, nor possibly even in France, during these years. Bacteriology, of course, was not a component of medical education prior to the 1870s.

Nineteenth Century Medical Training in the United States

Medical training in the United States during much of the 19th century was strikingly similar to that in the previous century. Though the number of medical schools was increasing—twenty-five by 1830, catering to some 2200 students—few were worthy of the name.[5] Clinical work was minimal, and experimental approaches were almost nonexistent. Most of those wishing to become physicians were trained as apprentices. Actual schooling was minimal, and largely involved paying a fee for the privilege of attending such schools. Coursework consisted almost entirely of lectures by practicing physicians; if a student wished clinical experience, he—physicians were nearly all males at the time—had to initiate the process on his own. It goes without saying that nothing resembling a course in bacteriology existed. Once the student received his degree, he was free to set up a practice. Even with this minimal training, for most interested in the medical field, learning through an apprenticeship remained the primary means of training physicians. If a student wished to improve or modernize his skills, he was forced to travel to Europe, primarily Paris; during the 1830s, some two hundred American students did exactly that.[6]

The earliest reform in American medical education began with the establishment of the American Medical Association. In 1845, Dr. Nathan Davis presented a resolution before the New York state medical association calling for a national meeting to discuss the poor state of medical education in the country. The national meeting, held in Philadelphia in 1847, and attended by 300 physicians, resolved "that it is desirable that a uniform and elevated standard of requirements for the degree of M.D. should be adopted by the medical schools of the United States."[7]

Implementation of suggested reforms was delayed by political infighting, particularly concern about competition from "diploma factories" if requirements were too strict, as well as the Civil War which began slightly more than a decade later. Changes began, albeit slowly, in the immediate aftermath of the war. In 1867, at the association meeting in Cincinnati, Davis again introduced a resolution "that every medical student be required to study four full years, including three regular annual courses of medical college instruction, before being admitted to an examination for the degree of doctor of medicine; that the minimum duration of a regular annual lecture term, or course of medical college instruction, shall be six calendar months; that every medical college shall embrace in its curriculum the following branches, to be taught by not less than nine professors, namely: descriptive anatomy, including dissections; in organic chemistry, *materia medica*, organic chemistry and toxicology; general pathology, therapeutics, pathological anatomy and public hygiene; surgical anatomy and operations of surgery; medial jurisprudence and medical ethics; practice of medicine, practice of surgery, obstetrics, and diseases of women and children; clinical medicine and clinical surgery."[8] Few schools chose to follow the guidelines. In 1870, fifty medical schools were granting degrees, a number which doubled by 1880, and more than doubled again by 1890. Many of these institutions were dubious as far as training in modern medicine, and included schools of homeopathy or eclectic medicine. As William Welch, then a student, but a future member of the Johns Hopkins faculty described the situation, using the word of fellow students, "There is no use of attempting to do anything here.... I do think that the condition of medical education here is simply horrible."[9]

Among the few schools which did implement the proposed guidelines during the 1870s and 1880s, discussed in greater detail in subsequent chapters, were the University of Michigan, the newly established Johns Hopkins, Harvard and medical schools in California. The University of Michigan, for example, expanded the number of laboratory courses, and even instituted a Ph.D. program in chemistry. Chapter 10 addresses the changes at Michigan instituted by Drs. Victor Vaughan and Frederick G. Novy. A significant number of the faculty at Johns Hopkins received training in Germany, and were familiar with German clinical and research methods. Included in this category were Franklin Mall, professor of anatomy, John J. Abel, professor of pharmacology who, in addition to his work in Baltimore, established the Department of Pharmacology at the University of Michigan, his *alma mater*, and William Welch, professor of pathology (see Chapter 7).

A significant number of these reforms, whether simply proposed or newly implemented, were modeled on the German schools. In 1880, bacteriology was not among the proposed additions, but that would begin to change early in that decade as the germ theory became more established. As we will see in subsequent chapters, much of that change would result from the training American students and future faculty received in Germany, and in particular, the laboratory of Robert Koch.

Medical Training in Germany and France

Unlike the situation in the United States, entrance to a university program in medicine by the 1830s in both Germany and France required a diploma from a preparatory school, a *gymnasium*; an apprenticeship was not a viable path in itself to a medical degree. In 1830, over six thousand students were enrolled in German programs, approximately half in university medical schools, of which there were twenty-four, the remainder enrolled in other forms of schooling such as practical schools, of which there were thirty.[10] Students received an intensive education in a four-year curriculum: "botany, chemistry, physics, zoology, and anatomy in the first year; physiology, pharmacy, pathology, and pathological anatomy in the second; and concluding in the last two years with advanced pathology, surgery, midwifery, ophthalmology, and practical clinics in the university hospital."[11] In order to be licensed, both practical skills, learned largely through their work in clinics, and classical education were necessary. Emphasis was also placed on research. The changing political climate in Europe, and particularly in the German speaking portions of the continent, reduced those numbers significantly.

During these first decades of the century, and especially so after the political upheavals of the late 1840s ended, support by the governments of the German states—Germany would not be unified until the 1870s—resulted in the establishment of new or updated, modern universities: Berlin in 1810, Bonn in 1818, among others, with emphasis on adequate space, a varied medical curriculum, and perhaps most important, funding. Faculty at Bonn included the physiologist Johannes Müller, considered "father of scientific medicine" in Germany, psychiatrist Friedrich Nasse and anatomist A.C. Mayer.

In many respects, medical education in France was similar to that in Germany. In 1830, over 3500 students were enrolled in the three medical schools, located in Paris, by far the largest of the three, Montpellier and Strasbourg, twenty-two *écoles secondaires* (secondary school), and nine military schools.[12] As described by McCullough, many of these students, particularly in the first decades of the century, were Americans looking to broaden their education. The primary difference between the programs was the increased emphasis placed on laboratory instruction in German schools. Among the most important differences between schools in Germany and France, in contrast with those in the United States, was training with the use of cadavers, a practice which continued to be limited in America. Still, the actual number of American students in German schools remained small—fewer than twenty in 1850. The modernization of German medical schools, beginning at the midpoint of the century, and continuing for decades, resulted in increasing numbers of foreign students, including Americans, forsaking France and enrolling in German schools. Why? Thomas Bonner, a historian of the period, has suggested it was a combination of the German laboratories, "its objective and serious atmosphere, its exciting sense of standing on the frontier of medical discovery, its discipline and devotion to the spirit of science ... the exhilarating sense of freedom."[13] Paris was fine for several weeks of touring, but it was in Berlin and other German university towns that scientific excitement was to be found.

In the opinion of Bonner, the "scientific output" and influence of German universities reached its maximum in the 1870s.[14] The list of faculty and researchers in German universities, which included that in Strasbourg following the French surrender, reads like a "Who's Who" of scientific investigation and achievements: physiologists Carl Ludwig and Felix Hoppe-Seyler; pathologists Rudolf Virchow, Friedrich von Recklinghausen, Julius Cohnheim, Ludwig Traube and Edwin Klebs; and Theodor Billroth in surgery.[15] National standards were established for licensing physicians: a diploma from an approved *gymnasium*, four years of study, which included experience in medical and surgical clinics, and passing of a rigorous national examination. The examination itself was not limited to a written test, but included demonstrative clinical expertise. "Students were assigned the care of six patients— two each in medicine, surgery and gynecology—for a period of eight days, during which he was quizzed about his diagnoses, recommended treatments and prescriptions, and knowledge of surgical procedures."[16] The testing included the dissection of a cadaver. Nowhere in the United States, or anywhere else for that matter, was a medical program as rigorous. The results could speak for themselves; Germany was the center of scientific research during a significant portion of these decades.

France, in turn, in part to compensate for the defeat in the war, made an attempt to modernize their training programs. Medical schools were established in Lyon, Bordeaux and Lille were expanded or established, with greater emphasis on laboratory instruction—for some students. Only in 1878 was laboratory instruction, including the fields of physiology, pathology, anatomy and histology, mandatory for all students. An increase in funding by the French government was included as well. Nevertheless, with exception of "stars" such as Louis Pasteur and his colleagues, French scientific training and research was a poor second to that in Germany.

The changes in German medicine during the period roughly bracketed by 1840 and 1870 reversed the trend of study carried out by American students. This book describes and explains some of those trends by focusing on one scientific discipline: bacteriology. Chapters 1 and 2 deal with the man himself: Robert Koch, his background and education, and in the basic research which he would apply in the study of etiological agents of disease. The understanding of germ theory was not the result of a "eureka moment," but required growing insight into the association of these microscopic agents with pathological changes in the infected host. Laboratory research was critical in this endeavor, an area sorely lacking in American laboratories and training in that early period—i.e., pre-1880. A more comprehensive view of the state of instruction of bacteriology in the United States is described in Chapter 3, which includes contributions from some of the early pioneers in that subject.

Chapter 4 focuses on the Cartwright Lecture of 1883, largely a platform for Dr. William Belfield, a member of Rush Medical College in Chicago, in addressing the skepticism of Dr. Henry Formad as to Koch's identification of the etiological agent of tuberculosis. Formad was not the only such skeptic, but his position in the Philadelphia medical community provided him with a credibility on the issue one might argue he did not deserve. Formad appears again in Chapter 8, in the debates over the same issue, but with Dr. Edward Shakespeare. The Cartwright Lecture also provides insight into the thinking and experimental approach of scientists of the time.

Chapter 5 describes Koch's pedagogy and on-hands approach in training of a generation of bacteriologists. As repeatedly emphasized in this story, an increasing number of American students traveled to Berlin for a first-hand look at the work carried out by Koch and his colleagues. Their stories provide a direct account of their experiences in learning the methodology of a new discipline. The remaining biographical chapters, 6 through 11, address the experiences of the major individuals who subsequently instituted programs in bacteriology in their respective schools. Both the education and background of these persons are described, followed by their impact once these programs were established. All were males, with one notable exception: Lydia Rabinowitsch-Kempner. Unlike the rest, she was trained in Germany, with Koch, and applied her learning to development of the new bacteriology discipline in the Woman's Medical College in Philadelphia. Finally, Chapter 12 provides a summary of the impact the institution of Koch's methods had on the changes implemented in the medical programs which ultimately incorporated this work in their respective curricula.

1

Robert Koch
His Life and Role in Bacteriological Research

"The more or less constant presence of animal forms during disease does not prove they are the cause.... We feel sure the ultimate conclusion will be that bacteria are only incidental to disease and death."[1]

Robert Koch (1843–1910)

In order to understand the attraction largely specific to the laboratory of Robert Koch for those interested in the new field of bacteriology, it helps to begin with the story of the man himself. Heinrich Hermann Robert Koch was born December 11, 1843, in Clausthal in the province of Hanover, a mining area located in the southwestern portion of the Harz Mountains; Koch's birthplace is still present though the house is a private residence. The town had already been home to the Koch family for several generations, several members of which had been employed by the Prussian government.

Robert was the third of thirteen children—eleven sons and two daughters—born to Hermann Koch and Mathilde Julie Henrietta Biewend; Robert's two older brothers died in infancy, leaving him as the oldest surviving male. The father, Hermann, was a well-known mining engineer, even being honored with the title *Bergrath* by the Prussian government for his expertise in that field. Robert's primary interests as a youth were in the subjects of biology and photography, the latter likely due in part to the influence of his uncle, Eduard Biewend, his mother's brother whose hobbies included photography.

His earliest schooling was at the Clausthal *Gymnasium*, where Koch excelled in athletics, as well as developing an interest in the natural sciences; his hobbies including the collection of plants and minerals. During walks with his father and, on occasion, with his Uncle Eduard through the mountains, Koch also developed interests in geology and zoology, maintaining these interests throughout his life.

Koch's original career goal, or at least the one supported by his father, was in the field of commerce. During these years in mid–19th century, cities such as Hamburg and Bremen were increasingly becoming centers for worldwide trade. That, coupled with his father's governmental connections, pressured him first in that direction following his graduation from the *gymnasium*. However, his strong interests in the natural sciences, and for a time, the limited finances of his father, led him to a career either in teaching or, if the financial situation improved, in medicine.

In 1862, Koch enrolled at the University of Göttingen, initially with the goal of becoming a teacher. The choice of the university proved to be fortunate, as the faculty included a significant number of important scientists. The organic chemist Friedrich Wöhler, in 1828, had synthesized urea in the laboratory, as well as being co-discoverer of several new elements in nature. In 1836 he joined the faculty at Göttingen. Among the other faculty were the pathologist Wilhelm Krause, who had recently joined the university and would become well-known for his work with muscle and nerve structure, and physiologist George Meissner. But the most important member of the faculty, the man who would have the greatest influence on the young Koch, was the physician and anatomist Jacob Henle, and whose work would help lay the basis for what would become the germ theory.

After completing courses in mathematics, physics and botany during his first semester at the university, Koch's interests in teaching were replaced by the decision to make a career in medicine. During the following semesters, Koch enrolled in courses taught by Henle, Wöhler, Karl Ewald Hasse, professor of special pathology as well as medical director at the university, and Meissner, whose experimental work on animals would shortly result in a memorable experience on the part of Koch.[2]

In 1865, Koch entered a competition established by the medical faculty at the university, the topic being the structure of the uterine nerves. Carrying out this work under the direction of Krause, now the director of the Pathological-Anatomical Institute, including the museum, Koch, along with a second student, Adolf Polle, was awarded the monetary prize of 30 ducats. The thesis, entitled "Ueber das Vorkommen von Ganglienzellen an den Nerven des Uterus"—"On the Presence of Ganglion Cells on the Nerves of the Uterus"—was dedicated to his father. Koch used the prize money in traveling to Berlin to attend the 49th Congress of the *Gesellschaft Deutscher Naturforscher und Arzte* (*Society of Naturalists and Physicians*), where, among others, he had the opportunity to meet Rudolf Virchow, among the most important figures in the field of public health during that era.[3]

In July 1865, Koch was appointed assistant to Krause at the Pathological Museum, using the opportunity for greater training in pathology. Concurrently, he began a study under the direction of Meissner at the Physiological Institute on excretion of succinic acid by animals fed diets high in protein and fat. In the fashion of the day, Koch himself served as a guinea pig, eating a half pound of butter a day, and measuring the output of succinic acid in his urine. The experiment lasted five days; as a result of the hot summer days, he was unable—literally—to stomach the high fat diet for longer than that. The experiment was completed with less sensitive animals. The work was subsequently published in the journal established by Henle, *Zeitschrift für rationelle Medizin* (*Journal for Rational Medicine*).[4] In January 1866, the topic also served as the dissertation, delivered in Latin by Koch, for his doctor's degree. In March of that year, Koch passed the state examination, now officially entering the practice of medicine. Though Henle's ideas were forerunners in the germ theory as it subsequently became part of the discipline of bacteriology (see Chapter 2), there is no evidence that Koch had any training in that particular subject from him while enrolled at Göttingen. In fact, Henle's instruction was in the subject of anatomy, not bacteriology.[5]

Other changes also were taking place in Koch's life during this period. Soon after Koch passed his medical examination, he became engaged to Emmy Fraatz, the daughter of an official in a church in his home town of Clausthal. They would have one child, a daughter Gertrud, in a marriage which would ultimately fail years later. But that was long in the future. For now, Koch would need a steadier income if he was to support a family—he and Emmy would marry in July 1867. During the summer of 1866, he accepted a position as medical assistant in the Hamburg General Hospital. The position paid poorly, and he would serve in that capacity only some three months. But during this time he obtained significant experience in dealing with infectious diseases such as an epidemic of cholera, which had broken out in the region that summer.

In October 1866, Koch found a more suitable position, accepting an offer to serve as physician at the Asylum for Idiots (as it was then called) in the small town of Langenhagen, located near Hanover. At the same time, he was able to develop a private practice, purchasing a horse and buggy for transportation in the surrounding area. He would remain there until July 1868, moving initially to Niemegk, and then in 1869 to Rakwitz.[6]

It was while living and practicing in Rakwitz that Koch had an opportunity to develop his skill in that profession. Certainly it was not sufficiently financially rewarding to act on his wishes for travel. Intellectually, however, in his spare time—such as it was for a country physician—Koch was able to pursue his interests in natural history as well as a hobby in beekeeping. On a lighter note, Koch also served as a drinking companion for the mayor and local pharmacist.[7]

In July 1870, France declared war on the North German Confederation, consisting primarily of the Kingdom of Prussia—a unified Germany under Otto von Bismarck would not appear until after the German victory a year later—in a conflict known as the Franco-Prussian War. Koch, initially exempt because of near-sightedness, nevertheless enlisted as a physician in a battlefield hospital. It was during his brief service in this capacity, primarily in Neufchateau and Orleans in northeastern France, that he had the opportunity to observe and study sepsis associated with battle wounds.

Writing to his father, Koch observed that he learned more during this period than he would have in a surgical clinic.[8] Nor was Koch the only future contributor to the germ theory to serve as a military physician in that conflict. Edwin Klebs, among those who later identified the etiological agents of diphtheria and typhoid fever, carried out over 100 autopsies at a Karlsruhe military hospital during the three month period of August to October in 1870, observing bacteria in nearly all of the battle wounds. "I found rod-shaped bodies, so-called bacteria, which did not move and were frequently

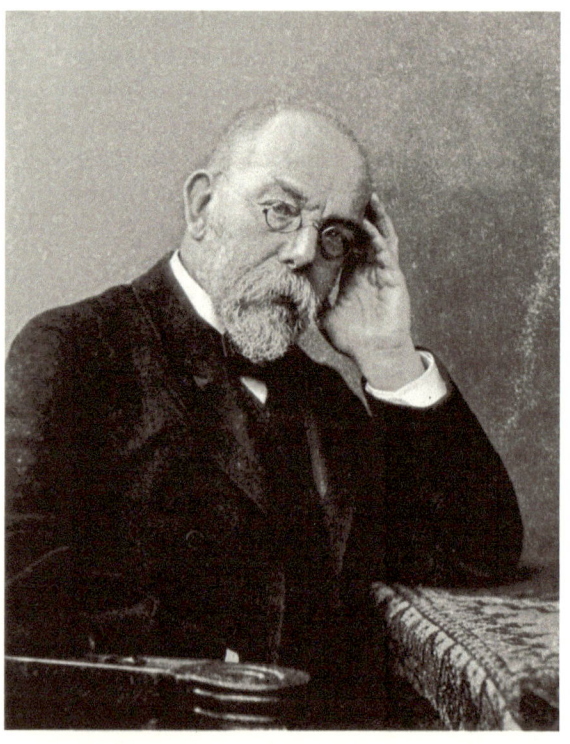

Robert Koch (1843–1910). A German physician, Koch was arguably among the most important researchers in bacteriology during the latter 19th century. He is credited with the identification of the etiological agents of tuberculosis and cholera among his many contributions to the field, and he was awarded the Nobel Prize in Physiology or Medicine in 1905 (National Library of Medicine).

attached to others in rows, so that they formed long articulated threads; also numerous microspores, shiny and extremely small bodies whose diameter might be half a micromillimeter at most [significantly less than half the size of the bacilli described by Klebs], and these lay unattached by themselves and then made oscillatory movements or else were clustered together in groups (zoogloeaforms or lined up in rosary-like threads [perhaps spores]."[9] Believing these organisms represented stages in the life-cycle of identical bacteria, Klebs termed the organism *Microsporon septicum*. Though mistaken in his interpretation (see below), Klebs' zoogloeaforms study became a key component in explaining the association of micro-organisms with infections—particularly infections associated with wound sepsis—and in their role as etiological agents of disease.

The contribution by Klebs in the development and evolution of Koch's Postulates was only one of the applications from this work. (See Chapter 2.)[10] Neverthelesss, Klebs' interpretation of his observations was handicapped by the prevailing theory of the time, that most microscopic agents were variations of the same organism. This idea, termed pleomorphism by the botanist Ernst Hallier (1831–1904), originated with the latter's observations on fungi, and the varied life cycles of those specific classes of organisms. However, Hallier's studies of fungi were subsequently extrapolated to those of all microorganisms, including bacteria. The varied shapes and sizes of bacteria were assumed to represent different stages in the lives of identical organisms. Hallier's ideas, as applied to widespread pleomorphisms, were soon disproved, particularly as they applied specifically to the bacteria. But for a time they had a significant influence in the interpretation—including that by Klebs—of the presence of different forms of bacteria in wound infections.

Koch and Anthrax

> "If anyone wore a garment made from tainted wool, his limbs were soon attacked by inflamed papules and foul exudates, and if he delayed too long to remove the material, a violent inflammation consumed the parts it had touched."[11]

Koch's career in the military was short-lived. He was needed back in Rakwitz, and returned there shortly after the end of the year. While Koch was well respected as the local country doctor in the town, his ambitions—both monetarily as well as professionally—were to lead him elsewhere. He had earlier applied to take the examination for promotion to *Kreisphysikus*, the district public health officer, only to be interrupted by military service.

Following his return, Koch applied for and passed the examination early in 1872. A position soon opened in Wollstein, a small city of 3000 persons, and was offered to Koch. In April 1872, Koch moved with his family to the city.

The position of *Kreisphysikus*, while important, was still limited in its scope. The salary of 900 marks still required an element of budgeting in managing a household. For example, one choice he was forced to make was whether to purchase a carriage for making house calls in the county, or purchasing a microscope for research studies. His choice was the microscope, a Hartnack, among the best of the time.[12] The ability to maintain a private practice would be critical, as the professional role of the *Kreisphysikus* primarily involved the issuance of death certificates, maintaining records of (smallpox) vaccinations, and the investigation of epidemics.[13] But it was during his eight years there in which Koch began to establish his role as a researcher of disease.

During fall 1875, Koch took the opportunity to travel through Germany and Austria, both to attend scientific meetings—the *Deutsch Gesellschaft für öffentliche Gesundheitspflege* (German Society for Public Health) in Munich, and the *Gesellschaft Deutscher Naturforscher und Ärtze* (Society of German Natural Scientists and Physicians) in Graz—and to observe scientific research in several laboratories. Among the laboratories he had the opportunity to visit was that of Max von Pettenkofer, among the most important hygienists of the day; Koch would someday have profound disagreements with von Pettenkofer about the etiological agent of cholera.[14]

Anthrax is an ancient disease, among the earliest to be definitively identified. Some Biblical historians have attributed the 5th Pharonic plague—sometimes described as a "murrain"—primarily on the basis of affecting a variety of species, typical of anthrax, but also characteristic of other infections as well. Not all historians agree with that interpretation. More definitively was the description provided by the Roman poet Publius Virgil in the agricultural *Georgics* (ca. 29 B.C.E.), as quoted above. The disease, as described by the author, affected both sheep and humans; the relationship to "tainted wool" is nearly identical to what was referred to as Woolsorter's Disease in more recent centuries, a respiratory illness contracted from live bacteria or spores which contaminated the wool obtained from infected sheep.

Descriptions of outbreaks in more recent centuries depict a devastating disease. During the mid–18th century, an epidemic killed half of the sheep in Europe. In 1864, a period contemporary with that of Koch, over 72,000 horses died in Russia from the disease. Before the end of that decade, another 56,000 horses, cattle and sheep died. The number of deaths included over 500 persons as well.[15] Anthrax clearly had an economic impact in a region. But it was also a potentially fatal disease in humans.

Suspicion as to the etiological role played by bacteria in anthrax did not begin with Koch. Among others, the Frenchmen Casimir Davaine and Aloys Pollender had observed rod-shaped micro-organisms termed *Bacteridia* in the blood of animals dead from anthrax during the 1850s. (See Chapter 2.) Davaine had already demonstrated that transfer of a small volume of blood from a diseased animal into a healthy one would induce the disease. What was difficult to explain at that time—the 1850s—was why soil on which a diseased animal had grazed could also be a source of the disease in a healthy animal.

In 1873, an outbreak of anthrax occurred in Bomst, within the district in which Koch served as *Kreisphysikus*; Koch began his investigation of disease in March of that year through the microscopic examination of blood obtained from infected sheep. A more detailed description of Koch's work with anthrax is presented in Chapter 2 in the context of the development of his postulates. It is useful, however, to describe Koch's methodology in the understanding of the role spores played in the life cycle of the bacterium, and the significance of their presence in soil.

In April 1874 he observed the critical feature in the life cycle of the organism: the formation of spores. The German botanist Ferdinand Cohn (1828–1898), among the founders of modern bacteriology, had previously reported spore formation by the hay bacillus, now known as *Bacillus subtilis*, suspecting that a similar stage might be exhibited by the etiological agent of anthrax, a disease to which Cohn also referred as splenic fever. The existence of spores, a dormant stage which explained how the bacterium survived adverse conditions in soil, provided the explanation for why contaminated soil continued to be a source of the disease.

As Brock has pointed out in his biography of Koch, the conceptual leap from understanding the life cycle of *Bacillus anthracis*, to its role as the etiological agent of anthrax was no easy task. Koch's continued interest in both the natural sciences as well as the human quality of maintaining household pets—available now as experimental animals—played key roles in the process.[16] Among the problems Koch encountered, was the necessity of maintaining proper temperatures for his studies—in the absence of electricity, a kerosene heater was employed. His home-made incubator consisted of flat dishes filled with sand, with filter paper placed on top, and the kerosene lamp placed below to maintain the warm temperature. His slide cultures were then placed on top. The setup seemed to work—temperatures were said to vary no more than 1 to 2 degrees centigrade each day. The water-jacketed incubators currently in use in some modern teaching laboratories are no more efficient.[17]

In order to confirm a role for the bacterium as a pathogen, foreshadowing the postulates, it was necessary to test the ability of the organisms to cause disease in an experimental animal. Since cattle or sheep, the usual victims of an anthrax outbreak, were at a premium in the Koch household, Koch used wild house mice, captured in their horse barn, for this portion of the study. Captured mice were kept in a tall glass jar, fed and cared for by his wife, Emmy. When the mouse was needed, Koch used a bullet extractor brought home from his service in the war (Koch's mouse forceps) to remove the mouse from the jar.[18]

"It has not been possible for me to observe the multiplication of the bacteria directly in the animal. But multiplication can be inferred from the inoculation experiments which are described below. I have used the mouse as my experimental animal, as it is simple to use.... In most experiments I inoculated the mice at the base of the tail, where the skin is loose and covered with long hair.... I have made a large number of inoculations in this way, using fresh anthrax material, and in every case I have had a positive result, and I believe therefore that the success of the inoculation can be used as an indication of the viability of the bacilli inoculated.... Partly in order to always have available fresh material, and partly to discover if the bacilli would change into another form after a certain number of generations, I inoculated a number of mice in series, one after the other, each time using the material from the spleen of a mouse which had just died. The longest series of mice

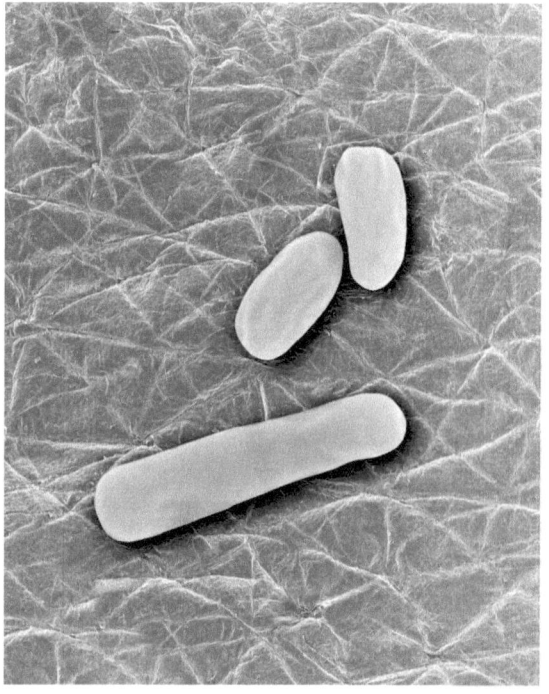

Bacillus anthracis with spores. Though Koch was not the first to observe this bacillus in animals with anthrax, his work firmly identified the organism as the etiological agent. In the course of observing the organism, he discovered the presence of spores, a dormant stage in the life cycle of the bacillus (image copyright Dennis Kunkel Microscopy, Inc.).

treated in this way was twenty.... In all animals the results were the same. The spleen was markedly swollen [hence the alternative designation of splenic fever] and contained a large number of transparent rods which were very similar in appearance and were immotile and without spores.... A small number of bacilli could always develop into a significant mass of individuals of the same type."[19]

And what of the significance of spores as a means of infecting animals grazing on contaminated soil? Koch had carried out his laboratory studies with mice. But what was true in mice was likely equally valid in ruminants, an extrapolation he quickly made. "We thus see that anthrax tissues, regardless of whether they are relatively fresh, putrefying, dried, or years old, can produce anthrax when these substances contain bacilli capable of developing spores of Bacillus anthracis. Thus, all doubts regarding Bacillus anthracis as the actual cause of the disease must be dispelled. Bacillus anthracis is indeed the contagion of anthrax. The transmission of the disease in fresh blood occurs rarely in nature, only in persons who come into contact with blood or tissue juices while killing, cutting and skinning animals infected with anthrax.... But, the great percentage of infections are produced only by the penetration of the spores of Bacillus anthracis into the animal body. For the spores can survive in an amazing manner for many years. When these spores have once formed in the soil of a region, there is good reason to believe that anthrax will remain in this region for many years.... A single cadaver, handled improperly, can furnish almost innumerable spores.... If it would be possible to discover how the spores of Bacillus anthracis were disseminated, and the conditions under which the contagion renews itself *de novo*, it might then be possible to prevent the growth of the bacillus and therefore reduce the incidence of disease or perhaps even exterminate it entirely."[20] If indeed the presence of spores explained the reappearance of the disease among cattle and sheep, Koch recognized the implications—that is, burying animals dead from anthrax in shallow graves would result in continued contamination of the soil.

Koch's conclusion that he had observed a spore stage in the life cycle of the bacilli, an observation previously made by Cohn as alluded to above, was still subject to other interpretations. "I [Koch] wanted to continue my studies for longer before publishing them, but just at that time a well-known botanist declared that the rods associated with anthrax were crystalloids, so it seemed to me that I should publish my observations."[21] The botanist to which Koch referred was likely German pathologist Otto von Bollinger. Bollinger (1843–1909) was already known for his observations on the transmission of anthrax using blood from infected animals, but was skeptical about the existence of spores. Since Bollinger was an authority on the subject, it was necessary for Koch to confirm his own observations in front of Cohn himself.

On April 22, 1876, Koch sent a letter to Cohn, by then a professor at the University of Breslau, summarizing his work on the life cycle of the bacillus. The letter included his interpretation of the importance of the sporulation process in maintaining the etiological agent in soil, and his interest in showing his work directly to Cohn and his colleagues:

> Honored Professor!
>
> I have found your work on bacteria, published in the *Beiträge zur Biologie der Pflanzen*, very exciting. I have been working for some time on the contagion of anthrax. After many futile attempts I have finally succeeded in discovering the complete life cycle of Bacillus anthracis. I am certain, now, as a result of a large number of experiments, that my conclusions are correct. However, before I publish my work, I would like to request, honored professor, that you, as the best expert on bacteria, examine my results and give me your judgement on their validity. Unfortunately, I am not able to send you preparations which would show the various developmental stages, as I have not succeeded in conserving the bacteria in appropriate fluids. Therefore, I earnestly request that you permit me to visit you in your Institute of Plant Physiology for several days, so that I might show you the essential experiments. If this request is agreeable to you, perhaps you might inform me of a suitable time that I could come to Breslau.
>
> Very sincerely yours,
> Dr. Koch, Kreisphysikus[22]

Cohn was "greatly delighted" when receiving the letter, and immediately invited Koch—yet an unknown country physician—to the institute at Breslau.[23]

Beginning on April 30, and continuing for three days, Koch demonstrated his technique that first afternoon to Cohn and his assistant Eduard Eidam (see *n*17), by growing samples of anthrax bacilli obtained from a guinea pig dead of splenic fever (anthrax) in sterile blood serum and in the aqueous humor of a cow. "Fresh anthrax blood from a guinea pig was diluted with fluid of the eye cavity from the eye of one calf and placed in several batches in the incubator, with or without the magnifying glass for 10–12 hours at a temperature of 35 degrees.... In one preparation consisting of the serum of guinea pig blood on a concave slide [the hanging drop technique], masses of bacteria in long threads had developed.... The threads that were located at the edge of the cover slip were longer and better developed and showed at their extremities regularly arranged strongly light-refracting grains that remained behind in formation when the threads fell apart and disappeared."[24]

By the third day of Koch's visit, the results of the demonstration were disseminated throughout the university. Among Cohn's colleagues who came to observe the results was Julius Cohnheim (1839–1884), director of the Institute of Pathology at the university, and well-known for his studies of inflammation.²⁵ Following his observation of Koch's demonstration, Cohnheim was said to be so excited, that "he rushed back to the Pathological Institute, called his assistants together [including Dr. William Welch, working in Cohnheim's laboratory while visiting from America] and told them to stop their work and hasten to the Botanical Laboratory where they could see the demonstration for themselves."²⁶

Koch had indeed correctly described the role of the spore in the life cycle of *Bacillus anthracis*, as well as establishing its likely role as the etiological agent of anthrax. However, Cohn too had observed spore formation among a "sister" bacillus of the organism, *Bacillus subtilis*. If these were actually separate species, it would be necessary to show that the latter organism, neither the vegetative cell nor its spore, could cause anthrax. Koch demonstrated its lack of pathogenic potential, serving it as a control in the experimental model. Koch's work was quickly prepared for publication, which became the fifth in a series of papers dealing with bacteria published in *Beiträge zur Biologie der Pflanzen*, the journal established by Cohn himself.

With the publication of his manuscript, Koch's experimental work on anthrax was largely completed. He did return to Breslau in October 1877 to again demonstrate the pathogenic potential of the organism in rabbits, as well as its process of sporulation. This time the "audience" was Dr. John Burdon-Sanderson (1828–1905), Jodrell Professor of Physiology at the University of London and among the early advocates of the germ theory of disease.²⁷

An additional application of this work would play a significant role in his future research. Koch had been among the first to utilize the relatively new oil immersion lens and Abbe condenser in his microscopic studies. One handicap in publicizing his earlier work was the necessity for using hand drawings to illustrate his observations. However, by the time Koch's first paper had been published, the technology involved in photomicroscopy had developed sufficiently enough to allow actual photographs of bacteria to be produced. Koch purchased the requisite supplies and materials, and though it required a year or so of practice to produce images sufficiently resolute, by late 1877 he was able to produce quality prints for publication. Among the first such images captured by Koch was that of the bacterium *Bacillus anthracis*.²⁸

Etiological Agents of Wound Infections

By the late 1870s, Koch had begun the evolution from serving as a local small-town physician, into a research scientist with a developing national reputation. Of particular importance to his future in the field, was his growing interest in the wider significance of what he had accomplished with his anthrax studies—the role played by micro-organisms in wound infections.

Any understanding during the early 1870s of the role played by micro-organisms in development of pyaemia (internal spread of abscesses), septicemia (also known as sepsis or blood poisoning, the spread of bacteria through blood) or traumatic infections, was muddled to put it mildly. Was the presence of micro-organism the source of the sepsis, or "merely" the result of pathological changes occurring in the host? Some believed the presence of similar organisms in healthy individuals was evidence for the latter. Casimir Davaine, the French scientist who was among the first to observe the agent of anthrax, had demonstrated as early as 1872 that blood from a patient with septicemia could be serially transferred through as many as 25 rabbits without losing any level of virulence.[29] Klebs, of course, had observed a variety of micro-organisms in the tissues from autopsies he had performed. His mistaken interpretation—that these represented varieties of the same microbe, *Microsporon septicum*—had yet to be disproved. And what about the possible role of a toxin, perhaps even independent of any microbes? In 1856, the Danish physiologist Peter Ludwig Panum (1820–1885) had described a toxin, a "putrid poison," present in filtered putrefying solutions from decomposing meat; unrecognized at the time, the solutions originated from bacterial growth on the meat. Infusion of the solutions into dogs resulted in collapse and death of the animals; the rate at which symptoms developed was a function of the dose to which the animals were exposed.[30] Panum considered two possibilities for the nature of the poison: microbial, likely a form of vibrio, or an actual toxin. Neither possibility seemed to support the data—the sometimes long delay seemed to rule out a fast-acting toxin, while the resistance to boiling seemed to rule out microbes.

Advances in bacteriology during the following decades—most notably the developing germ theory of disease—resulted in Panum republishing his work in 1874. This time Panum favored the idea of a bacterial toxin, even proposing the possibility that the presence of bacteria resulted in toxin production. "Maybe this poison is produced through the life process of bacteria, or to be more explicit probably through the small rods named Bacterium termo *Cohn*, and it seems to be produced in a way analogous to ergotine. [alkaloid similar to LSD, produced by certain fungi]."[31] It is likely that the "vibrios" which Panum had observed were Gram-negative rods, though as pointed out by Kolmos, development of the Gram stain would not occur for another decade. If so, what Panum had provided was the first description of bacterial endotoxin.

The importance of Panum's 1874 report, *vis-à-vis* Koch's subsequent work on traumatic infection, was not the description of a likely toxin, but in the confusion it engendered in the arguments as to whether pyaemia, septicemia, etc., towards the significance of microbial infection or contamination. It was with this context in the background, that Koch began his final area of research while living in Wollstein.

Koch's approach was straightforward (stated simplistically). He applied the expertise he had developed in microscopy with the newly evolving techniques in bacterial staining—procedures resulting in large part from the work by his colleague in Breslau, Carl Weigert, using aniline dyes. The initial question to be addressed, the control observation, was whether the bacteria observed in wound infections were unique to those situations. Or were these organisms merely part of the background flora; that is, were bacteria present in normal tissues?

It was in addressing this question that Koch's experience played a significant role. "I have, on many occasions, examined normal blood and normal tissues using methods that ensure that such organisms are not overlooked, and I have never, in a single instance, found bacteria. *I therefore conclude that bacteria do not occur in the blood or tissues of normal animals or humans.*

"On the other hand, some of the objections to the conclusion that bacteria do cause traumatic infective diseases are well founded. In order to prove that bacteria are the cause of traumatic infective diseases, it would be absolutely necessary to show *that bacteria are present without exception and that their number and distribution are such that the symptoms of the disease are fully explained*" [all italics in original].[32]

Rather than investigating infections in humans, Koch carried out his study in mice and rabbits, reasoning that any results would be analogous to those in humans. Six forms of disease were investigated: septicemia and destruction of tissue in mice (gangrene), while in rabbits he studied spreading abscesses, pyaemia, septicemia and erysipelas, a rash-like infection now known to be associated with streptococci.[33] Koch was able to demonstrate that the infections in animals under all circumstances required the presence of bacteria, and that these infections were in most cases completely analogous to those found in humans. As summarized by Gradmann,[34] confirmation of the bacterial etiology for these diseases required the fulfillment of three important criteria: (1) disease resulting from inoculation of small quantities of infectious material must "preclude a confusion with poisoning"; "For the infection was produced by such small quantities of fluid (blood, serum, pus, etc.) that the result cannot be attributed to a merely chemical poison,"[35] and (2) the presence of bacteria must be demonstrated in all cases, a requirement later incorporated into his postulates, and "there has to be a different and well-distinguishable form for each different disease"[36]; and (3) the quantity and physical characteristics of the bacteria must show a relationship with the disease with which they are allegedly associated. Each of these criteria was fulfilled.

Koch was able to develop several significant conclusions. Despite the inability to grow these bacteria in pure culture outside of the animal body at that time, a procedure he would develop several years later, Koch concluded the animal body itself would produce a pure culture of the organism. In all cases of distinct diseases which he observed in the animal—whether mouse or rabbit—the appearance of the micro-organisms remained constant. Furthermore, the appearance of the micro-organism associated with one form of the disease was generally distinct from that in other forms of disease. "The bacteria found [in animals which died from traumatic infectious disease] were identical with those which were present in the fluid used for inoculation, and a definite form of organisms corresponded in every instance to a distinct disease.... Even in the small series of experiments which I was able to carry out, one fact was so prominent that I must regard it as constant, and, as it helps to remove most of the obstacles to the admission of the existence of a *contagium vivum* for traumatic infective diseases, I look on it as the most important result of my work. I refer to the differences which exist between pathogenic bacteria and to the constancy of their characters. A distinct bacteric form corresponds, as we have seen, to each disease, and this form always remains the same, however often the disease is transmitted from one animal to another. Further, when we succeed in reproducing the same disease *de novo* by the injection of putrid substances, only the same bacteric form occurs which was before found to be specific for that disease."[37] In addition to the medical significance described by Koch, three technological advances were also presented in the publication: "(1) Staining of bacteria in diseased tissues with aniline dyes; (2) Introduction of the Abbe condenser; and (3) First use of the Zeiss oil-immersion lens."[38]

Director of a Bacteriological Laboratory

Koch's 1876 demonstration, before Cohn and others at the University of Breslau, of the life-cycle of the anthrax bacillus, and the publication two years later of his investigation of sepsis in non-human animals, in which he provided evidence for the role played by different types of bacteria, significantly enhanced his reputation before that portion of the medical community. The argument could be made, of course, that what had been demonstrated in these animals may not be directly applicable to that in humans. But within a few years, the Scottish surgeon Alexander Ogston (1844–1929) described two similar appearing micrococci in samples of pus obtained from infection: chains of cocci previously termed streptococci by the Austrian surgeon Theodor Billroth, and a different species of micrococci arranged in clumps, which Ogston termed as staphylococci. Koch's observations were now extended to infections in humans.[39]

For now—late 1878—Koch continued his in role as *Kreisphysikus* in Wollstein, spending most of his time on his medical practice at the cost of continuing in any significant research capacity. Things began to change the following January. The medical faculty at the University of Breslau had been duly impressed by this young researcher who had produced significant results while working under less than optimal conditions in a laboratory largely developed on his own. As a result, the faculty presented a nomination to the German Minister of Culture, that Koch be appointed as *ausserordentliche* professor of hygiene at the university. The position itself, roughly the equivalent of a professorship, though without most of the benefits, was meant to be temporary while a new Institute of Hygiene was established.[40] Unfortunately, the timing of the offer was not ideal, as the actual position had yet to be established. The authors of the nomination—the dean and rector of the university in addition to the faculty, including Cohn himself—had made the offer in good faith. Koch's professorship was to be within a new Institute of Hygiene. Establishment of the Institute was postponed, and would be for years. Instead, the faculty moved to what future administrators might call a "Plan B." Koch was offered a position as *Gerichtsarzt*, Municipal Physician, for the city of Breslau, similar to that which Koch held in Wollstein, but with an increase in salary. Koch accepted the offer, and moved to Breslau in July 1879.[41] The increased duties and need for establishment of a new medical practice convinced Koch the move was an error, and in October he and his family returned to Wollstein.

During the years immediately following the unification of the German states under Otto von Bismarck in 1871, a *Kaiserliche Gesundheitsamt* (Imperial Health Office) was established and headquartered in Berlin. The first director appointed to head the office was Dr. Heinrich Struck (1825–1902).

The primary duties of the office included the monitoring of consumer protection for the populace, including that of food safety and public hygiene. Initially serving only in an advisory capacity, the sixteen members of the council were subsequently encouraged to establish a research program. Struck's influence was particularly important in this matter, which significantly expanded the purpose of the office. Two laboratories were established for that purpose: in chemistry, directed by Dr. Eugen Sell, and hygiene, headed by Dr. Gustav Wolffhügel.[42]

Late in 1879, a position on the council became available when a member, Dr. Karl Finkelnberg, resigned and Koch—likely through the result of support from Cohnheim—was nominated as Finkelnberg's replacement.[43] Koch was officially offered the position by Struck in April 1880. "By the selection of this man, I have in mind not only his extensive experience in medical practice, but his high skill in experimental pathology and in microscopy. The lack of such experience at the *Gesundheitsamt* is serious. It is therefore a happy accident that Herr Koch, one of the most experienced researchers in this area, and a competent, hardworking, and dedicated scientist, can be easily attracted to such a position."[44] The appointment of Koch would fulfill the need for a researcher in the new science of bacteriology.

While the offer certainly recognized the growing recognition of Koch as a researcher, the position was still largely honorary. Koch had already uprooted his family and moved once—to Breslau—only to return, in part the result of a limited salary for that position. He had no desire to repeat the same mistake unless a proper salary was included with the offer. Struck requested such a salary for Koch through the Minister of Culture, the request was accepted, and in July 1880 Koch moved to Berlin as the newest member of the *Amt*, with the title of *Regierungsrath* (Government Councilor).[45] To paraphrase a quote from the movie Casablanca, "this was the beginning of a beautiful friendship."

Koch quickly assembled a series of associates, complementing his colleagues at the Amt, some of whom constituted a "Who's Who" of late 19th century bacteriology: in particular Georg Gaffky and Friedrich Loeffler. Within little more than a year, Koch had completed and published six articles: four under his own name, including a method for growing bacteria in pure culture, one article with Wolffhügel as co-author, and another with Gaffky and Loeffler as co-authors. These works were considered by some to represent the end of the first portion of Koch's professional life—the "inventive period."[46] During his decade of work ending in 1881, Koch had established the role of a spore stage in the life cycle of the anthrax, providing an explanation for the long-term danger of land in which infected cattle or sheep had grazed. He had applied the new technology of improved lens systems for observations of bacteria, as well as developing photomicroscopy for production of permanent images. In the medical field, Koch demonstrated the significance of bacterial presence in wound infections and similar forms of trauma, and their role in subsequent septicemias. Initially Koch found the establishment of pure cultures difficult, a necessity in assigning an etiological role to specific species of bacteria. By the close of this decade, however, Koch had developed a means to do so—initially using the surface of a potato, but graduating to gelatin (and later replacing gelatin with agar, a method developed by Koch's associate Walther Hesse).

For much of the remaining professional life of Koch, a period of nearly three decades, his work consisted largely of the application of the methodologies which he had worked out. His two most important scientific achievements were accomplished within the decade of the 1880s: certainly the isolation and identification of the etiological agent of tuberculosis, the purpose of his being awarded a Nobel Prize in 1905, and, arguably, his identification of the cholera bacillus.

Koch began his research in Berlin during the summer of 1880. Within little more than a year, March 1882, Koch announced his identification of the tuberculosis bacillus, work aided in no small part by his development of a staining mechanism for observation of the agent. Koch's work is described in greater detail in the following chapter, within the context of both the germ theory of disease as well as what became known as Koch's postulates. Some of the controversies surrounding his interpretation of the results are addressed in Chapter 4.

In fact, Koch's achievement was even more remarkable in that his identification was accomplished in a period of some nine months. Koch was a member of the German delegation participating in the Seventh International Medical Congress, held in London during the summer of 1881. At that meeting, Koch's techniques of photomicroscopy were specifically cited by Joseph Lister. Though it was not cited, Lister apparently first became aware of Koch's plate techniques as a more convenient means of growing bacteria in pure culture during this meeting as well. After returning to Berlin, Koch began his study of tuberculosis.

In June 1883, an epidemic of cholera broke out in Egypt, killing an estimated 58,000 persons by the end of the year. Following closely on the establishment of commissions by both the French and British governments, a German commission was established in August of that year, with Koch at its head, and including Gaffky, Bernhard Fischer and Hermann Treskow, the purpose of which was to investigate the source of the outbreak, and recognize a possible etiological agent.[47]

Koch had limited success in Egypt, observing a possible etiological agent in the intestinal mucosa of cholera victims, but being unable to fulfill the postulates by transferring the infection to a test animal. Unknown to the investigators, few non-human animals are susceptible to the disease. In mid–November 1883, with the number of victims of the disease in Egypt decreasing, Koch and the rest of the German Commission traveled to India for further investigation. This time the Commission was more successful, examining 92 victims—52 upon autopsy, and 40 live patients—and observing a slightly curved, comma-shaped bacillus. In some cases, the organism was so concentrated in the diarrhea that it "was almost like a pure culture."[48] Koch again had difficulty in finding a useful animal model. But the prevalence of the same organism in nearly all cases of cholera, and its decreasing prevalence in convalescent patients, made a convincing argument that this was the actual etiological agent.[49] Koch was honored with the Order of the Crown by Kaiser Wilhelm I—father of the "villain" of World War I—following his return from India, as well as being awarded 100,000 marks.

The years at the *Gesundheitsamt* brought Koch international fame. In addition to identifying the etiological agents of tuberculosis and cholera, his postulates—granting that an argument can be made that his associate Loeffler should receive equal billing for developing the steps in the process—established a working means associating specific agents with disease. Loeffler, during this same period—the early 1880s—established the bacterium *Corynebacterium diphtheriae* as the etiological agent of diphtheria.

Koch's work had "brought a modern focus on the discipline of hygiene as a scientific study."[50] Specifically, he was among the first to integrate the emerging field of bacteriology with the science of hygiene, itself perhaps the first interdisciplinary field by integrating medicine with the other sciences and a role for the environment. The first Institute of Hygiene had been established by Max von Pettenkofer in 1878 (*n49*). But Pettenkofer was no supporter of the germ theory of disease, at least from the viewpoint that disease is an infectious process resulting solely from the presence of microorganisms. During the early 1880s, two additional Institutes of Hygiene were established, one at the University of Göttingen in February 1885, and another at the University of Berlin soon afterwards. In May 1885, Koch was offered a position at the Institute in Berlin, an offer which was readily accepted. The offer included the proviso that Koch could retain his affiliation with the *Kaiserliche Gesundheitsamt*, while being appointed professor of hygiene and bacteriology in the just established Institute of Hygiene at the University of Berlin.

Koch's Hygiene Laboratory in central Berlin was housed in a building which had previously served as a technical school. The Prussian government paid for an extensive renovation and equipping of the laboratory, which was ready for occupancy in July of that year.[51] In addition to his research program, Koch's professorial duties included developing and teaching courses both in the field of hygiene as well as in bacteriology, the first course specifically in that subject in the world. Three separate courses were developed that summer and fall 1885: Hygiene, both lecture and laboratory courses, only open to a select few students, and public lectures on Bacteriological Research Methods. The first such public lecture was offered that November.[52] A more detailed description of Koch's teaching, particularly that which involved students from the United States, is presented in a later chapter.

Koch's Later Career

The thesis of this book is Koch's influence on the development of bacteriology in the United States, a period which encompassed the years between 1885 and the early 1890s, when analogous, and quality, courses began to appear in American medical schools. During the years between the beginning of his professorship in 1885, and his development of what he had considered a "cure" for tuberculosis in 1890, Koch's research productivity remained at a level significantly below that which he had achieved during the decade between 1875 and 1885. The years were not unproductive, as Koch developed a cohort of students and professional associates—among the notables being the aforementioned Loeffler, Richard Pfeiffer, Emil von Behring and others—whose work provided significant contributions to the "Golden Age of Bacteriology."

In 1890, Koch made what many medical historians consider Koch's most significant mistake, the preparation and use of a mycobacterial extract called tuberculin, the preparation of which initially remained a secret. Koch himself believed tuberculin to be a cure for that disease. An extensive analysis of the reasons for Koch's development and use of the extract, including the psychological context which played a role in this work, is in the work by Gradmann.[53] It is sufficient to say that analysis of the results of any field trials was sloppy—for example, no controls were included—and the treatment gave no evidence it was capable of curing the disease.

Despite this setback in his career, Koch continued to be honored with further recognition of his contributions. In 1891, the Institut für Infectionskrankheiten (Institute for Infectious Disease) was opened in Berlin, with Koch as its first director. He remained in that position for thirteen years, until in 1904 he was replaced, at his own request, by his associate George Gaffky. During those years, Koch traveled to German East Africa where he investigated a series of tickborne diseases among cattle; Koch returned two years later as head of the Sleeping Sickness Commission, investigating outbreaks of that disease in the human population.

Koch's awards during this period, and there were many, included the Nobel Prize in Physiology or Medicine (1905). Even the beginning of cardiac failure early in 1910 failed to prevent Koch from attempting to continue his work. Koch died May 27, 1910.

2

Germ Theory of Disease
Origins of Bacteriology

> "*The more or less constant presence of animal forms during disease does not prove they are the cause. In medicine isolated facts do not prove anything.... We feel sure the ultimate conclusion will be that bacteria are only incidental to disease and death, and no more their cause than the higher forms of animal and vegetable life that feed and grow upon dying and decaying animal and vegetable matter the cause of their death and decay.*"[1]

Though Robert Koch might rightly be considered the "godfather" of the germ theory of disease, the result of his experimental process linking specific agents with specific diseases, his ideas were more representative of an evolution in the understanding of disease. Nor was he the only late 19th century figure to play a role in firmly establishing the concept of "germ theory." One cannot describe Koch's work without invoking that of the French chemist Louis Pasteur as well. The two were rivals during this period, both professionally as well as politically, with Koch a representative of Germany, and Pasteur of France. Certainly their work at times overlapped, as with their respective studies on anthrax, and later with cholera. However the underlying theme of research carried out by Koch was that of medical microbiology/bacteriology; that of Pasteur, chemistry, applied most clearly in his development of vaccines for prevention of anthrax and rabies. But the bacteriology portion of the story is primarily that of Koch's contributions, not Pasteur's, and only the occasional reference will be made of the latter.

This is not to imply that Pasteur played less than a significant role in development of the germ theory during the late 1800s. The importance of timing in scientific discoveries is often overlooked. As a simple example in modern times, the Hershey-Chase experiment, carried out in 1952, is often cited as an experiment in which DNA was confirmed as the source of genetic information (at least in bacteriophage). In the procedure carried out by Alfred

Hershey and Martha Chase, bacteriophage DNA was labeled with radioactive ^{32}P, and viral protein with ^{35}S. Following infection of *Escherichia coli* by the phage, it was primarily the radioactive DNA which entered the cell, not the protein. But if one studies the actual result, some 20 percent of the protein also entered the cell during infection.[2] Why then was there no "Aha moment," in which skeptics could argue that this supports the hypothesis of protein as genetic material? The answer was timing. Oswald Avery and his co-workers had already shown several years earlier that DNA was the source of genetic material.[3] In a sense Hershey and Chase confirmed what Avery had previously shown, albeit in a manner less definitive.

How did timing play a role in the contributions by Koch and Pasteur to the germ theory? There is a significant difference between an early hypothesis which attempts to explain experimental or other forms of observations, and development of the technology necessary to support that hypothesis. Centuries prior to the birth of Koch or Pasteur the Italian physician (and perhaps father of epidemiology) Girolamo Fracastoro (ca. 1476–1553) suggested disease might be passed between humans through invisible (at the time) "spores" or similar forms of entities; his hypothesis could explain the observation of the contagious nature of many diseases. Because there was no contemporary means to test his hypothesis—the microscope had not yet been developed—Fracastoro believed his spores or entities to be chemical rather than biological in nature.

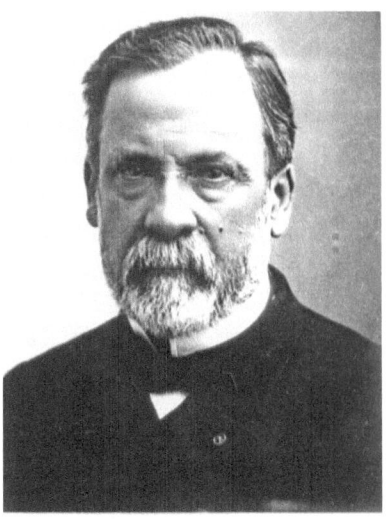

Louis Pasteur (1822–1895). A French chemist, Pasteur was initially recognized for his discoveries in fermentation, the identification of the agents in silkworm disease and in debunking of the theory of spontaneous generation. Among his contributions to the germ theory of disease, his work in bacteriology included development of vaccines against anthrax and rabies (National Library of Medicine).

It required the expertise of the Dutch draper, haberdasher and amateur lens maker (as well as the official wine taster for the city of Delft), Antonie van Leeuwenhoek (1632–1723) to make the "invisible" visible. Using a method involving carefully ground glass, van Leeuwenhoek was able to assemble a crude microscope, one capable of magnifying some 200X, sufficient to observe biological agents such as protozoa and larger bacteria. In approximately 200 letters and manuscripts sent to the Royal Society of London beginning roughly in the 1670s, van Leeuwenhoek described observations from various water sources, as well as using scrapings from his teeth, and even samples of his sperm.[4] Most of van Leeuwenhoek's observations were those of protozoa, and even these were not connected at the time with illness. But the applications using this technology became critical a century and a half later in linking his "infusoria" to disease.

Fermentation and Putrefaction

The link between the observations of microscopic "animals" and disease came about indirectly following the determination that fermentation by yeast and putrefaction reactions were biological in nature. The earliest descriptions of yeast from samples of beer were again provided by van Leeuwenhoek: "I have made [several] observations of the yeast from which beer is made and I have generally seen that it is composed of globules floating in a clear medium (which I judged to be the beer itself). Also I saw very plainly that each globule of the yeast consisted of six distinct globules [clumps?] of exactly the same size and shape as the corpuscles of our blood." Van Leeuwenhoek also described air bubbles emanating from the globules.[5] However, there was no suggestion on the part of van Leeuwenhoek that the yeast he observed was a living entity.

Independent observations by three individuals early in the 19th century produced the first evidence for the role of yeast in fermentation reactions: French physicist Baron Charles Cagniard-Latour (1777–1859), German physiologist Theodor Schwann (1810–1882) and German botanist Friedrich Traugott Kützing (1807–1893). In several publications during 1836 and 1837, Cagniard-Latour described the ability of yeast globules to undergo reproduction, confirming the living nature of the agent. He also proposed that production of carbonic acid and alcohol in fermentations was the result of vital activities by the yeast on sugar, observations confirmed and expanded on later in 1837 by Schwann, subsequently credited with the "germ theory of fermentation."[6]

It would fall to Pasteur to firmly establish the role of living organisms in fermentation or putrefaction reactions, at the same time playing a significant role in negating the concept of spontaneous generation—a concept supported by Schwann, among many others during those years.

Pasteur's initial foray into science dealt with the chemical nature of tartaric acid. Briefly (and simplistically), in times pre–Pasteur, it had been observed that racemic acid (paratartaric acid), lacking optical activity, failed to rotate a plane of polarized light, unlike other forms of the acid. Pasteur found racemic acid to be a mixture of dextro-rotatoty and levo-rotatory forms, each rotating light in opposite directions. From there he began an investigation of the rotation properties of fermentation products, asking the question of why they exhibited optical activity. His conclusion was that this demonstrated that fermentation reactions required life forms such as yeasts to take place.[7]

Pasteur spent much of the following two decades—1857–1870s—studying various forms of fermentation reactions, describing in the process concepts such as aerobic and anaerobic growth. His other work during these years, the role of micro-organisms in spoilage of wine and the protozoan silkworm disease pébrine, would be applied in the nascent germ theory of (human) disease.

Friedrich Gustav Jakob Henle

Though not universally accepted by any means, the application of the observations by Cagniard-Latour and Schwann that fermentation and putrefaction reactions were the results of vital processes, led to the idea that the disease process might have a similar basis. Several problems would have to be overcome in order to place this concept on a firmer basis. First was the element of size. To state the obvious, micro-organisms were small. How would something unable to be seen with the naked eye cause something potentially lethal in a large animal

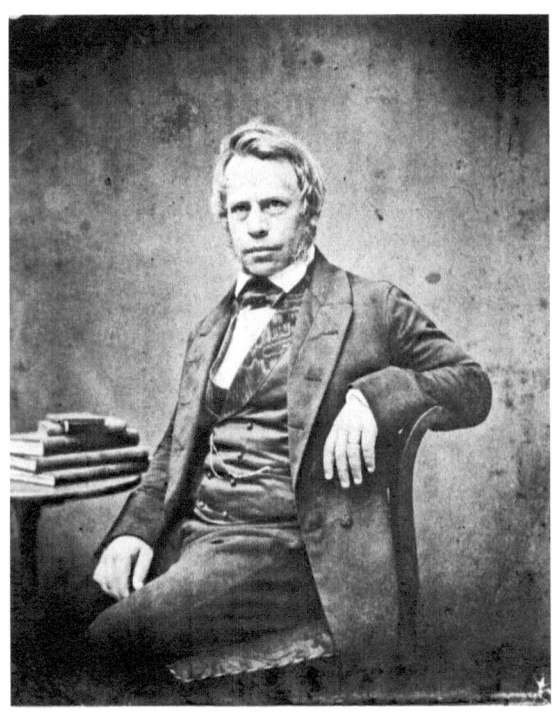

Friedrich Gustav Jacob Henle (1809–1885). A German physician, Henle during the 1840s proposed a series of experiments which could associate an etiological agent with a specific infectious disease. Preceding by a generation the germ theory, the testing of Henle's ideas was hampered by the inability to grow micro-organisms in pure culture (National Library of Medicine).

(including, of course, humans)? Second, the technology necessary to overcome this problem was insufficiently developed: microscopes in the 1830s were crude instruments unable to resolve organisms smaller than fungi, and not even readily available to most physicians. And third, even if one wished to study micro-organisms, there were few methods for isolation and growth in any form remotely resembling pure cultures.

Among the first to overtly link the fermentation and putrefaction processes carried out by living organisms with the disease process was the German physician and anatomist (and discoverer of the eponymous Loop of Henle) Jacob Henle. Henle was a close friend of Schwann's, and thus it would come as no surprise that he had been influenced by the latter's theories. Henle's most important contribution to understanding the basis of disease was in his work *Pathologische Untersuchungen* (Investigations of Pathology)(1840), more specifically in the portion entitled "Von der Miasmen und Contagien und von den miasmatisch-contagiösen Krankheiten" ("On the Miasmatic, Contagious and Miasmatic-Contagious Diseases").[8]

Henle was a realist in that he was aware experimental proof for his views on the etiology and contagious nature of disease would require actual isolation of the agents and growth in pure culture. In 1840 the techniques for doing so had yet to be developed, and Henle's ideas remained in the area of theory. Henle acknowledged the problem: "If it was possible with our present-day methods to solve the question of the nature of the contagium through direct observation, then the theoretical discussion which I have advanced as proof would be superfluous and unnecessary. Unfortunately it must be predicted that a rigid proof from positive observations is not yet possible."[9] Nevertheless, what could be rightly referred to as Henle's Postulates, to adapt a later vernacular, as we shall see, formed the foundation in associating an infectious agent with a specific disease.

As William Bulloch has pointed out in his history of bacteriology, among the competing theories explaining the cause of disease at the time Henle produced his work was what might be referred to as that of "contagia," arising spontaneously through derangement of the chemical properties in the body, and which then can spread in the form of gasses or droplets.[10]

Henle's reasoning was based on the premise that "the material of the contagium is not only organic, but also living, and indeed even has a separate existence, which is related to the diseased body in the way that a parasitic organism is related to it.... [Unlike the competing theory] it is not the disease, but the cause of the disease which reproduces itself."[11] Henle laid out three arguments in support of his theory: "(1) The ability to reproduce by the assimilation by foreign substances is an ability that we recognize only in living beings. No dead, chemical substance, organic or inorganic, can reproduce from the food of another." Henle went on to use the examples of fermentation espoused by Cagniard-Latour and Schwann in which they showed the process involves decomposition by fungi utilizing nutrients such as sugar; (2) "The action of the contagium may be compared with the fermentation in that the extent of the effect has no relation to the amount of the ferment used. [Using as an example the disease smallpox] A needle which is immersed in a solution of a grain of small pox material in a half dram of water is sufficient to cause an infection. This effect by such a small dose depends on the ability of the agent to reproduce itself, in the same way that such things occur in the fermentation or putrefaction, and is therefore a further proof for the living nature of the contagium"; (3) "The exactly constant course in the development of the miasmatic-contagious diseases, and the similarity in the course throughout an epidemic, speaks for a time-wise development of the disease inducer, in the same way that living beings develop."[12]

As alluded to above, Henle's arguments were purely in the realm of theory. "In order to prove that they are really the causal material, it would be necessary to isolate the animal seeds and animal fluid, the contagious organism and contagious fluid, and then observe especially the power of each one of these to see if they corresponded. This is an experiment which cannot be performed."[13] Henle's arguments—isolation of a contagium and growing it separately in the laboratory—represented the forerunner to what eventually evolved into Koch's Postulates, the series of steps linking a disease with a specific etiological agent. What Koch (or his associates) later included in the postulates, once the initial steps of isolation and growth became possible, was the follow-up experiment in which samples from a pure culture of the organism could induce the same disease in a healthy test animal.

Nor was Henle the only physician, prior to Koch, to suggest a mechanism to test the role of a (theoretical) etiological agent. In the 1860s, the French army surgeon Jean Antoine Villemin (1827–1892) demonstrated the infectious nature of tuberculosis. His work, *Etudes sur la Tuberculosis (Studies on Tuberculosis)* (1868), included experiments in which Villemin described the transmission of the disease from humans to rabbits and other animals using sputa from diseased patients. Other animals appeared insensitive to the material. Villemen's interpretation, that the cause of the disease was due to a living, reproducing agent, would be mirrored by Koch a decade later. "The inoculation of tuberculous material does not act by virtue of the visible and tangible matter, but because it contains a more subtle principle which escapes our sense [i.e., could not be observed with the naked eye].... We would be wrong to think that the affected organism has made the virus, since if we transfer from one organism to another a drop of vaccinal serosity, a drop of variolar or syphilitic pus, a fragment of tuberculous matter, etc., one reproduces in the inoculated subject a multitude of lesions which are similar to those found in the subject from which the inoculated material had been taken.... But the organism plays only the role of a medium in which the virus multiplies as a parasite.... We must establish a fundamental distinction between the virus and the substance that contains it. The latter is made by the organism under the prodding of the virus. The variolar virus is contained in the pus of the pustule but the pus is not the virus."[14]

Koch had a significant advantage which Villemin lacked when carrying out his own experiments—he was able to grow his agents in pure cultures and observe the actual organisms.

The failure to observe the physical entities coming to be known as germs, coupled with the inability to grow and study them in pure culture, still left Henle's and Villemin's hypotheses in the realm of theoretical. This did not mean that some physicians accepted and applied these ideas in their own work. Among the first in the mid-19th century to recognize the existence of a transmissible agent, albeit its exact nature being unknown by either, were Drs. Ignaz Semmelweis and Oliver Wendell Holmes, Sr. Semmelweis (1818–1865) was a Hungarian physician at the Vienna General Hospital's obstetric clinic during the 1840s, while Holmes (1809–1894), father of the famous jurist, was a physician practicing in Boston during the same period. Independently of each other, the physicians determined that puerperal fever, an often deadly disease which developed in women shortly after childbirth, was likely transmitted by the attending physicians themselves. Their solution was to require the physicians to wash their hands or clothing between patients—albeit the "soap" consisting of carbolic acid. Needless to say, the accusations that the physicians themselves were responsible for the suffering of these women were not readily accepted. However, when what today would be accepted hygiene— the routine washing of hands, unfortunately, not always followed in modern hospitals—was carried out, the incidence of puerperal fever dropped.

Puerperal fever is usually the result of infection by a common organism, *Streptococcus pyogenes*, which is also associated with infections such as erysipelas, a severe rash, and strep throat. In some cases, these infections among other patients may have been the source for puerperal fever. Neither Semmelweis nor Holmes would have known of the specific agent, and there is little reason to believe that at the time they carried out their studies, they would have even been aware of the role played by bacteria in any disease.

This was not the situation with the British physician and surgeon Joseph Lister. Lister (1827–1912), professor of surgery at the University of Glasgow during the 1860s, was all too familiar with the development of a contagion which commonly followed surgeries. It was not unusual for the patient to survive the surgery, only to die from sepsis—often referred to as "ward fever" or gangrene—in the days or weeks which followed. Pasteur's work on fermentation as the product of a vital force, and particularly his demonstration that micro-organisms were found in the air, convinced Lister that the source of the sepsis was contamination from airborne organisms. "To the question how the atmosphere produces decomposition of organic substances we find that a flood of light has been thrown upon this most important subject by the philosophic researches of M. Pasteur, who has demonstrated by thoroughly convincing evidence that it is not to its oxygen or to any of its gaseous constituents that the air owes this property but to minute particles suspended in it, which are the germs of various low forms of life long since revealed by the microscope and regarded as merely accidental concomitants of putrescence, but now shown by Pasteur to be its essential cause resolving the complex organic compounds into substances of simpler chemical constitution, just as the yeast-plant converts sugar into alcohol and carbonic acid."[15]

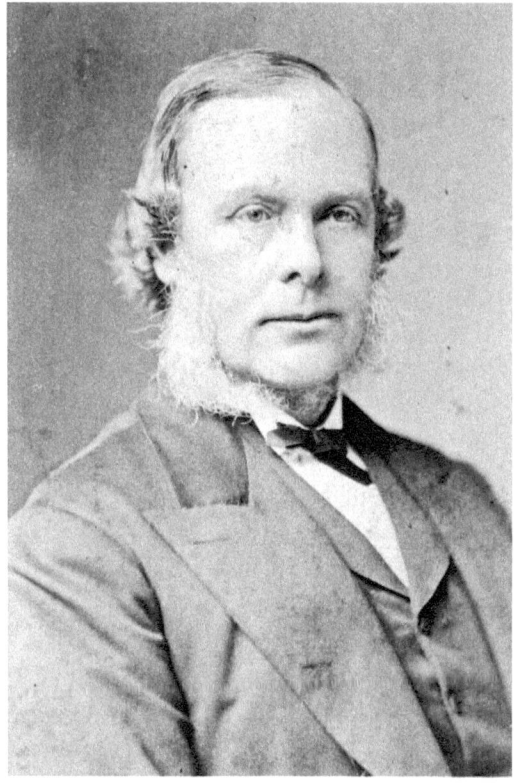

Joseph Lister (1827–1912). A British physician, Lister was the "founder of modern surgery" and considered among the first to apply the developing germ theory to antiseptic surgery. Prior to Lister's use of carbolic acid (phenol) as a sterilizing agent on surgical instruments and wounds, infections, often fatal, were almost inevitable. Lister also used his authority in requiring surgeons working with him to wash their hands in the carbolic acid solution (National Library of Medicine).

Since the actual infections could not be treated in that pre-antibiotic period, the only solution was to prevent the contamination in the first place. The answer appeared in the form of carbolic acid—phenol. A colleague of Lister's, Thomas Anderson, a professor of chemistry at the University of Glasgow, had informed Lister that carbolic acid was being used to treat sewage in the town of Carlisle. Not only did this eliminate odors, it also killed micro-organisms which were infecting the cattle. Upon investigation, Lister found this to be true, and decided to attempt the same principle in preventing post-surgical infections, reasoning that a similar process was involved in putrefaction and sepsis. Testing this idea, Lister soaked the dressings to be placed on the surgical wounds with carbolic acid. "Carbolic acid proved in various ways well adapted to the purpose. It exercises a local sedative influence upon the sensory nerves; and hence is not only painless in its immediate action on a raw surface, but speedily renders a wound previously painful entirely free from uneasiness. When employed in compound fracture its caustic properties are mitigated so as to be unobjectionable by admixture with the blood, with which it forms a tenacious mass that hardens into a dense crust which long retains its antiseptic [a term also coined by Lister] advantages."[16] Further additions to his surgical procedure included soaking ligatures in the same carbolic acid solution, and spraying a mist of carbolic acid over the patient.

While Lister is often credited with the first use of carbolic acid as an antiseptic, it is probable he had been preceded in this method of antisepsis by the Italian Enrico Bottini (1835–1903), who reportedly used the method during surgery at Novara, Italy, several years earlier.[17]

Lister has also been credited with developing a procedure during the late 1870s for isolation of a pure culture. Starting with a suspension of lactic acid producing bacteria, he diluted the sample such that it contained only a single cell. There were several obvious disadvantages to the method. First, the organisms would remain in suspension rather than on a solid medium, making it more difficult to observe contamination. Second, it only worked with the dominant organism in the culture, since it required the less numerous organisms to be diluted out. These problems would be solved within a few years, during which Koch developed a method for growing bacteria on a solid medium.

Casimir Davaine and Anthrax

Henle: "After it has been shown that the contagium is alive, there still remains the question of how the contagium works to bring about its damage. If it could be possible to prove that a contagium can be cultured outside the body, as in the observations of [Jean Victor] Audouin in the silkworm disease, then such a contagium could only be a plant or animal."[18] During the 35 years after Henle published his ideas, as a result of advances in laboratory methodology, medicine began to apply his concepts in identifying an etiological agent: the bacillus which causes anthrax.

The first observation of a micro-organism subsequently linked to a disease is often accredited to the French physician Casimir Davaine (1812–1882) and his mentor, Pierre Francois Rayer (1793–1867), who in 1850 observed a large rod-shaped organism termed *Bacteridium anthracis* in the blood of sheep dying from anthrax.[19] However, proper credit would arguably belong to the German physician Aloys Pollender (1800–1879), who, in 1849, observed what is now recognized as the agent of anthrax. Pollender was not associated with any formal laboratory, limiting his ability to publish his work, and consequently often overlooked in medical histories.

Regardless of whomever deserves credit for identification of the anthrax agent, it was Davaine wo carried out much of the early research on the subject. "I [Davaine] thought at that time I should be able, when the occasion arose, to check on the existence of those filiform infusorial bodies found in the blood of sheep which have died from anthrax and to find out if the development of these microscopic beings (rather like algae) was not the cause of deterioration in the blood and afterwards of the death of the animal.

"The occasion had not arisen and other work had prevented me from continuing active research when, in February 1861, M. Pasteur published his remarkable work on the butyric ferment, a ferment consisting of small cylindrical rods which possess all the characteristics of vibrios and bacteria. The filiform corpuscles that I have seen in the blood of anthracic sheep were much like the vibrios in shape and I was led to try and discover if this kind of corpuscle (or others of the same nature as those which determine butyric fermentation) when introduced in the blood of the animal would not act as a ferment."[20]

The logical next step in Davaine's research would be to determine whether the organisms he observed in the blood were actually the agents causing anthrax. The technology for growing the "corpuscles" in pure culture was not yet available, but Davaine addressed the question indirectly—whether the organisms were always present when the disease appeared. Using samples of blood from the sheep which had died from anthrax, he inoculated two rabbits and a rat. All three animals developed the disease and died. When Davaine transferred a sample of blood from the dead rabbit to a healthy one, that animal died as well. In a series of similar experiments, Davaine was able to build a strong circumstantial case that these organisms were the etiological agents of the disease: "(1) Anthracic blood is not infectious as long as the 'stick-shaped corpuscles' have not appeared; (2) He proposed the term *bacteridia* to designate these 'stick-shaped corpuscles'; (3) ... In pregnant females, the placenta acts like a filter retaining the *bacteridia* and thus protecting the fetus from the disease; (4) Putrefied anthracic blood caused in the inoculated animals a different disease, and in doing so he was already distinguishing septicemia from anthrax. [Here was the difficulty which resulted from an inability to grow the organism in pure culture. Putrefaction was the result of the presence of contamination by a different organism]; (5) Dried anthracic blood will remain virulent for a long time; blood kept dry for eleven months, then moistened and inoculated, still transmits the disease. [Davaine was unaware of the existence of spores, later observed by Koch]; (6) Birds and frogs appear to be refractory to anthrax; (7) ... The term 'spleen-blood' applied to anthrax is improper, since all the blood and not only the spleen blood is infested by bacteridia."[21]

Among Davaine's observations, was that the "malignant pustule," now called a black eschar, localized on the skin of a human, contained *bacteridia* identical to those found in the blood of sheep with the disease. Further experiments demonstrated that if he killed the organism by heating it at 52°C, the disease was no longer transmissible.[22] "These experiments prove that it is a living being, endowed as it is with a very complex organization, can be invaded and destroyed by a vibrio. In this fact will be seen, I hope, another argument in favor of the opinion I sustain on the nature of anthracic disease."[23] As Davaine's biographer pointed out, this was among the first experiments strongly supporting the *contagium vivum* theory, and demonstrating as well, that the infectious agent was not multicellular, as in the situation with mold or other fungal diseases. The agent was a unicellular microbe.[24]

In a more complex experiment, Davaine hoped to provide further support for his theory that the bacterium was the etiological agent by separating the organism from the medium in which it was grown, in effect producing what for the methodology of the time (1869) was a pure culture. Davaine placed a small quantity of anthracic blood in water, and allowed it to sit for 24 hours; the bacteria sank to the bottom of the solution. He then proceeded to inoculate one group of guinea pigs with a drop from the supernatant, and a second group with samples from the bacteria which sank to the bottom of the vessel. Only the second group of guinea pigs became ill with anthrax and died.[25]

Davaine's work could be considered a bridge between that of Pasteur and Koch. It was Pasteur's work on butyric fermentations which inspired some of Davaine's ideas about anthrax as well as some understanding of putrefaction. Davaine's name was invoked some 75 times by Pasteur in his own publications. "I [Pasteur] pride myself for having so often followed up your own learned research."[26] In 1876, Koch discovered the spore stage of the anthrax organism, which explained why contaminated soils retained the organism for years. (See below.)

Koch's Postulates

Jacob Henle's ideas, as constricted within the realm of theory as they were, and Davaine's experiments, laid the foundation for what would become known as Koch's Postulates, the experimental basis for linking an infectious disease and a specific agent. Whether Koch's own ideas which coalesced into the postulates were derived from Henle is unclear, as at the time Henle published this work—1840—the germ theory had yet to be developed. Koch himself appears to never have acknowledged Henle in that respect despite the latter's influence on his career. There is perhaps a stronger argument to be made that a contemporary of Koch's, Dr. Edwin Klebs, may have played a greater role in formation of the postulates.

Klebs (1834–1913), a Prussian-born pathologist, had received his initial training with Rudolf Virchow, with whom he worked until 1866. Following service as a military physician in the Franco-Prussian War, Klebs became a member of the faculty at the University of Bern in Switzerland as a professor of pathology, eventually moving first to Wurzburg (1872) and then to Prague in 1873. Much of his research in these years addressed the question of the role played by bacteria as etiologically agents of infection. In this area, he

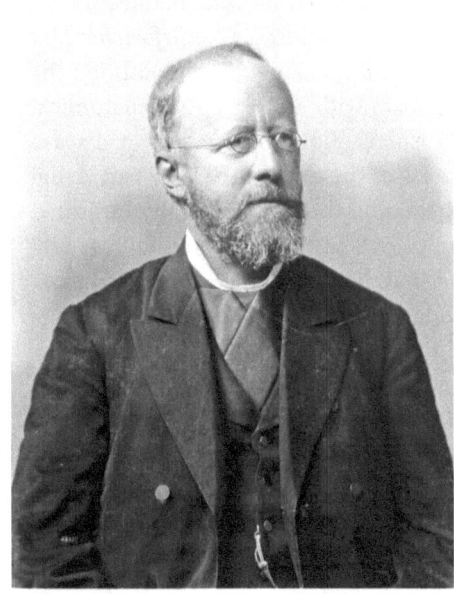

Edwin Klebs (1834–1913). A German physician and pathologist, Klebs used his expertise developed as a physician during the Franco-Prussian War to suggest a link between bacteria and wound infections. He and Friedrich Loeffler later identified the etiological agent of diphtheria. Klebs is also remembered for the eponymously named bacterial genus *Klebsiella* (National Library of Medicine).

became increasing estranged from the work of Virchow, who regarded disease as resulting more from changes in the physiological processes rather than from external infectious agents.

In 1872, Klebs published a work describing the pathology of gunshot wounds, likely an application of his role as a physician in the Franco-Prussian War. Koch reportedly considered this work to be "the first attempt to demonstrate a causal connection between bacteria and the infected wound diseases."[27] It was Klebs' belief that "tracing the invasion and the course of the micro-organisms can make causality probable, but the crucial experiment is to isolate the efficient cause and allow it to operate on the organism."[28] Klebs continued to pursue the same logic in his subsequent works. In an 1875 publication, he stated "inflammation and other reactive changes follow, step by step, the spread of the schistomycetes, then it is logical to infer a causal relation rather than a simple coincidence ... [it follows that] 'one must isolate substances from the body and use them to induce further cases of infection.'"[29] In 1877, in a presentation before the *Gesellschaft deutscher Naturforscher und Aerzte* (German Society of Naturalists and Physicians), Klebs outlined the methods necessary to associate an organism with a disease. "(1) anatomical investigations of diseased organs; (2) isolation and cultivation of disease germs; and (3) the initiation of new cases of the same disease by conveying germs to healthy animals."[30] Klebs touched on the same difficulty indicated by Davaine: growth of the organism in pure laboratory culture, followed by induction of the same disease. Beyond that, however, Klebs described most of the experimental steps for what today in basic microbiology courses is attributed to Koch.

While it was his work in which he determined the etiological agent of tuberculosis which led Koch to formalize his postulates, his studies of the etiological agent of anthrax laid the groundwork for his own application of the procedures. The reason why anthrax, a disease which while common during that time in animals but was relatively rare in humans, became a significant part of his research, is unclear. Thomas Brock, in his discussion of Koch's work, believed it to have been a "fortuitous" choice. Certainly there were advantages in choosing this particular disease and organism for study. As pointed out by Brock, the organisms were relatively large and easy to observe, they could be found in large numbers in the blood of diseased animals and were easily isolated, and even though anthrax was largely a disease of domesticated animals, humans did contract the disease.[31]

Koch's initial interest may have been triggered by an outbreak of anthrax in the district of Bomst in 1873, at the time a region of Prussia in eastern Germany. The following April, Koch described what were clearly spores which were forming among Davaine's *bacteridia*, isolated from the blood of sheep which had died from the disease. "The bacteria swell up, become shinier, thicker, and much longer. Slight bends develop. Gradually a thick felt develops. Within the long cells, cross walls appear and small transparent points develop at regular intervals."[32] This work represented the beginning of Koch's attempts to confirm the ideas of Davaine's—that the bacilli each had observed were indeed the agents of anthrax. In the process of studying the life-cycle of the organism, Koch not only produced an explanation for how the organism remained viable even while dormant, but demonstrated that a "relatively" pure culture of the bacilli would produce anthrax when inoculated into a susceptible animal.

Koch conceded that Davaine's ideas were not universally accepted. "Several workers have obtained experimental anthrax by inoculating blood containing bacteria, but have been unable to show the presence of bacteria in the blood of the diseased animals. Others have been able to induce anthrax by inoculation with blood which could not be shown to contain bacteria, but the diseased animals then had bacteria in their blood. Others have noted that anthrax is not derived solely from a contagium which is transmitted above ground, but that this disease is related in some way with conditions of the soil."[33]

Koch's colleague and mentor, Ferdinand Cohn, had observed spore formation by the hay bacillus, *Bacillus subtilis*, a year earlier, and it was logical for Koch to suspect a similar mechanism in maintaining viability by the anthrax bacillus, an organism similar in appearance (i.e., a filamentous rod). In order to address this question, Koch placed a sample of spleen obtained from an animal with anthrax on a microscope slide, and mixed it in either a small sample of beef serum or aqueous humor from the eye of a cow. After incubating the sample, Koch observed the presence of "light-refracting grains," what were obviously spores, as well as rod-shaped bacteria in different stages of a life-cycle. Further observations found the spores germinating, developing back into a filamentous form. When spores were inoculated into mice, the animals developed anthrax.[34]

As pointed out previously, the missing link was the requirement for growing the agent in a pure culture, preferably on a solid medium, and producing the disease in a susceptible animal. Koch's decision to observe spore formation by this bacillus in the liquid medium, followed by establishment of anthrax when injected into animals, was fortunate in that the likelihood of other organisms being present was small. But to be truly convincing, it would be necessary to ensure beyond a reasonable doubt that the organism was, in fact, a pure culture. By 1881, Koch was able to solve this problem.

Koch's initial idea for a solid medium was, in retrospect of course, almost obvious: the cut surface of a boiled potato. If the potato was first cooked, then maintained in a sterilized vessel, no bacterial colonies appeared. Such a potato slice, however, exposed to air and placed in a moist chamber, within several days gave rise to a variety of colony types. When examined with the microscope, the colonies consisted of different types of micro-organisms, including bacteria as well as molds. Since the surface was solid, individual colonies would be separated from each other. If one transferred colonies to another slice, the appearance would be identical to that of the source.

The method was limited to those organisms which grew on the potato. For the study of the more common organisms this approach worked well. Unfortunately, Koch discovered that many of the pathogenic organisms which he wanted to study failed to do so, and a different approach would be necessary. He found a substitute in nutrient gelatin—gelatin mixed with a nutrient liquid, poured over a watch glass or slide, and allowed to harden.[35] "Now it is only necessary to take a flamed needle and remove some blood from the opened heart or a convenient blood vessel and streak it a few times on the nutrient gelatin. There will occur growth in colonies of several types of micro-organisms, among which will be a greater or lesser number of pure, characteristically matlike and granular colonies which can be characterized under the microscope as those of the septicemia bacteria.... [If] the sought-for organisms were in the minority, it would still be possible to have success.... It is only necessary to dilute the bacterial mixture considerably

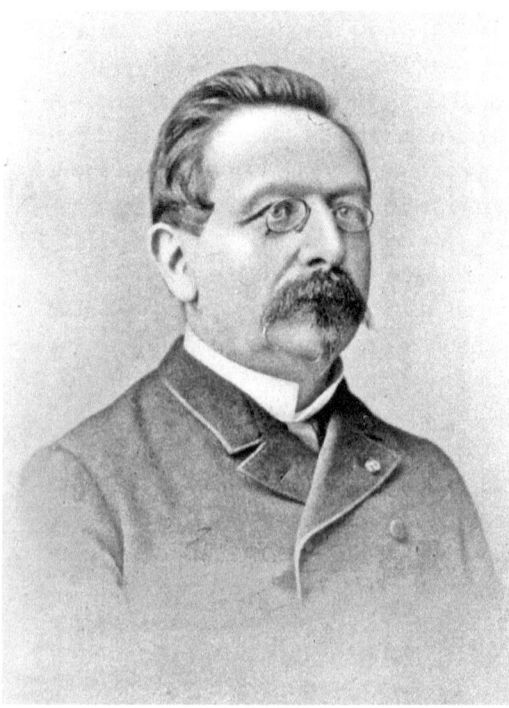

Jean-Antoine Villemin (1827–1892). A French physician, Villemin during the 1860s demonstrated the infectious nature of tuberculosis by transmitting the disease from humans to rabbits. Hampered by the inability to isolate and grow the organism in culture, Villemin was unable to definitely prove the contagiousness of the disease (National Library of Medicine).

and then make a large number of streaks. In such circumstances it is advantageous to inoculate into the still liquid gelatin, in order to spread the various germs over a wide area, and then pour it on the slides and locate the colonies which develop under the microscope."[36]

Koch's isolation and identification of the etiological agent of tuberculosis not only brought him significant fame—and a future Nobel Prize—it also represented the work in which he formally described the steps which would become known as his postulates. Tuberculosis, also known as consumption, the white plague, or phthisis—a term applied to the wasting of the body—was among the most dreaded of the 19th century diseases. It was associated with one-seventh of all deaths. During the 1860s, Jean Antoine Villemin had demonstrated the infectious nature of the disease (see above), as did others in subsequent years. Still, by the time Koch applied himself to studying tuberculosis, the etiological agent had yet to be identified. There was no shortage of physicians carrying out similar research. The major problems they encountered were two-fold: the organism, if indeed there was one, did not appear to grow on the laboratory media in use, and, in addition, the ordinary staining methods used in the laboratory failed to detect anything which appeared to be an infectious agent.

Like Klebs, the German pathologist Julius Cohnheim had received much of his training while serving as an assistant to Rudolf Virchow. As a professor of pathology at the University of Breslau in 1876, he was among those who observed Koch's demonstrations of the life-cycle of the anthrax bacillus. The following year, Cohnheim demonstrated that transfer of tubercular material into the anterior chamber of the eye of a rabbit would induce the production of tubercles, in effect providing support for the belief that tuberculosis was the result of an infectious agent. Cohnheim's choice of a culture medium, the liquid portion of the eye, would be repeatedly applied by Koch in his own work.[37]

Again illustrating the importance of timing, several advances in technology and methodology, some described in the previous chapter, played important roles in the ability of Koch to identify the tuberculosis agent: (1) aniline dyes, first discovered in the 1850s as coal tar derivatives, and used in the clothing industry to stain fabric, were also found to selectively stain bacteria, allowing the physician to differentiate the infectious agent from tissue; (2) use of the Abbe condenser, a system developed by the German physicist Ernst Abbe which allowed significantly better resolution by the microscope; and (3) application of the Zeiss oil-immersion lens. Though immersion lenses, including those which used oil, had been in use for decades, the lens developed by Zeiss in the 1870s was a significant improvement over its predecessors.[38]

On March 24, 1882, Koch presented his work before the Physiological Society of Berlin in which he identified the infectious agent. "The discovery of Villemin that tuberculosis can be transmitted to animals has been confirmed a number of times, but has also been opposed on seemingly good grounds, so that up until recently it has not been possible to state for certain whether tuberculosis is an infectious disease or not. Since then, [Julius] Cohnheim and [Carl] Salomonsen, and later [Paul Clemens von] Baumgarten, have achieved success by inoculation in the anterior chamber of the [rabbit] eye, and Tappeiner has been successful with inhalation [in dogs]. These studies have shown without a doubt that tuberculosis must be counted amongst the infectious diseases of mankind."[39]

Koch was able to visualize the tuberculosis bacilli using what could be referred to today as a differential stain—heated methylene blue, an aniline dye, in an alcohol solution made strongly basic with potassium hydroxide as the initial step, followed by the brown stain vesuvin. The tubercle bacteria appeared blue, while cell components stained brown. Other bacteria, with the exception of the leprosy bacillus, a member of the same genus as that of the tubercle organism, also stained brown. The significance of the use of a differential stain went beyond simply a means to observe the organism. The organisms were few in number, but plainly visible. "The bacteria visualized by this technique show many distinct characteristics. They are rod-shaped and belong therefore to the group of bacilli. They are very thin and are only one-fourth to one-half as long as the diameter of a red blood cell, but can occasionally reach a length as long as the diameter of a red cell. They possess a form and size which is surprisingly like that of the leprosy bacillus."[40] Koch provided an explanation as to why these organisms had not been previously identified. "The bacilli are extremely small structures, and are generally in such small numbers, that they would elude the most attentive observer without the use of a special staining reaction. Even when they are present in large numbers, they are generally mixed with finely granular detritus in such a way that they are completely hidden, so that even here their discovery would be extremely difficult."[41] The staining procedure developed by Koch allowed the investigator to observe the bacteria against the background of cellular or tissue material—in effect allowing the bacilli to stand out against an alternatively stained background. In his description of the organism, however, Koch described what he considered spores within some of the bacilli: "Under certain conditions ... the bacilli form spores even in the animal body. Individual bacilli contain several, usually two to four spores, oval in shape, and distributed at even intervals along the entire length of the bacillus."[42] *Mycobacterium tuberculosis* is not a spore-former. So what was Koch observing? Koch had of course observed spore formation in the anthrax bacilli which he had studied some years earlier. Indeed, spore formation was a significant part of the life cycle of that organism. Gradmann has provided an additional explanation. Since the methodology to stain spores did not exist at that time, their presence was sometimes inferred by their invisibility. If the sputum or caseous mass remained infectious even in the seeming absence of bacteria, the existence of spores provided a reasonable explanation. As Gradmann noted, "Koch's tuberculosis spores seemed to cease to exist later on."[43]

Indirect evidence supporting Koch's contention that he had identified the correct etiological agent was based upon the increased presence of the bacilli as the disease progressed, and their disappearance when the disease became quiescent. But Koch was also aware that if he was able to culture the organism in the laboratory, something which had eluded physicians until now, and produce the disease in a susceptible animal—in effect, following the postulates—the argument would be more convincing.

In order to produce a solid medium, Koch heated blood or sheep serum until it coagulated, placing it in a test tube and allowed it to harden at a slant. Coagulated blood or serum had proven superior to gelatin as a hardening agent. Unlike gelatin, serum did not liquify at temperatures above 30°C. The serum slants were inoculated with tubercles extracted from an animal dying from the disease, and incubated for one to two weeks. Similar solid media was prepared using agar as the hardening agent in a meat or peptone solution, and the same incubation procedure was followed. A minimum of one week's incubation was necessary to observe colony development.[44] Koch determined that whatever the source of the bacilli, whether from infected humans or other animals, the characteristics of the organisms were identical. Furthermore, inoculation of guinea pigs, among the few animals capable of developing, relatively quickly, a disease resembling human tuberculosis, with isolated tubercle bacilli resulted in a similar disease.[45] Use of guinea pigs as test animals served another purpose as well. The tuberculosis agent was a slow-growing organism, requiring a minimum of a week's incubation to be observed in culture. Contaminating organisms, such as found in the tissues prepared from human victims of the disease, would quickly outgrow the tuberculosis bacilli. The disadvantage was that in order to prove definitively the bacilli were the agents of human tuberculosis, it would be necessary to transfer extracts from the diseased organs in guinea pigs into humans, an experiment which could not be carried out, of course.

It would be two years before Koch outlined what clearly became known as his postulates. Despite the implication that the procedures were being applied to the agent of tuberculosis, it was his earlier work with anthrax which was outlined in the publication. The reason had to do with the step requiring exposure of a healthy organism to the agent, resulting in disease. To do so with tuberculosis required the use of a human subject, since the agent often grew poorly in non-human animals. Guinea pigs were an exception since exposure to the agent of human tuberculosis did result in disease. Even so, this was not necessarily sufficient to convince skeptics that Koch had indeed isolated the correct organism.

Koch's reasoning went as follows: "If the rod-containing blood of an animal which had died of anthrax was inoculated in an extremely minute quantity into another animal, this second animal always died of anthrax and its blood contained the characteristic rods, the so-called anthrax bacilli. However, this has not proved that through the inoculation of the rods, the disease was transmitted, because not only the rods were inoculated, but also the other formed and unformed elements of the blood. In order to decide whether it was the bacilli or some other substance of the anthrax blood which causes anthrax, the bacilli must be isolated from the blood and inoculated by themselves. The most certain way of isolating the bacilli is through continued pure culture. For this purpose, a small amount of blood containing bacilli is placed on a solid medium on which the bacilli are able to grow, such as nutrient gelatin, or boiled potato. On these they begin to reproduce quickly and soon are present in large numbers, while the other substances of the blood, the red and white cells and the blood serum, remain unchanged. After two or three days when the bacilli have formed a dense mass of sporulating filaments, a very small amount of this white mass is taken and streaked again on nutrient gelatin or boiled potato.... Already in this second culture there are no traces under the microscope of the other elements of the blood.... Now if the culture is transferred twenty or fifty times, then it can be assumed with complete certainty that the bacilli no longer are associated with even the slightest amount of disease products from the body.... The anthrax bacilli in pure culture in this way have therefore no relationships with the first organisms that came out of the blood, or with the disease products which belong to the metabolism of the animal. In spite of this, they are able to induce fatal anthrax as soon as they are inoculated into a healthy animal.... Also, in its blood appear the characteristic anthrax bacilli in countless numbers. From these facts no other conclusion can be drawn than that the anthrax bacilli are the actual cause of this disease, and not merely an attendant phenomenon or symptom."[46]

In this manner, Koch for the first time stated what microbiology students in the future would memorize as Koch's Postulates:

1. Observe the presence of the organism when the disease is present;
2. Isolate and grow the organism in pure culture;
3. Inoculate the organism into a healthy animal, causing the same disease;
4. Observe the presence of the same organism following induction of disease.

Ironically, it was not Koch who formally listed the steps of the postulates as they are routinely described, but his associate Friedrich Loeffler. Loeffler (1852–1915), an assistant in the Imperial Health Office in Berlin, worked with Koch between 1879 and 1884. In 1884 he (and Klebs) confirmed the identity of the etiological agent of diphtheria. The disease had been described by the French physician Pierre Bretonneau in the 1820s, including the presence of a pseudomembrane in the throats of victims. But the observance of a variety of organisms in the throat, coupled with the difficulty in transmitting the disease to animals, made it difficult to determine the specific etiological agent. In December 1883, Loeffler stated the requirements necessary to confirm the role of an infectious agent in the disease. The work was published shortly thereafter. "If, then, diphtheria is a disease caused by a micro-organism, three postulates must be fulfilled:

1. The organism typical in form and arrangement must be consistently demonstrated in the diseased area;
2. The organism which by its behavior appears responsible for the pathological process, Must be isolated and grown in pure culture;
3. A specific experimental disease must be produced with the pure culture."

Loeffler then described the difficulties in fulfilling these

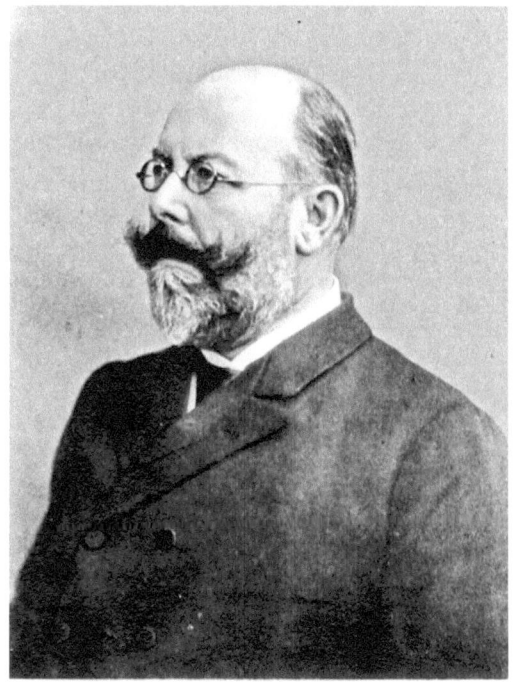

Friedrich August Johannes Loeffler (1852–1915). A colleague of Robert Koch's, Loeffler and Edwin Klebs identified the etiological agent of diphtheria. His description of the steps necessary to link an agent with a specific disease preceded, and largely mirrored, what became known as Koch's Postulates (National Library of Medicine).

postulates in the study of diphtheria, including the absence of bacteria in affected organs—as we are now aware, it is the toxin produced in the throat which results in the pathology—and the presence of other bacteria. Once the agent, *Corynebacterium*, was grown in pure culture, these problems were solved.[47]

This period, very roughly the two decades between 1875 and 1895, has been referred to as the "Golden Age of Bacteriology." The period began with the confirmation by Koch of *Bacillus anthracis* as the etiological agent of anthrax (1876), ending with the isolation of the plague bacillus independently by the Swiss-born physician Alexandre Yersin and the Japanese physician Kitasato Shibasaburō (1894). Each had trained for a time with Koch, though Yersin made his identification under the auspices of the Pasteur Institute. In between those years, the etiological agents for major diseases such as gonorrhea (Albert Neisser in 1879), leprosy (Hansen in 1880), pneumococcal pneumonia (George Sternberg and Pasteur, independently, in 1881), tuberculosis (Koch in 1882), cholera (Koch in 1883), diphtheria (Klebs and Loeffler in 1884) and tetanus (Shibasaburō in 1891) were identified. The postulates were not applied for every disease—even Koch was unable to transmit cholera to healthy animals—but the theory underlying those ideas was a defining feature for medical advances during that era.

3

Bacteriology in 19th Century United States

Medical training in general, and teaching or training in the new field of bacteriology in particular, were of minimal quality in the United States even as late as the last decades of the 19th century. It would not be an exaggeration to state that if one wanted to become a physician, all it required was minimal schooling—often without any training in anatomy—and perhaps an apprenticeship. There were a few exceptions by the 1880s, most notably the medical schools associated with Johns Hopkins University and the University of Michigan. But even these schools lacked any sort of bacteriology program prior to that decade. When bacteriology was finally incorporated into a medical program it was usually included within a department of hygiene. Those individuals who wanted further training, or simply better quality medical training, traveled to Europe for those purposes.

The improvements in technology, which included better microscopes, and advancement in culture techniques now available for the study of pure cultures, were European, mainly German, in their origin. By the 1880s, Pasteur had long proven the presence of micro-organisms in the air, negating the idea of spontaneous generation, and had demonstrated that rabies was a microbial disease (albeit due to an unseen filterable agent). Koch had identified the tubercle bacillus; other physicians had likewise linked specific microbes with disease. The concept of the germ theory was generally accepted in Europe, though as we have seen with individuals like von Pettenkofer, acceptance was not universal. The theory continued to be more controversial in the United States, the following quote being an example. Schenck presented other arguments as well in attempting to negate the germ theory: "It is said these diseases are dependent upon microscopic life, because their origin, progress and diffusion cannot be accounted for by any other theory. Granted—and neither can they by this. A few months ago I waited upon Mrs. M. in labor. She lived upon the high prairie, with no near neighbors. There was no child-bed fever or erysipelas among my patrons, and none in the neighborhood, yet upon the second day she developed puerperal fever, and barely escaped with her life. Whence came the micrococci? In this and thousands of similar cases they must have been original creations."[1]

Nor was this disagreement in the United States unique to Schenck. Dr. Charles Winslow Dulles, lecturer on the history of medicine at the University of Pennsylvania and secretary for the College of Physicians in Philadelphia, went so far as to argue that rabies in humans was not an infectious disease but was the result of "a form of hysteria based upon dread of the disease,"[2] and that he was "inclined to the view that there is no such specific malady" in that in the sixteen years in which he investigated that disease he "failed to find a single case on record that can be conclusively proved to have resulted from the bite of a dog or any other cause."[3]

How might one account for the lack of acceptance, indeed almost the lack of interest, among physicians in the United States. Medical "inertia," the refusal to accept anything which contradicted the professional beliefs of the individual, might account for part of the reason. A major contributor to this was the seeming absence of evidence to the contrary. How, for example, might one differentiate between the probability that these microscopic agents were indeed the etiological agent of the disease, from the (real) possibility that their presence was merely incidental to the process. This is where Koch's (and to do justice, Henle's and Klebs' as well) Postulates came into play, and where Henle's ideas remained in the area of theory: the ability to isolate and grow the alleged agent in the laboratory, and by exposing a susceptible organism to the agent, produce the identical disease. Koch's inability to find suitable test animals, other than humans, for this important third step after identification of the etiological agents for cholera and tuberculosis, would for a time serve as evidence among those opposed to his theories.

An additional reason for the slower acceptance of the germ theory in the United States was the lack of access to scientific writings on the subjects, more specifically the absence of English language texts and journals. The few scientific journals which did exist at the time of Koch's discoveries were written in either French or German, languages with which the American physicians likely were not familiar. Few attended international meetings. The first original English compendium on the subject was written by the British histologist and bacteriologist Dr. Edward Klein, whose *Microorganisms and Disease* was published in 1884.[4] In 1886, English physician and bacteriologist Dr. Edgar Crookshank published *An Introduction to Practical Bacteriology Based on the Methods of Koch*, and a year later, *Photography of Bacteria*, two texts which provided significant access to the ongoing work in Europe.

The first American physician who could arguably be considered a bacteriologist was Dr. George Sternberg (1838–1915). Sternberg, a Union army physician captured during the Civil War, was already well-known by the early 1880s for his work with the Yellow Fever Commission in Havana investigating transmission of yellow fever—the Spanish physician Dr. Carlos Finlay suspected a role played by the mosquito, later confirmed by a commission headed by Walter Reed. Sternberg in 1881 also identified the pneumococcus as the cause of bacterial pneumonia. In 1880, Sternberg translated from French into English the published work of Dr. Antoine Magnin (1848–1926), *Les bactéries* (1878), published in English as *The Bacteria* (1880), one of the first books attempting to compile the then current knowledge of the subject.[5] Sternberg produced a revised edition of the book in 1884. He subsequently produced two publications of his own on the subject: *Manual of Bacteriology* (1892), the first major work published in the United States, and *Textbook of Bacteriology* (1896). Sternberg served as Surgeon-General from 1893 to 1902.

It was during these years that the first scientific journals devoted largely to bacteriology also appeared, though in a language foreign to most American physicians: *Jahresberichte (Annual Reports)* in 1885, *Zeitschrift für Hygiene (Journal of Hygiene)* (1886), *Centralblatt für Bakteriologie (Source for Bacteriologie)* (1887) *and Annales de l'Institut Pasteur* (1888).[6]

A third reason American physicians were often skeptical of the rumors or published reports coming from Europe was the inability to reproduce some of the observations. Equipment such as microscopes and even glassware was at a premium. In the absence of any sort of manufacturing of these basics in the United States until about 1890, physicians were forced to import any sort of apparatus needed for such work. Even the basic technique of staining could be a challenge. Because of their unusual lipid content, the tubercle bacilli reported by Koch required an unusual staining procedure in order to even be observed.

Still, discoveries made by Koch did receive recognition in the written media of the period. Koch's identification of the tubercle bacillus, for example, made headlines in major newspapers. Even if physicians were not familiar with the details of his work, they were likely aware of the reports on the methodology and observations which came from his laboratory. "[John] Tyndall on Koch's Work: Parasites Found to Transmit Tubercular Disease.

"On the 24th of March, 1882, an address of very serious public import was delivered by Dr. Koch before the Physiological Society of Berlin. [See previous chapter] It touches a question in which we are all at present interested—that of experimental physiology—and I may, therefore, be permitted to give some account of it in the [*London*] *Times*. The address ... is entitled

"The Etiology of Tubercular Disease." Koch first made himself known by the penetration, skill, and thoroughness of his researches on the contagium of splenic fever. By a process of inoculation and infection he traced this terrible parasite through all the stages of development and through its various modes of action. This masterly investigation caused the young physician to be transferred from a modest country practice, in the neighborhood of Breslau, to the post of Government Advisor in the Imperial Health Department of Berlin.

"From this department has lately issued a most important series of investigations on the etiology of infective disorders. Koch's last inquiry deals with a disease which, in point of mortality, stands at the head of them all. If, he says, the seriousness of a malady be measured by the number of its victims, then the most dreaded pests which have hitherto ravaged the world—plague and cholera—must stand far behind the one now under consideration. Koch makes the startling statement that one-seventh of the deaths of the human race are due to tubercular disease, while fully one-third of those who die in active middle age are carried off by the same cause. Prior to Koch it had been placed beyond doubt that the disease was communicable; and the aim of the Berlin physician has been to determine the precise character of the contagium which previous experiments on inoculation and inhalation had proved to be capable of indefinite transfer and reproduction. He subjected the diseased organs of a great number of men and animals to microscopic examination and found, in all cases, the tubercles infested with a minute rod-shaped parasite which, by means of a special dye, he differentiated from the surrounding tissue. It was, he says, in the highest degree impressive to observe in the centre of the tubercle cell the minute organism which had created it. Transferring directly by inoculation the tuberculous matter from diseased animals to healthy ones, he in every instance reproduced the disease. To meet the objection that it was not the parasite itself, but some virus in which it was embedded in the diseased organ, that was the real contagium, he cultivated his bacilli artificially, for long periods of time, and through many successive generations. With a speck of matter, for example, from a tuberculous human lung, he infected a substance prepared, after much trial, by himself, with the view of affording nutriment to the parasite. Here he permitted it to grow and multiply. From this new generation he took a minute sample and infected therewith fresh nutritive matter, thus producing another brood. Generation after generation of bacilli were developed in this way without the intervention of disease. At the end of the process which sometimes embraced successive cultivations extending over half a year, the purified bacilli were introduced into the circulation of healthy animals of various kinds. In every case inoculation was followed by the reproduction and spread of the parasite and the generation of the original disease."[7] As noted in the previous chapter, the only portion of what became his postulates which was lacking in Tyndall's report, was the inability to infect the normal hosts—human beings—with bacilli from the isolated cultures. Nevertheless, neither the lay reader in America, nor, certainly, American physicians—skeptics such as Schenck and Dulles aside—could simply ignore the evidence provided by Koch as to the agent of tuberculosis.

Even among those familiar with, and accepting, the germ theory, mistakes were made. Dr. Henry Formad (1847–1892), pathologist at the University of Pennsylvania, during the fall of 1882 instituted a class on the subject of bacteria and their role in disease. (See below.) Formad had traveled to Koch's laboratory that summer, and again during the fall of 1883, for training in the techniques which Koch had developed. While considered a competent pathologist who at times also served as coroner, Formad's knowledge of bacteriology did have its limits. In one particular example, Formad mistakenly associated a micrococcus with an outbreak of diphtheria in Michigan in 1882.[8] In a collaborative work with Dr. Horatio Wood, Formad carried out an investigation of an outbreak of diphtheria in the spring of 1881 in Ludington, located on Lake Michigan on the western side of the state. Wood and Formad had previously observed micrococci within the pseudomembranes formed in the throats of victims, usually children, of diphtheria. Their investigation of the Ludington outbreak resulted in similar observations. "Almost all the children had had it, and one-third of them were said to have died. Dr. Formad examined a large number of cases, obtained a supply of diphtheritic membrane, and brought home pieces of the internal organs of a child on whom he had made an autopsy. In every case the blood was found more or less full of micrococci, some free, others in zooglea masses, others in the white blood corpuscles. The organs brought home also all contained micrococci, which were especially abundant in the kidneys, where they formed numerous thrombi, choking up and distending the blood vessels.... Experiments were now made with the Ludington material upon animals. Inoculations were practiced under the skin, deep in the muscles, and in the trachea. In all cases the results were similar. A grayish exudation appeared at the seat of inoculation, along with much local inflammation, the animal sickened, and in the course of a few days death occurred.... The blood examined during life or after death was found to contain micrococci precisely similar to those found in the Ludington cases, and in a few instances micrococci were found in abundance in the internal organs.... In the diphtheritic membrane the micrococci exist frequently in balls, and it is plain that these collections are merely leukocytes full of the plant." Wood and Formad continued their experiments, testing whether the micrococci grown in culture would continue to produce disease in rabbits. Something else they observed may provide a clue as to with which organisms exactly they were working. "*We cultivated micrococci from the surface of ordinary sore throats* [italics added], from furred tongue, from cases of mild diphtheria as we commonly see it in Philadelphia and from Ludington cases. We found, in the first place, that there were no differences to be detected in the general or special appearance of the various micrococci, and no constant differences in size.... We conclude, therefore, that as no difference is detectable between the micrococci found in ordinary sore throat and those of diphtheria, save only in their reproductive activity, they are the same organisms in different states.... We have made many inoculations with cultivated micrococci [in rabbits] and have succeeded in producing diphtheria.... This success ... seems to us sufficient to establish the fact that the micrococci are the *fons et origo mali* [source and origin of evil] of diphtheria."[9] From their description of the organism—cocci which were also present in ordinary sore throats, and their appearance as "balls," neither being characteristic of Corynebacteria—suggests they were actually observing either streptococci or staphylococci. The internal appearance of the organisms would also suggest a systemic infection of some sort, not typical with diphtheria, but in accordance with infections by the either streptococci or staphylococci.

Formad also was among those skeptical with Koch's assertion that he had identified the agent of tuberculosis, a topic discussed in greater detail in the next chapter. Koch himself had conceded that the leprosy bacillus stained in the same manner as that of the tuberculosis agent, which we now understand is the result of the two organisms being structurally similar. But Formad also alleged that other bacilli also stained in a manner similar to that of the tubercle bacillus using the Koch procedure. Since there is no available record for analysis of Formad's own staining procedure, his allegations cannot be tested.[10]

Bacteriology Instruction in the United States

As the germ theory of disease acquired greater acceptance, American physicians and scientists—the professions were largely synonymous at the time when applied to medical science—were at a disadvantage. Since most of these reports were published in French or German, few were familiar with the discoveries coming out of Europe beyond what might be reported in the news media. Until the early 1880s, bacteriology courses were not included in medical education. Even when basic equipment such as microscopes had been available, training in the techniques and methodology to observe or study micro-organisms was minimal.

The solution to the issue of incorporating bacteriology in the medical curriculum in the last decades of the 19th century, was for American physicians to travel to Europe to learn necessary laboratory techniques. Most made their sojourn to Germany, with a large proportion of those traveling to Berlin to work with Koch or his associates. Among the first was William Welch who in 1876 and 1877 traveled to Strassburg and Leipzig for training, returning to Bellevue Medical College in New York to establish a medical laboratory modeled after those he observed in Germany. In 1884 Welch returned to Berlin in hopes of working directly with Koch, world famous by now for his discovery of the tubercle bacillus. After briefly traveling elsewhere in Germany, Welch, along with Dr. Harold Ernst from Harvard and Dr. Theophil Mitchell Prudden from Columbia University, in 1885 became the first Americans to study directly under Koch. Welch returned to Baltimore where he was appointed to the new Johns Hopkins School of Medicine. Several years later he became dean of that program. A more expansive description of Welch's professional career is provided in a later chapter.

Beginning in the fall of 1885 at Harvard, Ernst (1856–1922) developed a course consisting of six lectures in bacteriology. He became a professor of bacteriology in a newly established department at Harvard in 1895, carrying out work in disparate areas such as immunization against rabies, and studies on the presence of tubercle bacilli in milk. Prudden (1849–1924) established the first course in bacteriology for students at Columbia, the first such course in the city. Included in the laboratory portion were lessons on staining bacteria within tissue sections, and the use of solid media for growth of microorganisms. Prudden's research included the study of bacteria found in air and water, producing several monographs on that subject. Prudden also was instrumental in producing the first commercial diphtheria antitoxin in New York during the 1890s.[11] More detailed discussions of Prudden's career, and his training in Koch's laboratory, are found in later chapters.

While the most notable teaching and research efforts in the nascent field of bacteriology were being carried out in Europe during this period, it would be a mistake to ignore those "home-grown" American scientists, some in the medical field, others in different areas of biology, who also made contributions in the 1880s and 1890s. Described in a rough chronological order, the most notable of these individuals were located in the east and Midwest.

Dr. Thomas Jonathan Burrill (1839–1916) was a botanist and plant pathologist at the University of Illinois who, in the late 1870s, identified the etiological agent of the plant disease pear (fire) blight. The agent had initially been thought to have been a fungus. However, Burrill noticed that while samples of infected tissue were often free from fungus, masses of rod-shaped bacteria were invariably present. Burrill separated samples of the bacteria which he used to inoculate fresh plants, repeatedly inducing the disease. The organism, which he named *Micrococcus amylovorus*, now known as *Erwinia amylovorus*, was the first bacterium shown to be the etiological agent of a plant disease.[12] Burrill was among the first American instructors to include discussion of bacteria in his courses, publishing a sixty-five-page pamphlet, *The Bacteria: An Account of Their Nature and Effects, Together with a Systematic Description of the Species* (1882), in which he described the current state of bacteriology. Included in his pamphlet was the classification scheme of bacteria recently published by Ferdinand Cohn in Germany. At the time of his death, Burrill was president of the Society of American Bacteriologists.

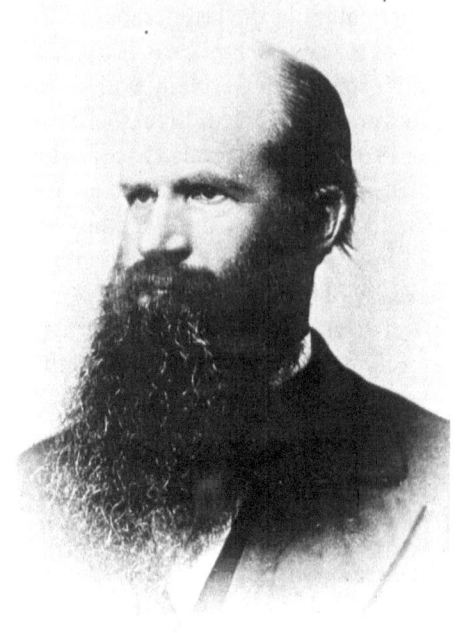

Thomas Jonathan Burrill (1839–1916). A professor of botany at the University of Illinois, Burrill discovered the first bacterium shown to be the agent of a plant disease, pear blight. He was among the first university professors to include the study of bacteria in his courses, publishing *The Bacteria: An Account of Their Nature and Effects, Together with a Systematic Description of the Species* (1882), a description of the status of the subject (National Library of Medicine).

Dr. Henry Formad, during the fall of 1882 instituted a class at Harvard on the subject of bacteria and their role in disease. As noted above, Formad had twice traveled to Koch's laboratory, once that summer, and again during the previous fall, for training in the techniques which Koch had developed. Among the topics Formad included in his class, was the methodology for staining and observing the tubercle bacillus in the sputum of suspected victims. In addition, his classwork included staining procedures for bacteria, and methods for cultivating bacteria.[13]

Despite his skepticism about Koch's identification of the tubercle bacillus, Formad was an early advocate of the germ theory of disease, a topic included in his lectures. Among his notable pupils was Dr. David Bergey. His interests in medicine were not confined to himself, as Formad's sister, Marie Formad, a graduate of the Woman's Medical College in Philadelphia, became the first woman granted membership in the Obstetrical Society of Philadelphia.

Dr. Alexander Crever Abbott (1860–1935) was a member of the generation of bacteriologists which studied under George Sternberg. Born in Maryland, Abbott received his medical degree from the University of Maryland in 1884. That same year he joined Sternberg's laboratory at Johns Hopkins University, where he received his first training in bacteriology. After Dr. William Welch became director of the Pathological Institute, Abbott joined him as his assistant in the instruction of that subject. Abbott and Welch subsequently confirmed Loeffler's identification of the etiological agent of diphtheria. In 1892, Abbott joined the faculty at the newly established Laboratory of Hygiene at the University of Pennsylvania, offering a course in bacteriology not only to medical students at the university, but to others who wanted such training for their own professional careers. In 1892, Abbott published the first edition of *The Principles of Bacteriology*. The text remained a staple for students for decades. Abbott later became chief of the Bureau of Health in Philadelphia, during which time he instituted chlorination of water supplies for elimination of water-borne diseases such as typhoid. In 1899, Abbott, Dr. Herbert Conn of Wesleyan University, and Dr. Edwin Jordan from the University of Chicago, were members of a volunteer committee, the recommendation of which led to the founding of the Society of American Bacteriologists. Abbott was elected to be the first vice-president of the organization.

Abbott's wife, Georgina Osler, was a niece of Sir William Osler, for whom their son, William Osler Abbott,

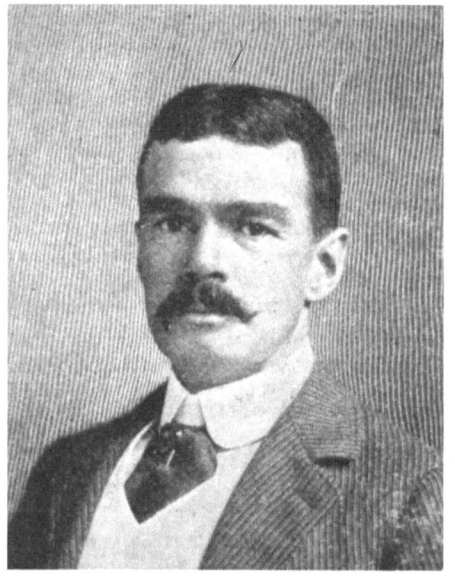

Alexander Crever Abbott (1860–1935). Abbott was among the first faculty members joining the newly established Laboratory of Hygiene at the University of Pennsylvania. His text, *The Principles of Bacteriology*, became a primary source for several generations of medical students at the school. Along with Drs. Herbert Conn and Edwin Jordan, Abbott was a founding member of the Society of American Bacteriologists (National Library of Medicine).

was named. William Abbott became a prominent physician as well, noted for development of the Miller-Abbott tube, used for decompression of the small intestine.

A program in bacteriology at the University of Wisconsin during this same period (mid-1880s) was instituted by Dr. William Trelease. Trelease (1857-1945) was a member of the faculty there for only a short period—roughly 1881 to 1885—after which he received an appointment as Engelmann Professor of Botany at Washington University in St. Louis. The course in bacteriology which he taught during the years 1881-1883 is considered by some to have been the first in the United States, though technically it had only been incorporated into his botany course. In 1889, he was appointed director of the Missouri Botanical Gardens in St. Louis, a position he held until 1912. Trelease's field was that of botany—his doctoral thesis at Wisconsin was published as "Observations on Several Zoogloeae and Related Forms." But while carrying out this work, the role he played in bacteriology at the university primarily lay first in including the subject of bacteriology in his instruction, and second in his influence with others.[14]

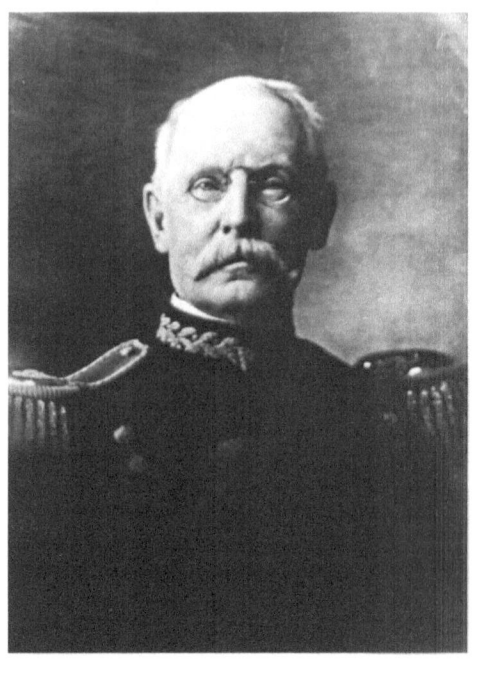

George Miller Sternberg (1838-1915). Considered the first American bacteriologist, Sternberg wrote *Manual of Bacteriology* (1892), the first American-produced text on that subject. In 1893, he was appointed to the position of surgeon-general by President Grover Cleveland, serving in that position for nine years (National Library of Medicine).

Following Trelease's departure in 1885, Dr. Edward Ashael Birge (1851-1950) replaced him as the instructor in bacteriology, establishing the first formal course dealing entirely with that subject. Trelease had already arranged for the purchase of materials for the course, ordering the supplies from Germany.[15] As was the situation with Trelease, Birge's field was other than bacteriology, in his case, limnology. Much of his career at the university was as an administrator, serving first as director of the Wisconsin Geological and

Natural History Survey, and later as president of the university. Birge continued the teaching of bacteriology until 1893, when he was replaced by one of his own students, Dr. H.L. Russell. Though a Congregationalist and teacher of Bible classes in his personal life, Birge was a strong believer that the study of evolution and the Bible were compatible. During the 1920s, he and William Jennings Bryan, an advocate of a more literal translation of Scripture, had strong disagreements over the subject.

Joining the faculty at Wisconsin in 1893, Harry Luman Russell (1866–1954) was the first titled professor of bacteriology at the university. After training in bacteriology under Trelease and Birge for his graduate work, Russell spent two years in Europe—in Paris at the Pasteur Institute, in Robert Koch's laboratory in Berlin, the same time in which Koch announced the application of tuberculin (early 1890s), and subsequently in Naples, for further studies (see Chapter 5). Returning to the United States in 1892, he earned his Ph.D. at Johns Hopkins while working under William Welch. Russell entered the program as assistant professor of bacteriology, with a joint appointment to the staff of the Agricultural Experiment Station in 1893. Later that year he replaced Birge as chair of the Department of Bacteriology. In 1897, he was promoted to full professor. Russell's area of research focused largely on the role of bacterial contamination in the milk and milk product industries, including bovine tuberculosis.[16]

Dr. Hermann Michael Biggs (1859–1923) was a major figure in the evolution of public health in New York City during the early 20th century. In 1883, after receiving his medical degree, he was appointed house surgeon at Bellevue Hospital Medical College, following which he traveled to Berlin where he received further training in Koch's laboratory. His work with Koch included experience with the staining procedure for identification of the tuberculosis bacillus, perhaps the first physician in New York City to have the expertise in that technique. In 1887, he identified the cholera bacillus among emigrants to New York, helping to prevent an outbreak in that city. During these years, Biggs instructed a generation of students in the techniques of bacteriology, basing his teaching both from his own knowledge and experience, as well as that which he had learned from Koch. Biggs advocated the establishment of a municipal diagnostic laboratory, following which he was appointed as its first director. Koch himself commended the laboratory as a model others should follow. As a result, tuberculosis joined a list of notifiable diseases. In 1902, he was appointed General Medical Officer for Health, a post he held until 1913.[17]

When French physician Dr. Emile Roux, bacteriologist and associate of Pasteur's, at the Pasteur Institute, described a method in 1894 for creating diphtheria antitoxin using serum from immunized horses, Biggs and Prudden petitioned the New York City Board of Estimate for funds to purchase horses for production of their own serum, but were refused. Instead, they purchased their own horses, for production of antitoxin. The treatment proved effective, becoming the first effective treatment of an infectious disease in the United States.[18]

Dr. Louis Hermann Pammel (1862–1931) was another of the more prominent students to have been trained in bacteriology under Trelease and Birge. He was graduated with a bachelor's degree with honors for his work on parasitic fungi from the University of Wisconsin in 1885, the first to earn a Bachelor of Agriculture degree from that institution. After earning his doctorate at Washington University in 1889, Pammel joined the faculty of Iowa State University as professor of botany. In the spring of 1889, Pammel offered a course in bacteriology to the veterinary students at the school. Among students Pammel taught during his first years at Iowa State was George Washington Carver, later to become well-known for his work in agriculture at Alabama's Tuskegee Institute.

Dr. Hermann Knapp (1832–1911) was an ophthalmologist and founder of the New York Ophthalmic and Aural Institute in 1869. Though not a bacteriologist, Knapp had spent time in Berlin during the 1880s, returning with supplies necessary for a bacteriological laboratory. In 1882, Knapp was appointed Professor of Ophthalmology at New York University School of Medicine. A colleague, Dr. John Elmer Weeks (1853–1949), taught a course in bacteriology from 1885 to 1887. In 1886, Weeks isolated a bacterium associated with conjunctivitis, proving Koch's Postulates by inoculating himself with the bacillus and developing that infection. At the same time Weeks was isolating the agent, Koch himself independently observed the same organism in cases of conjunctivitis. Now identified as *Haemophilus aegyptius*, it is also known as the Koch-Weeks bacillus.

Dr. Heinrich Janssen Detmers (1833–1906) joined the Ohio State faculty in 1885, transferring from Iowa State College and becoming the first professional veterinarian on staff. From 1885 to 1895, Detmers was chair of the School of Veterinary Science in Columbus. Born in what is now Germany, Detmers was trained at the Royal Veterinary Colleges in Hanover and Berlin. Detmers came to the United States in 1865. His first faculty appointment was at the Illinois Industrial College, now the University of Illinois, in 1869. Detmers moved to the Kansas State Agricultural College in 1872, where he remained for two years. Among the other faculty was his daughter, Jennie Detmers, who taught both chemistry and German. During the interim before moving to Iowa, Detmers engaged both in private practice, as well as working with the Department of Agriculture Bureau of Animal Industry. Among his colleagues was Dr. Daniel Salmon, with whom he studied the problem of hog cholera which he termed swine plague. Detmers mistakenly believed the etiological agent was a bacillus he isolated, naming it *Bacillus suis*. Only later was the agent determined to be a virus.[19]

While at Ohio State, he oversaw the teaching of veterinary science and veterinary medicine, but beginning in 1886, also instituted a course in bacteriology for senior veterinary students.[20]

Dr. Bayard Taylor Holmes (1852–1924) received his medical degree from the Homeopathic Medical College in Chicago in 1883. After interning at Cook County Hospital, in 1888 he developed a course in bacteriology for students at Chicago Medical College, now Northwestern University School of Medicine. The following spring of 1889 he was appointed to the position of professor of bacteriology in the Postgraduate Medical School of Chicago. In July of that year Holmes was appointed secretary of the College of Physicians and Surgeons in Chicago, now the University of Illinois at Chicago College of Medicine. As professor of bacteriology and surgical pathology, Holmes developed a lecture and laboratory course in bacteriology for the medical students.[21]

The names of Drs. Victor Vaughan and Frederick Novy were nearly synonymous at the University of Michigan during the late 1880s and 1890s. Vaughan was dean of the medical school from 1891 until his retirement in 1921. Novy began his medical career as a student of Vaughan's, eventually serving as chair of the Department of Bacteriology. During these years, the two collaborated in much of their work, even traveling at the same time to Berlin where they gained experience working in Koch's laboratory. In 1889, they developed the first formal course in bacteriology at the University of Michigan. A more complete discussion of their scientific achievements is provided in a later chapter.

Dr. Herbert William Conn (1859–1917) received a Ph.D. at Johns Hopkins University in 1884 for his study of animal morphology and physiology. While at Johns Hopkins he developed an interest in bacteriology while studying with the pathologist Dr. William Councilman. In 1884 he joined the faculty of Wesleyan University in Middleton, Connecticut, becoming professor of biology in 1887, and subsequently chair of that department. Dr. Conn's interest in research was agricultural bacteriology, with emphasis on bacteriology of milk and soil. His teaching included instituting a course in bacteriology. In 1899, Conn was among the founders of the Society of American Bacteriologists, the forerunner of the American Society for Microbiology. Conn first served as secretary, and in 1902 became president of the society.

Dr. William Thompson Sedgwick (1855–1921) received his Ph.D. in biology from Johns Hopkins University in 1881, remaining at the university as an associate in biology for two years. In 1883, he joined the biology faculty at the Massachusetts Institute of Technology, where he remained for much of his professional career. Many consider him to have been a founder of modern public health in the United States as a result of the structured programs in that subject which he instituted. His earliest research at the Institute involved collaborations with the chemist Dr. William Nichols in physiological studies of gas poisoning. However, in 1886, while traveling in Berlin, Nichols suddenly died, and when his effects were returned to MIT they included gelatin tubes from the laboratory of Robert Koch. Their application to bacteriology stimulated an interest in the subject on the part of Sedgwick, who, during the academic year 1888–1889, developed the first formal course in bacteriology at the university for students in the civil engineering program.

In 1891, Sedgwick was promoted to professor of biology,

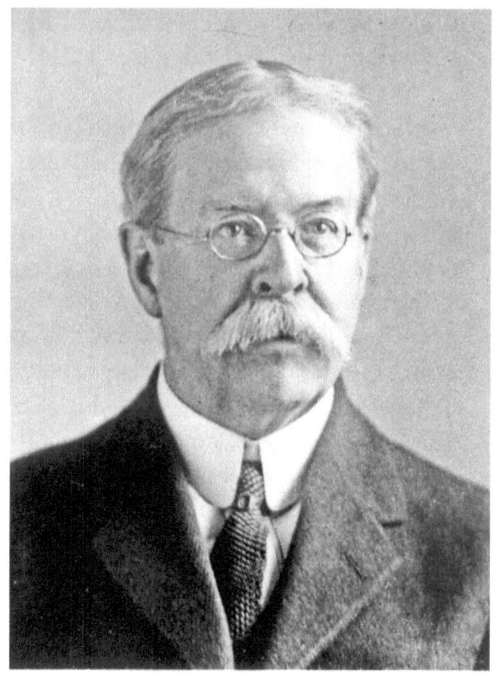

William Thompson Sedgwick (1855–1921). A bacteriologist and member of the faculty at the Massachusetts Institute of Technology from 1883 until his death, Sedgwick in 1888 developed the first formal course in bacteriology at the university for students in the civil engineering program. He was a founding member of the Society of American Bacteriologists, serving as the organizations first president in 1899. Much of his professional career dealt with the study and institution of changes in the field of public health (National Library of Medicine).

and subsequently to chair of the Department of Biology. Under his guidance the department became known as Biology and Public Health. In his honor, the Sedgwick Memorial Medal was established by the American Public Health Association in 1929, which became a yearly award for distinguished work in the area of public health.[22] Sedgwick was also a founding member of the Society of American Bacteriologists, being elected as the first president in 1899.

Dr. Joseph MacFarland (1868–1945) received his medical degree from the University of Pennsylvania in 1889. He received further training during a visit to the laboratory of Dr. Carl Fraenkel, an assistant to Robert Koch, in Berlin. In 1892, MacFarland was appointed to a lectureship at the University of Pennsylvania Medical School, where he developed a bacteriology course for second year medical students. In addition to instruction in the standard, by then, methods for isolation and staining of bacteria, MacFarland paid particular attention to staining methods for identification of the tubercle bacillus, using techniques he had learned while spending time in the laboratory with Fraenkel.[23] MacFarland's later professional accomplishments included appointment as bacteriologist for the Philadelphia Board of Health, chair of the Department of Pathology and Bacteriology at Medico-Chirurgical College, and professor of pathology at Woman's Medical College.

Dr. William Hallock Park was among the dominant figures in New York City public health during the first decades of the 20th century. Receiving his medical degree from Columbia University, College of Physicians and Surgeons in 1886, he received further training in 1889 and 1890 at the University of Vienna. Upon his return he carried out a private practice until in 1894, when he was appointed director of the Bureau of Laboratories of the New York Health Department. He became professor of bacteriology and hygiene at Bellevue Hospital and the Medical College of New York University in 1897. In these positions he carried out the teaching of bacteriology within the medical programs. Until the time of his death in 1939, Park was appointed to numerous positions within the city, state and federal public health programs, including the New York State Department of Health (1914), consulting bacteriologist for the United States Quarantine Service (1921), and served as president of the American Public Health Association (1923).

While there were others who contributed to the development of bacteriology programs during these years, the aforementioned individuals played dominant roles in instituting what, by the beginning of the 20th century, was a vital portion of medical education. A common feature among most of these young students of medicine, or who carried out studies in other areas of biology, was that significant training for the study and teaching of bacteriology was obtained in Europe. As a result of that training, these individuals instituted their own programs at their respective colleges and universities, preparing the next generation of physicians and scientists with knowledge in that field.

Society of American Bacteriologists

> "[Dr. Edwin Jordan,] Why don't you bacteriologists have a society of your own? I just met [Alexander C.] Abbott also wondering around like a lost soul."[24]

If one were to demarcate the development of bacteriology in the United States between the early 1880s, when an understanding of the importance played by bacteria in disease was evolving in Europe, and the end of the 19th century, two features would be described.

The first—the training of physicians and other scientists who would initiate the recognition of that field as a separate branch of medicine—was described above. The first courses which dealt specifically with bacteriology as a branch of biology on its own, rather than as a sub-category of hygiene, were introduced beginning about 1880. By the late 1890s, the germ theory of disease had been accepted by most medical personnel, and the importance of bacteria in other branches of biology such as soil or agriculture, was being recognized. Given that scientists in most fields had by then formed societies among like-minded investigators, it was no surprise that bacteriologists would do the same. The result was the formation of the Society of American Bacteriologists in 1899.

The impetus to establish the society appears to have begun with the above quote from Dr. Franklin Mall, professor of anatomy at Johns Hopkins University, to Dr. Jordan at the Christmas 1898 meeting in New York of the American Society of Naturalists. The society had been founded in 1883, one of the first professional societies dedicated to science in the United States. Mall's joking comment—whether the result of too much Christmas "spirit" is unknown—spurred Jordan to confer with his colleagues Abbott and Herbert Conn as to whether such a professional organization of bacteriologists had merit. The result was Jordan and Conn authored a letter, sent to some forty bacteriologists in the United States and Canada the following October, to determine the interest in such an organization: "An attempt is being made to organize a society of American bacteriologists upon the lines followed by the ... affiliated societies with the Society of American Naturalists. It is thought that such an association will conduce to unification of methods and aims, will emphasize the position of bacteriology as one of the biological sciences and will bring together workers interested in the various branches into which bacteriology is now ramifying.

"It is hoped that you will be willing to aid in this undertaking. Should you be willing to cooperate in the formation of such a society will you kindly communicate with Prof. H.W. Conn, Wesleyan University, Middleton, Ct. before November 1st."[25]

Most responded favorably to the idea of this new society, and an organizational meeting was scheduled for December 28 at Yale Medical School in New Haven. The first session was presided over by Dr. William Sedgwick, with approximately thirty prospective members present. A committee consisting of Drs. Abbott, Conn, Jordan, Theobald Smith from Harvard Medical School, and Wyatt Johnston from McGill University in Canada was established to draw up the constitution. Sedgwick was elected first president, with Abbott as vice-president and Conn as secretary-treasurer. There were sixty charter members of the SAB, a "Who's Who" of bacteriology, which included not only Abbott, Conn, and Jordan, but prominent figures in the growing field such as Vaughan, Novy, Park, Welch, Simon Flexner and Ludvig Hektoen.[26] In 1960, the name of the society was changed to the American Society for Microbiology, reflecting the increased focus and representation among its members.

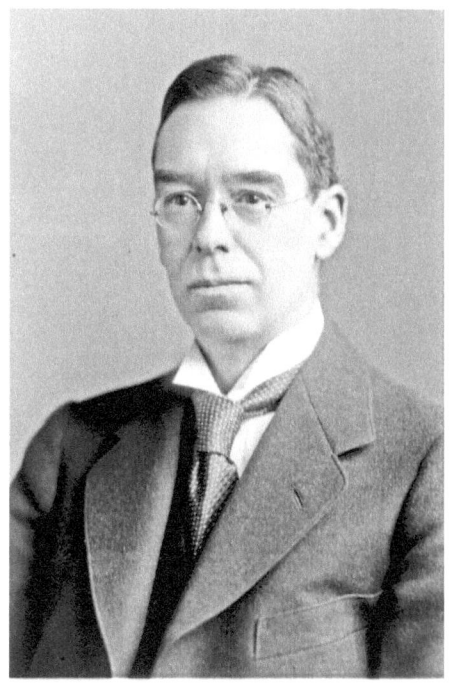

Edwin Oakes Jordan (1866–1936). Jordan helped establish the new program in bacteriology at the University of Chicago in 1893, one year after the institution itself began. The course was called Sanitary Science. He was also a member of the committee which helped found the Society of American Bacteriologists (National Library of Medicine).

The SAB was not the only professional organization established during this period with an emphasis on bacteriology. In 1901, Drs. Harold Ernst and William Welch organized the American Association of Pathologists and Bacteriologists, with an emphasis on medical sciences rather than clinical medicine. In 1976, the AAPB merged with the American Society for Experimental Pathology, becoming the American Society for Investigative Pathology.

4

The Cartwright Lecture
Belfield vs. Formad

"*Who are you going to believe, me or your lyin' eyes?*"[1]

The slow, but growing, establishment of programs of bacteriology in medical schools was not the only recognition of what would become its own field of study during the 1880s. A bequest in the will provided by Benjamin Cartwright of Newark, New Jersey in 1877, to the Alumni Association of the Columbia College of Physicians and Surgeons, provided for a yearly lecture, "modeled after the Lettsonian or Croonian lectures of England," for dissemination of medical knowledge. The first of these lectures was presented in 1881 by Dr. Robert Bartholow of Jefferson Medical College in Philadelphia, who described his research on motor excitability of the human brain. The lecture series continued semi-annually until ended in 1916, when what became World War I was raging overseas. The series was re-instituted in 1974. Among the most prominent physicians presenting these early lectures were Drs. William Osler (1886), Welch (1888) and Henry Fairfield Osborn (1892).[2]

In February 1883, the Cartwright lecture was presented by Dr. William Belfield (1856–1929), lecturer in pathology at Rush Medical College in Chicago. The title of his lecture was "Relations of Micro-organisms to Disease," one of the first such lectures presented in the United States on the topic of bacteria as etiological agents of disease. Material described in his lecture could be considered as a realistic depiction of the state of knowledge of the subject, circa 1883. Belfield drew much of his material from the work of Koch, Pasteur, and their European contemporaries, not surprisingly, since in the years following his 1877 graduation from Rush Medical College, Belfield had studied for a time with Koch.[3]

Belfield began his lecture with a brief review of the general characteristics of bacteria, first drawing on the observations of Leeuwenhoek, and progress-

4. The Cartwright Lecture

ing to the work of Pasteur in the 1860s which negated the idea of spontaneous generation. Joseph Lister was to apply the knowledge that bacteria were ubiquitous in the air to development of aseptic surgery. This, as well as the germ theory of disease, is discussed in greater detail in a later chapter.

Classification of bacteria was still in flux, as demonstrated by Belfield's comparison of the French school, based largely on Pasteur's fermentation work, in which the three major groups were vibrios, monads and torulaceae (fungi), with the more recent classification by the German Ferdinand Cohn. Reflecting what could be considered modern—21st century—nomenclature, Cohn placed bacteria into four major morphological categories: micrococci, or spherical; "oblong" bacteria; bacilli; and spirilla, or spiral shaped.[4] Belfield also acknowledged Cohn's working definition of bacteria, as "cells devoid of chlorophyll, of spherical, oblong or cylindrical, sometimes sinuous or twisted form, which reproduce themselves exclusively by transverse division and live either isolated or in families."[5]

Once again drawing upon the (then) recent work of Koch, Belfield summarized what would shortly evolve into Koch's Postulates demonstrating the infectious nature of disease. The reader here should be reminded, that Belfield's lecture took place early in 1883; while the theory underlying what would become Koch's postulates had been outlined by this time, it was in the following year—1884—that Koch described the actual steps of the postulates. Most researchers, when growing cultures of bacteria, still used either cultivation in flasks, or growth in tubes, each of which utilized a liquid medium. "The chief objection to flask or tube-cultivations, however, one which renders them utterly unsatisfactory as attempts at isolation, is the impossibility of detecting with certainty the presence of foreign organisms. Some varieties, it is true, indicate their presence macroscopically, but the absence of them does not prove the absence of others. One is compelled to remove the cotton [something the modern student likely has never encountered since the advent of plastic caps], withdraw a drop of the liquid, and submit it to microscopic examination—a procedure perilous to the purity of the culture. But even in this way no certainty can be assured, for the one drop may be free from intruding organisms, which may nevertheless be present in the flask. More than that; since many varieties, at least many bacteria growing under different circumstances, are morphologically indistinguishable, one is not always certain that the organisms found are really the offspring of those planted rather than morphologically identical intruders...

"A source of possible error in these methods, not always recognized, is the necessary assumption that apparent community of form among bacteria proves identity of function.... In 1875 even Cohn pronounced the harmless bacillus subtilis of hay infusion morphologically identical with the bacillus anthracis."[6] Even Koch was challenged in attempting to maintain pure cultures in liquid media.

Belfield presented the solution to this problem, a result of his experience in Berlin. "Three years ago there was introduced—thanks to the ingenuity of Koch—a method which avoids, theoretically and practically, the difficulties inseparable from previous attempts at isolation of a given bacterial species found in an animal, both from other varieties and from the accompanying animal juices. The essential feature of this method consists simply in the substitution of a solid—transparent when possible—for the liquid material adapted to the nutrition of the organism.

"The general plan is as follows: a solution of gelatin, beef-extract, peptone; or blood serum, the relative proportions of the various ingredients varying with the species to be cultivated, is sterilized by repeated heating and then spread as a thin layer upon a disinfected slide and allowed to dry or coagulated by heat. A previously heated needle or scalpel is then dipped into the material containing the bacteria—septic mouse blood, for example—and drawn lightly over the surface of the culture substance on the slide.... The slides so prepared are then transferred to the incubator or placed under a bell jar; or, if they are to be long preserved, in a thoroughly disinfected vessel closed with cotton. A disadvantage of this method, like that with liquid media, is the uncertainty of sterilizing the nourishing media."[7] Belfield was clearly familiar with the technique developed by Koch for isolation of bacteria in pure cultures.

But more than simply providing a description of Koch's use of solid media, Belfield also anticipated the steps which, within a year or so, would become known as the postulates. "The burning question in pathology today is, in what degree are the various species of bacteria, present in human tissues during certain morbid conditions, to be regarded as the cause of the morbid processes with which they are respectively associated?...

"Before admitting the causal relation of a bacterium to the disease, we must be convinced not only that all observed phenomena can be easily reconciled with such assumption, but also that they can be as plausibly explained by no other assumption. The evidence of such causal relation must establish, therefore, (1) the competence of the observer and the accuracy of the observation; (2) the presence of a constant bacterial form in every case of the disease, and in numbers sufficient to explain the morbid phenomena [*Step one of the postulates*]; (3) the demonstrable isolation of the bacteria by successive cultures [*Step two of the postulates*]; (4) the induction of the disease in numerous healthy animals by inoculation with the isolated organisms [*Step three of the postulates*]; (5) the reproduction of the same bacterial form in the inoculated animal [*Step four of the postulates*]."[8] Belfield provided several examples in which the etiological agent was established using the aforementioned phenomena, most notably anthrax and tuberculosis. In presenting the methodology necessary to link a specific etiological agent with a disease, Belfield was among the first, if not the actual first, American physician to describe what would be known as Koch's Postulates.

In the second of his series of lectures before the association, Belfield presented the growing evidence linking the presence of micro-organisms and sepsis, particularly as an aftermath of surgery—a confirmation of the germ theory of disease. "A new path of investigation had been opened by Pasteur's demonstration that the putrefaction of animal tissues is a phenomenon incident to the vital activity of certain bacteria—facts established incontestably by the researches of Pasteur, Tyndall, [Moritz] Traube, [Oscar] Brefeld, and their pupils. The determination of the relation between the bacteria and the diseases caused by the putrid products of their vital action soon became the object of most patient and careful investigation. [Leon] Coze and [Victor] Feltz found vibrios intra vitam [during life] in the blood of animals infected with putrid fluids; and similar organisms post-mortem in the blood of a patient dead of putrid infection. With this blood they inoculated a rabbit, which then exhibited septic symptoms, and whose blood was found to contain similar vibrios.... The work of Klebs on 'Gunshot Wounds' (1872) [during the recent war with France] opened the new epoch in pathological investigation. The examination of numerous gunshot wounds, both before and after death, showed that the organs and tissues exhibiting morbid changes due to such wounds were populated by bacteria; serous surfaces, both those opened by the bullet and those which, while still intact, lay adjacent to an abscess or to the track of the missile; the walls of blood vessels, not only those which had been the seat of secondary hemorrhage, but also those which, while not ruptured, showed beginning thrombus formation; metastatic abscesses in liver and lung; leukocytes in and near the track of the bullet—all contained colonies of bacteria."[9]

Belfield then continued with additional examples of the alleged role played by bacteria in wound sepsis, concluding with the application to aseptic/antiseptic surgery, the methodology developed by Lister a decade earlier. "Antiseptic surgery, then, is not comprised in the spray and carbolic acid [methods utilized by Lister]; it is not simply a question as to the relative antibacterial properties of this, that, and the other so-called antiseptic agents. It is an attempt to prevent the entrance into, as well as the formation within, a wound of all substances, organized and unorganized, which can interfere with cell nutrition. It comprises, first, the exclusion or removal of all putrefiable materials—blood, pus, necrosed tissue (a point to which the Listerian school seems inclined to ascribe a subordinate place)...; second, the exclusion of all ferments, bacterial or other; and, since neither of these can always be accomplished, since even under the most perfect Lister or other dressing [gauze soaked in carbolic acid and wrapped around wound], both putrefiable materials and bacteria may be present; third, the establishment of conditions incompatible with bacterial development. The most complete antisepsis is evidently not that which sees in bacteria the sum and substance of all surgical evil, but that which recognizes and endeavors to avoid all possible sources of infection."[10]

Belfield likewise addressed the problem of fulfilling criterion 4 above, step 3 in the postulates—the transfer of the disease to a healthy animal—using gonorrhea as an example. Several years earlier, Albert Neisser had isolated the etiological agent of gonorrhea, the genus of which—*Neisseria*—was named in his honor. The inability to infect and induce the disease in non-human animals with the organism left its identification in some doubt. "In 1879 Neisser made the assertion, based upon numerous examinations, that there is present in the purulent discharge of gonorrhea, whether from urethra, vagina, or conjunctiva, a micrococcus not found in other pus, distinguished by its size, shape and mode of reproduction. Neisser's previous work entitled this assertion to respectful consideration, and it was at once subjected to extensive tests. The reports have been, with one exception, unanimous in corroborating Neisser's assertions in all its details. I may mention especially [Paul] Ehrlich, a most expert and experienced, yet conservative and trustworthy observer; [Georg Theodor] Gaffky, a pupil and present assistant of Koch; [Emanuel] Aufrecht, of Magdeberg.... The only dissenter, so far as I know, is Dr. Sternberg, who asserts that this micrococcus form is widely distributed, and is, in fact, the same as that which Pasteur has shown to cause fermentation of urea."[11]

"Several attempts have been made to inoculate human subjects—since animals are not susceptible to the contagion—with the isolated micrococci ... [Max] Bockhart, having cultivated the organisms on gelatin, inoculated with the fourth culture a paralytic hospital patient [one assumes with permission], and observed a typical gonorrhea on the sixth day. Sternberg cultivated micrococci from gonorrheal pus in flasks, and observed only negative results in each of five patients inoculated therewith. Thus far, therefore, it is not decisively established that the bacterium associated with gonorrhea is the cause of the disease. Dr. Sternberg's present experiments, like all his previous work, evince great care, skill, and a sincere desire for truth that cannot be too much admired; yet his deductions would be far more convincing *if he would substitute a solid for the liquid culture medium*" [italics added].[12]

That not every test animal, including even humans, was equally susceptible to infection also posed a potential problem in explaining the infectious nature of disease. "We are not all equally susceptible to any one of the infectious diseases; even the most malignant cholera or yellow fever attacks only a portion—usually a decided minority—of the community. Explain it as we may, there is a something which we may call predisposition, by virtue of which only certain individuals yield to infection by cholera or by tuberculosis; and the facts is, that the number susceptible to tuberculosis seems smaller than to any one of several other infections. Comparatively few of us attain maturity without having had measles, scarlet fever, and whooping cough at least; yet six-sevenths of us complete our pilgrimage without exhibiting evidences of tuberculosis. That this is not mere accident is shown by experiment: guinea pigs and rabbits rarely, dogs and cats usually fail to respond with general tuberculosis to inoculation with tuberculous material. Even the deadly anthrax usually fails to destroy carnivorous animals, although the most virulent material be introduced; and it was long ago pointed out by [Auguste] Chauveau, and often confirmed, that although sheep are very susceptible to this disease, yet some [albeit Algerian, and not French] sheep resist all experimental attempts at inoculation, even when large quantities of fresh anthrax material are injected into the animal. Dogs enjoy in general immunity against infection by anthrax; yet young dogs are often successfully inoculated. Infection implies, therefore, not simply a virus capable of propagation in an animal, but also an animal capable of permitting such propagation. All variations of this relative adaptability may be exhibited between animals of the same species and a given virus. To affirm, then, that a disease—anthrax or tuberculosis, for example—is infectious is to assert that it can be communicated by the diseased to *a* healthy animal, not to *all* healthy animals [both italics in original], even of the same species. Herein lies evidently our security against tuberculosis, as well as against many other infec-

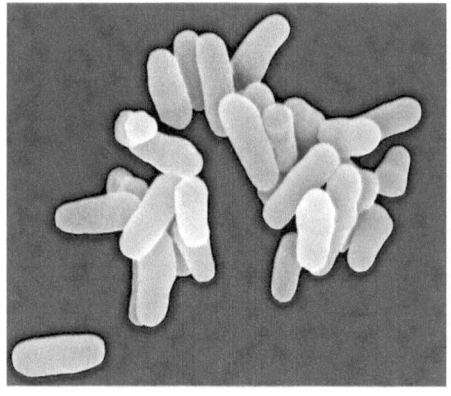

The etiological agent of *Mycobacterium tuberculosis*. Koch's identification of the organism resulted in his being awarded a Nobel Prize in 1905 (image copyright Dennis Kunkel Microscopy, Inc.).

tious diseases. The general principle—the survival of the fittest—seems to have been for generations at work in eradicating this disease from the human family, by removing those members of it susceptible to tuberculosis; the great majority of us now living are as safe from tuberculosis as most dogs are from anthrax."[13] Belfield once again illustrates his likely familiarity with the work of Charles Darwin with the assertion that a selection mechanism has taken place, in that survival was largely restricted to those less susceptible to tuberculosis.

Belfield's familiarity with Koch's procedures extended beyond the latter's use of solid media for isolation of pure cultures. He had firsthand knowledge of what may have been his most important discovery. In March 1882 Koch announced his isolation of the tubercle bacillus. Belfield happened to be in Vienna at the time, and described the work in several letters sent to the *Chicago Medical Journal and Examiner* between May and July that year. When he returned to Chicago that summer, he demonstrated the diagnostic technique used for detection of the bacillus in the sputum of tuberculosis victims before an audience at both Cook County Hospital and the Chicago Pathological Society.[14]

Belfield was well aware that there remained some skeptics about Koch's announcement, even in the presence of strong experimental support. Some of these counterarguments were addressed in his presentation. Dr. Henry Formad, among those who spent time in Koch's laboratory and, as noted earlier, developed the first bacteriology course at Harvard University, was among those skeptics. (See also Chapter 8 for more information about Formad.) Dr. William Hunt, in an address before the Philadelphia College of Surgery in January 1883, presented some of those counterarguments from Formad. "Formad admits the bacillus, but denies the claim for it as a cause, and right well, by experiment and reason, does he sustain his propositions."[15] Formad is not the only opponent of Koch's report Hunt cited. "Dr. H.D. Schmidt ... now of New Orleans ... [wrote,] 'Just now I am very busy in preparing a paper on the bacillus tuberculosis of Koch, with which I have been occupied the past three months. I have made extensive microscopic researches on this subject, during which I prepared and examined several hundred sections of tuberculous lung tissue taken from a dozen fresh cases, besides other fresh sections which I had on hand from my studies of the military tubercle during last fall and winter, and I can say now that Koch's bacillus tuberculosis appears to be nothing else but a fat crystal formed from the fat globules in the degenerating tubercular cells. I have found this pseudo-bacillus even in pathological neoplasms containing fattily degenerating cells.'"[16]

Belfield's response to these and other different interpretations followed in his Chicago presentation. It begins with a comment which would be completely apropos to arguments in the 21st century regarding the evidence for evolution, or the association of vaccinations with autism. "There are those who will not or do not take into consideration the demonstrations attained by accurate experimental methods, and whose opinions rest upon distorted deductions from necessarily inaccurate clinical observations. Yet while those who are pleased to regard pathology as something extrinsic to practical medicine are still discussing the clinical proofs of the infectiousness of tuberculosis, it is quite otherwise with pathologists and clinicians whose opinions are founded upon knowledge without prejudice. One after another the German and French pathologists (who are not infrequently clinical teachers as well), honest in their previous conviction that the communicability of tuberculosis was not proven, honestly recorded their convictions as succeeding proofs were furnished, that the case was reversed; so that three years ago [Julius] Cohnheim said, 'Today there scarcely exists a pathologist who would deny that tuberculosis is a communicable disease.'"[17] In Hunt's presentation in attempting to refute Koch's claims, Hunt stated, "It is the fashion now for writers and thinkers to express their ideas by epigrammatic generalizations thus, Formad (agreeing with most recent pathologists)—'No inflammation, no tubercle.' Koch—'No bacillus, no tubercle.'"[18] Belfield retorted with "Dr. Wm. Hunt leads us to infer that 'most recent pathologists' agree in regarding tuberculosis as the result of a simple inflammation. Will he [Hunt] kindly name *one* [italics in original] pathologist who now holds this opinion, and mention the pertinent publication?"[19]

Belfield continued to single out Formad as one of the primary antagonists of Koch's theory, while attempting to separate the concepts of the bacillus as etiological agent, and the contagiousness of tuberculosis. In doing so, Belfield emphasized the "backward" nature of bacteriological research then being carried out in the United States, using observations on the subject as reported from Europe. "A popular impression ... saddles upon Koch the paternity not only of the bacillus, but also of the infectiousness of tuberculosis. Dr. Formad, for example, says, 'An analysis of Koch's experiments shows that he has not proved the parasitic nature of tuberculosis, so that the infectiousness of tubercular disease is still *sub judice*'. It is apparent from the facts which I have endeavored to summarize that the communicability of tuberculosis was established years before the well-known publication of Koch's discovery. Dr. Formad says, 'The supreme question before the medical world is now, whether the disease under consideration is really infectious.' This statement may represent faithfully that portion of the world bounded by the city limits of Philadelphia; the supreme question before that portion of the medical world including Virchow, Cohnheim, Billroth, Bamberger, Weigert,

Villemin, and the other German, French and Austrian pathologists and clinical teachers is, not whether tuberculosis is infectious, but whether the bacillus of Koch is the infective agent. For them the two questions are quite independent—the former established, the latter awaiting confirmation."[20]

Belfield then summarized Koch's methodology, and the subsequent announcement of his results, contrasting that, by implication, with Formad's own method of dissemination. "Koch's statements are so familiar to all, that detailed repetition would be superfluous; they may be summarized in the assertion that the active agent in the induction and propagation of tuberculosis is a distinct species of bacterium, a bacillus; that tuberculosis does not occur without the presence of this organism; that conversely all those anatomical changes and only those should be called tuberculosis whose point of departure from the normal condition is the presence and vital activity of this bacillus.... The evidence in it favor is first the experimental work of Koch himself, and then the unanimous confirmation of those of his statements which have been already tested...

"That Koch appreciated the situation is shown by his course in the matter; having discovered the bacilli in tuberculous tissue, he did not send an announcement to the Academy of Sciences nor blazon it through the medical press; he kept it to himself, satisfied himself that this was a constant, not an occasional or accidental association; that the same bacteria were present in the spontaneous tuberculosis of animals...; then he devised, by experimentation, a proper medium, *solid* [italics in original] of course, for cultivating the organisms outside of the animal body under constant microscopic supervision, comparing them with fresh bacilli from tuberculous tissues; ... found that while vaccination of the rabbit or guinea-pig with fresh tuberculous matter induced the disease, inoculation with such material after lying in alcohol for a month or dry for two months, was impotent to cause the disease, and *contained no living bacilli* [italics in original]; found that the bacteria were often, not always, present in the sputum of tuberculous patients, but never, so far as examined, in that of others...

"Having spent two years in the completion of this work, amid all the facilities of the imperial laboratory; having meanwhile permitted himself no public intimation of the same, Koch quietly announced his results at a regular meeting of a medical society.... I would call your attention to the fact that Koch's assertion embodies not a theory, but simply an ocular demonstration. If a man is seen to plunge a knife into the heart of another the killing is a fact, not a theory; if Koch saw tuberculosis invariably follow the introduction of isolated bacilli [grown on solid media], the relation of cause and effect is a *fact, not a theory* [italics in original]...

"If we accept Koch's observations as accurate, there is only one conclusion—that these bacilli cause tuberculosis. For here the conclusion and the observation are identical; this is not a deduction, but a demonstration.

"And how shall it be decided that this work is or is not free from errors of observation? Certainly not by saying that it cannot be so; not by exhuming [Felix von] Niemeyer's buried argument that tuberculosis is not infectious; but simply and solely through the repetition, by competent observers, of the same work."[21]

Belfield, in front of an American audience, summarized Koch's justification for his bacillus being the etiological agent of tuberculosis. While not stating such—as noted earlier in this chapter, the postulates had yet to be formalized—Belfield still invoked the steps of the postulates in linking the organism with the disease: the bacillus could be identified in (nearly) all cases of the disease, a fact confirmed by others (in Germany, at least); Koch grew the organism in pure culture on solid media; when inoculated into animals, tubercles, if not the disease itself, would appear; the organism could then be re-isolated.

But Belfield was not finished with addressing the critics, invoking humor as a means to humble those adversaries of Koch. "The subject might be properly left here; but I deem it advisable to briefly review two recent publications, not because they demand consideration by one familiar with the facts, but because they may have influenced some who derive their information chiefly from American literature.

"A few months ago there was heard a scream of exultation from a Western journal, soon echoed on many sides. The attention of press and public alike was attracted to the jubilant cry that Koch, bacillus, and bacteria were to be annihilated; that the 'bacillary craze' of German pathologists; the absurd fancy that a small organism could harm a large one; the comical idea that an experienced mycologist should know more about bacteria than a practicing physician; the barbarous doctrine that our loved ones could be subject to infectious disease; all these and similar absurdities which pseudo-scientists had vainly attempted to foist upon our superior intelligence would be forever buried. The American eagle, that implacable devourer of microscopic poultry, would consent to leave for a brief time its favorite swamp at the 'delta of the Mississippi,' and by a single act of deglutition [swallowing] would teach our terrified friends, 'the micro-pathologists,' to 'take their eyes from their mounted specimens,' and engage in less disreputable pursuits. So ran the widely advertised programme [sic]. After weeks of joyous anticipation the appointed day arrived; a distinguished microscopist, whose skill in mycology had been amply indicated by his failure to detect the bacilli always present in leprous tissue, appeared in the arena armed with the startling discovery that if caustic potash solution be added to fattily degenerated tissue, crystals of fatty acid appear! The announcement was greeted by the audience of assembled experts with rounds of applause—Sic transit bacteria,' etc. Again has free America repelled the assaults of effete Europe."[22]

Belfield's reference to the "German bacillary craze" was from a phrase presented in Hunt's article in the *Medical News* when making reference to the germ theory in general, and to Koch's discovery in particlar.[23] "It is truly astonishing how the medical, and the German medical mind especially, is impregnated with this subject. It really does seem to be a bacillary craze." Nevertheless, Belfield was proven to be correct in his defense of Koch. Hunt conceded that the light diffraction characteristic of his crystals was different from the diffraction observed with the bacilli, indicating they were not identical to each other. Schmidt, the New Orleans physician (see above), required more direct evidence to be convinced. "After [Belfield] reading his article, I sent him a slide of sputum containing the bacilli; in his reply he says, 'From what I understand now the minute crystalline rods which I discovered are not identical with Koch's bacilli,' and later, 'the failure with which I met in my attempts of staining the bacillus tuberculosis, appears to have been due to the worthless aniline oil which I have used....' This entire matter can hardly fail to teach far more effectively than lectures, that trustworthy investigations on this subject demand not only skill and experience in pathology, which Dr. Schmidt undoubtedly possesses, but also acquaintance with the special methods involved. "[24]

Belfield had more to say concerning Formad's ideas. "A paper called 'The Bacillus Tuberculosis' by Dr. Formad opens with the announcement that the author 'will bring forward some points from researches of my own, which will check the acceptance of the doctrine of the parasitic origin of tuberculosis ... my anatomical researches will also surely throw grave doubts upon the correctness of Koch's views on the etiology of tuberculosis.'[25] The author [Formad] fails to discriminate between the bacillus and the infectiousness of tuberculosis, which is in this article, however, a matter of little consequence, *except as an index to the general accuracy of the publication* [italics added].

"The original researches which are to destroy the 'parasitic theory' consist, curiously enough, in the time-honored demonstration that tuberculosis often occurs in certain animals (notably the rabbit and guinea-pig) after simple wounds, the irritation caused by glass, etc.; especially if the animals be carefully confined in a pathological laboratory where many others have died of this disease. As Dr. Formad has seen 'more than one hundred rabbits, out of five or six hundred operated upon,' die of tuberculosis, we may infer that in his laboratory there was no lack of tuberculous material for infection.[26]

"There is, however, one original feature in this work as reported by Dr. Formad. Actuated doubtless by a commendable high-tariff spirit of protection for American industry, while quoting copiously his own students, he resolutely ignores the work of [John] Burdon-Sanderson,[27] Cohnheim, and a dozen others who have, during the last fifteen years, performed the original experiments of which his own are repetitions; and neglects to state that Cohnheim and Fränkel found that while these experiments succeeded admirably in the Berlin laboratory where many animals had long been confined, no tuberculosis occurred in a subsequent repetition in a private dwelling. On the same principle, perhaps, he neglects to state that for such reasons as these, such experiments as his own were years ago abandoned to amateurs, while the battle for infectiousness was fought and won in the eye, the lung, and the intestine, as above stated. Perhaps Dr. Formad will kindly explain how he came to deny the infectiousness of tuberculosis merely on the strength of these long since abandoned experiments, without a solitary experiment, or even reference to an experiment, on the eye, etc.

"Because in his experiments no tubercular matter was 'intentionally or knowingly' introduced, he maintains that nothing could have entered; that the disease is therefore not specific nor infectious.... Formad says: 'I can positively prove that true tuberculosis may be produced without the bacillus in question.' The only proof adduced for this important statement is the experiment with glass, etc., in which the disease occurs without any 'conscious or intentional' introduction of the bacillus, and the *assumption* [italics in original] that the organisms were therefore absent; if, however, the parasites be nevertheless present in such cases, this assertion is evidently unwarranted. We are not informed on this point in the paper, although we may infer their presence from the following statement [by Formad]: 'Koch has discovered that tubercle tissue is *always* [italics in original] by bacilli, and this is correct. [Belfield includes a note here, that Koch did not make this statement.] To secure definite information, I [Belfield] addressed to Dr. Formad some months ago, three separate letters enclosing stamps, requesting him to state for incorporation in these lectures whether he had examined these cases of tuberculosis following wounds, mechanical irritation, etc., to ascertain the presence or absence of the bacilli, and if so, with what result. To these letters I have received no reply.

"As to the association of the bacilli with tuberculosis, Formad's limited observations seem to agree with Koch's statements."[28]

While the focus of Belfield's Cartwright Lecture dealt with the developing germ theory of disease, tuberculosis being the primary example, a significant portion addressed one of the primary American critics of Koch's work: Dr. Henry Formad; indeed, Formad was particularly singled out for that reason. Though Formad subsequently was forced to concede the bacillus isolated by Koch *may* have been the etiological agent, he remained unconvinced of how the disease was disseminated. He repeatedly argued that the evidence in favor of tuberculosis being contagious was limited, and that arguments in support of that idea were often biased. The following November 1883, in an address presented before the Philadelphia County Medical Society, and again in March 1884, nearly two years after Koch had announced his discovery, and concomitant with Koch's description of his postulates, Formad continued to express his skepticism about the contagiousness of, the etiological agent. "The contagiousness of consumption is the subject of some sensible remarks by Dr. Formad, of Philadelphia, who has given much time and patience to the investigation of consumption. He finds himself unable to coincide with the conclusions of Dr. Koch, the noted German investigator of what may for short be called the germ diseases, that consumption is caused by the germs or bacilli that are found in connection with it. The bacillus to which Koch imputes its origin is present in all cases of consumption, says Dr. Formad. It may be one of the causes of tuberculosis [Formad finally conceded], but still it cannot yet be said that its presence in consumption proves that to be a contagious disease. A contagious disease can have but one cause, and this observer declares himself, as the result of repeated observations, to be firmer than ever in his former conclusions that consumption may result from other causes than the presence of the germ which Dr. Koch has brought to notice. Dr. Formad concedes that the germ may on account of its irritating effects be one of the causes of the disease, but it is not the cause—at least it has not been proven to be such. The fact that people are known to be predisposed to consumption stands in the way of the acceptance of the bacillus theory. Dr. Formad believes that he will be able to show that consumption is not a contagious disease. The bacillus of Koch and Krebs [sic] is present as one of its symptoms. But bacilli and similar organisms are present in health. They may alter in disease; they may serve as carriers of disease, but they are not, in the case of consumption at least, the primary and sole cause of it, as they must be to sustain the claim that by their agency consumption is infectious."[29]

Formad's aforementioned lecture before the medical society was published in April 1884 in greater detail. In this presentation, and in the subsequent published work, Formad discussed in significant detail the reasoning underlying his disagreements with Koch and Belfield concerning not only the contagious nature of the disease, but also whether Koch had even correctly identified the sole etiological agent. In doing so, Formad, in effect, argued that the postulates—not yet formalized at this time—had not been fulfilled. He did not state so overtly, not surprising since Koch had not yet "officially" described them. But in his reasoning, Formad presented arguments contradicting several of the important steps of the postulates which did not appear to have been fulfilled. "The bacillus discovered by Koch, of Berlin, as is well known, is a vegetable organism, and belongs, according to Cohn's classification, to the group of filamentous bacteria (Desmo-bacteria), variety Bacillus."[30]

After a detailed description of the bacilli Koch observed in the sputum of patients diagnosed with tuberculosis—methodology which he—Formad—had himself learned during his time in Koch's laboratory, Formad laid out the requirements necessary to link those bacilli with the disease, and then the reasons those requirements had not been fulfilled. "After reading most of the numerous compilations in reference to the present standing of the tuberculosis question, it would seem that Koch has established that his tubercle-bacillus is always associated with tuberculosis, and with the diseased products and the various excreta in this disease—and in this disease alone. Since Koch's publication appeared, a number of observers, authoritatively and otherwise, assert the invariable presence of the bacillus in *all* tubercular products; and, further, it is claimed as a proved matter that the bacillus is found in the beginning of the disease—viz., in the youngest tubercle-tissues.

"*This is, however, not in accordance with the facts* [italics in original]. Neither in Koch's own publication, nor in the records of any microscopist (when the original papers are examined), is the invariable presence of the bacillus in tuberculous lesions or excretions, and its absence in non-tuberculous matters, either clearly shown or proved. Moreover, the authors of nearly all the literary productions are in favor of the contagiousness of tuberculosis, and they disregard, as a rule, the negative evidence."[31] Formad is arguing here, that reports by other investigators to the contrary, the alleged agent is not present in all tuberculous tissue; nor, by implication, is it invariably absent in non-tuberculous tissue. Both would be required to fulfill, in a literal manner, the first step of the postulates. Formad implied bias on the part of those investigators who reported otherwise—ignoring negative evidence in order to support their conclusions.

If indeed Koch was correct in his observations and conclusions, particularly with respect to the significance of those observations, a number of criteria would have to have been fulfilled. Formad continued with a listing of these criteria, and the evidence both in their favor as well as observations in opposition:

The examination of tissues affected by tubercular disease for the bacillus; and, if present, the time of its occurrence.... Tubercle-bacilli have been detected quite often in the various forms of tubercles of lung, and in scrofulous and tuberculous lymphatic glands; and likewise, although not so frequently, in tubercles of the various serous cavities; and in tubercular ulcerations of the mucous membranes and the skin. But it must be noted that only a few microscopists have recorded examinations of tubercle-tissue for bacilli, and among these there was *not one* [italics in original] who did not meet with a case or a certain number of cases in which tubercle-bacilli were either totally absent in the tissues, or only present in some of the tubercles. The great bulk of bacillus work done comprises merely examinations of sputum.

The facts concerning bacilli in tissues are as follows: Koch found bacilli in the majority of tuberculous lesions he examined, but still not in all, as he states himself; he only *supposes* [italics in original] that his bacilli, even if they escape observation, are still present in all cases and in all tubercles. His proposition, however, that in some tuberculous lesions only unstained spores of tubercle-bacilli are sometimes present, or that bacilli may be invisible, and not taking the staining when dead, or even may be absent if the tuberculous process comes to a "stand-still," is, of course, purely hypothetical. There is still another good reason for the assumption that the proportion of non-bacillary tubercles may be much larger in Koch's own examinations. As Koch says himself, he preeminently recognizes only such structures as tubercular which contain his bacillus, regardless of their morphology otherwise; it is therefore possible that he may have innocently excluded a number of non-bacillary tubercles from the list of his tubercle records.

As far as examination of tubercle-tissues for bacilli is concerned, only the following observations besides those of Koch are recorded (so far as is known to the writer), and with the following results:

Dr. George M. Sternberg, U.S.A., who is a man recognized as a competent mycologist, here as well as in Europe, failed to find tubercle-bacilli in the lesions of several cases of tuberculosis.

Heneage Gibbs also failed to discover bacilli in a number of tubercles, particularly in the reticular form; in fact, he had met several times with non-bacillary tuberculosis. Gibbs states that "he had examined the lungs of guinea-pigs which had become tuberculous after being kept in the air-shafts of the Brompton Hospital for Consumptives [London, England], and had found no bacilli in them; and he knew of an instance in which a guinea-pig, inoculated with sputum from a case of phthsis, presented a glandular abscess in the thigh which abounded in bacilli, whereas the internal organs, although full of tubercles, did not yield a single bacillus..."

"T.M. Prudden [see previous chapter], of New York, who made extensive and excellent morphological studies in reference to the occurrence of the bacillus in tuberculous lesions *failed to find bacilli in any part of the body in three cases of profuse tuberculosis* [italics in original]." Formad provided some dozen additional examples in which physicians failed to observe any traces of tubercle bacilli in patients with the disease. "The direct conclusion to be drawn from the total evidence relating to bacilli in tissues just quoted is, that tubercle-bacilli are not invariably present in even typical tubercle lesions; furthermore, that none of the investigators brought forward any proof or evidence that the bacilli are present or appear in the beginning of the disease. On the contrary, the results of the investigations of all observers, including those of the discoverer of the bacillus himself, point plainly towards establishing the fact that tubercle-bacilli inhabit preeminently disintegrated tissues...."[32]

"Examination of products discharged or eliminated with the excretions by individuals suffering from tuberculosis has been practiced quite extensively, and by a number of observers especially in reference to phthisical sputum.... Koch does not claim that sputum from every phthisical case contains bacilli; he met with cases without bacilli in sputum. He did not find, however, bacilli in cases said not to be tubercular. Ehrlich records twenty-six cases of phthisis in which bacilli were invariably present in the sputum; in other lung affections similar bacilli were not found." Formad continued to describe (literally) dozens of examples in which bacilli were invariably present in the sputum of tuberculosis patients.[33] Further examples included the fact several physicians observed the quantity of bacilli present in sputum reflected the prognosis of the case—when the patient began to recover, the level of bacilli was reduced. From these observations, Formad came to several conclusions: "First, that the presence of bacilli is a valuable diagnostic sign of tubercular disease of the lung; Second, that the quantity of bacilli found does not, as a rule, indicate the degree of the disease, and hence is not a prognostic sign; and third, that the absence of tubercle-bacilli is no proof whatsoever of the absence of tubercular disease."[34]

Whether or not tuberculosis, a disease primarily affecting the lungs, is contagious would hinge in part on isolation of the bacilli in the air. Formad summarized some of the work in which investigators analyzed the air in the sick-rooms of hospitals. Results were mixed. Charles Theodore Williams, a leading British figure in pulmonary diseases, suspended glycerin plates in the air shafts of Brompton Hospital; he found bacilli in "fair abundance." Other investigators were able to isolate bacilli from the breath of some patients, but not all. In some instances, no bacilli at all were detected. In a prescient manner, the Italian physicians Sarmoni and Marchifava, though unable to detect bacilli in the breath of tuberculosis patients, suggested that contagion might be mediated by "dried, powdered sputum, which floats as dust in the air. [During the 20th century, droplet nuclei would indeed be implicated in the respiratory spread of the bacilli.] … Surveying now the whole question of the habitat of the bacillus tuberculosis, it becomes evident that Koch's dilemma—that only that is tuberculosis, and everything is tuberculosis, where his bacillus is found—is overdrawn and cannot bear criticism. It would be much safer to reverse this proposition, and to *consider that bacillus alone a tubercle-bacillus which inhabits evident tubercular lesions* [italics in original] or their products,—e.g., sputum, and nothing else. For we have no difficulty in diagnosticating under the microscope a tubercle without the bacillus; but *a dilemma arises at once if we see questionable bacilli without the tubercle, or outside of sputum*" [italics in original].[35]

Formad then addressed the question of the contagiousness of tuberculosis, a topic with which he would appear to have been obsessed. Since he had trained with Koch some years earlier, even going so far as to acknowledge the expertise on the subject he had obtained there, one is forced to wonder exactly why he so strongly disagreed with the latter's thesis on the etiological agent and spread of the disease.

> It has been shown that the clinical evidence [i.e., bacilli in sputum] in reference to the contagiousness of phthisis is so meager that assertions as to its parasitic origin are unwar-

ranted.... This being the case, it would seem as if experimenters are trying to prove that which is not the reality...

Having arrived, from my own experiments, at conclusions different from those of Koch, I thought it at present timely to announce at least the results of my observations, as my detailed report cannot appear for some months to come.... The total evidence *pro* and *contra* gives me the impression that the doctrine of the contagious character and parasitic causation of tuberculosis can not be sustained.... For the establishment of a theory in regard to a parasitic origin of a disease by means of experiments on animals, etc., the following propositions must be affirmatively decided:

1. The disease produced experimentally in animals by means of inoculation with products of the human disease, must be proved to be identical with the disease occurring spontaneously in man.... In favor of the identity of human tuberculosis with that produced experimentally in animals there has been brought forward the fact that the products in both contain identical bacilli. But this surely does not prove the identity, because similar bacilli may be found in the lesions of various kinds of processes, resulting in cheesy products. Besides, there are many spontaneous and artificially-induced tubercular lesions in which bacilli could not be demonstrated. Hence, we can not rely upon the bacilli as a proof for the identity of the lesions.

Koch, and those who imitated his experiments, diagnosticate and declare all those artificially induced lesions as tubercular which occur in nodes and in which they found the tubercle-bacillus, without taking (so far as I know) into consideration any structural peculiarities or other conditions. Now, tubercle-bacilli will surely be found in the lesions, whatever these may be, as they were introduced into the animal in those experiments. Further, in the opinion of these gentlemen nothing is tubercle where there are no tubercle-bacilli. Therefore, how can we rely upon their statements as to what the lesions they induced in animals really were?...

In many instances where the experimenters have produced, by means of tuberculous materials, within two to eight days after the operation, a military eruption, it is not probable that those military nodes were tubercles, and were due to the effects of bacilli, which are known to grow extremely slowly, and it is not certain that the experimenters took pains to distinguish them from true tubercle, or were competent in all instances to do so. This is eminently true of the inhalation tuberculosis.

Tappeiner's induced inhalation tuberculosis of dogs [see previous chapter], so much relied upon by Koch and others for the establishment of the mode of the spreading of phthisis, and partly of the bacillus doctrine itself, has been proved to be a fiction. Tappeiner, as so often quoted, subjected dogs to an atmosphere heavily charged with phthisical sputum, so that the dogs were nearly bathed in the latter (known to contain bacilli) for weeks. But, in spite of this, the animals grew fat, if anything, and, after the lapse of a certain time, acquired local pulmonary affections in the form of nodules, not likely to have been tubercular in nature, of which only in one case were some observed in the liver and kidneys...

Although, judging from my own experiments, there is to my mind no doubt that some forms of artificially-induced tuberculosis in animals acquire gradually characters which make them identical with the spontaneous tuberculosis in man or beast, yet I do not think it is at all proved that the lesions so rapidly arising from the effects of the inoculation with the bacillus of Koch are identical with tuberculosis in man. The proof, then, upon this point, the supreme one for the settlement of the question of the nature of tuberculosis, is yet to be furnished.

2. There should be some evidence showing that inoculation in men is followed by the same result as follows the inoculation of the same material in animals, and that the disease is really contagious.[36] The idea of inoculating humans with a potentially—indeed, likely—

lethal organism would be anathema to medical scientists even in the nineteenth century. However, Formad does relate several such instances, one involving an accidental exposure, the other using a volunteer near death from an unrelated illness. The first example was that of a surgical intern who was likely exposed while carrying out a post-mortem examination; some time later he developed tuberculosis. The latter example involved a fifty-five year-old man dying from gangrene. His leg was intentionally inoculated with sputum obtained from a patient with tuberculosis. The man died some two months later from the initial infection; his lungs were found to contain numerous tubercles.[37]

3. There should be found a definite parasite at the beginning of the diseased process, and in sufficient quantity to account for the changes in all cases, and in all tissues involved by the disease.... Klebs, Toussaint, and Schüller have observed *micrococci* to be constantly present in tuberculous lesions and products (and have induced artificially the disease with the isolated micrococci), and no one has proved anything to the contrary; while Koch and Baumgarten discovered *bacilli* in the same lesions.... The reports of some competent microscopists and pathologists (when the originals are examined) show that the tubercle-bacillus is not invariably present in all cases and all products of tuberculosis; and, if present, it is often both seen in sufficient quantity to ascribe to it the claimed significance; and, furthermore, it is, as a rule, not present at the beginning of the disease...

The truth of the matter appears to be, and, indeed, from my daily observations in the laboratory upon a large quantity of material, I regard it as a fact, that the tubercle-bacillus of Koch is a mere concomitant of cheesy disintegrated materials, even if it be preeminently of tuberculous cheesy materials.[38]

Criterion number 4, as proposed by Formad, is analogous to the second step of Koch's Postulates: the isolation of the organism in pure culture, followed by the demonstration of its role in establishment of disease. Formad began by acknowledging the "capability" of the bacillus in induction of the disease, but continued to argue against its role as the sole agent *of* the disease.

There is no doubt that Koch's tubercle-bacillus, *when isolated and cultivated for many generations* [italics added] and then inoculated into certain animals, is capable of inducing tuberculosis, or a nodular eruption not distinguishable from it, more readily than other irritants, so far as tried.... Thus it appears that the above proposition could be answered for tuberculosis and the bacillus in the affirmative if only the following points were proved:

1st. That the nodular lesion thus induced is really tuberculosis, identical with the human disease.

2d. That this bacillus is the only bacterium or the only irritant capable of inducing tuberculosis; and,

3. That its action is specific,—i.e., that the bacillus is the only agency or factor at work, the sole cause of the disease.

The first point is not proved, as probable as it may appear.... [Regarding the other points] It has been proved that in tuberculosis micrococci, as well as bacilli, are causal, the evidence being "strong" for either "parasite"; whereas the bacillus alone should be the causal factor. As long as not disproved, Klebs,' Toussaint's and Schüller's investigations (in relation to the micrococci as causal factors) have as much claim as Koch's. The method of cultivating those tubercle-micrococci, as practiced by those investigators, was one not favorable for the development of the tubercle-bacilli. Further, Watson Cheyne's assertion that bacilli must have been present in the cultured materials with which those investigators inoculated successfully, is altogether a gratuitous assumption ... and, in fact, neither prove nor disprove anything...

> Koch has not proved that his bacillus is the only agency at work in the production of tuberculosis. Although he undoubtedly inoculated the pure bacillus [Re: Step 2 in the postulates], he ignored the specific reaction of the soil [lung tissue]; and it is the latter [i.e., response by the tissue] which I hold plays the most important role in determining the formation of tubercle. In introducing the bacillus into the animal organism, another factor—the injury inflicted, and its effects upon the living cells of the body—must be taken into consideration.
>
> In some animals all the tissues of the body react equally upon the introduction of irritants; in others only some one of the tissues responds, such as the serous [surface membranes, as associated with alveoli in lungs] membranes. This surely demonstrates the specific action of the soil [tissue]...
>
> It appears that the bacilli by themselves have no effect upon the healthy organism or the normal tissues. A predisposed soil [i.e., lung tissue] is the chief factor and is pre-eminently necessary for the production of tuberculosis; while, on the other hand, it is not proved at all that the bacillus is invariably necessary for the production of tuberculous lesions. Although the tubercle-bacillus is more liable to excite tuberculosis in an already inflamed and ill-nourished soil than all other simple irritants so far tested, it (the bacillus) might be readily substituted by other irritants ... a general fear of the bacillus tuberculosis as a contagion is unjustifiable, and that the ordinary dust suspended in the air is to certain persons as dangerous as the bacillus.[39]

Formad is arguing here, that it is not the bacillus *per se* which induces the disease, but rather the irritation established by its presence. In support of this thesis, Formad is providing examples in which administering a variety of irritants results in the induction of tuberculosis. The assumption, of course, is that it is truly tuberculosis which is the result, not simply production of a lesion which resembles the tubercle of the disease. Since many of these investigators had experience in pathology as well, one might expect they would be capable of differentiating between the tubercle characteristic of tuberculosis, and that of other forms of nodules resulting in pathological changes of serous tissue.

Formad's fifth criterion is analogous to the third step of the postulates—that

> the specific lesions of a disease resulting from the inoculation of a specific parasite must also contain that parasite, and have the specific properties of reproducing the same disease when re-inoculated in other animals.
>
> Koch claims that the products obtained in animals by inoculation with bacilli are capable of producing tuberculosis when inoculated into a second animal, while the products obtained by inoculation with innocuous substances do not have this effect. The former proposition is true, but the latter, I hold, is not in accordance with the facts. In my own experiments ... tubercles produced by inoculation with innocuous material under antiseptic precautions were likewise capable of producing tubercles when inoculated into other animals, having thus the same action as the innocuous material primarily used...
>
> Wherever inoculation with innocuous substances [by a variety of investigators] was followed by positive results, the over-zealous germ-theorists call it *"accidental tuberculosis"* [italics in original]. They say that at the time of former experiments the communicability of tubercle by a mediate contagion was not recognized, and as the precautions necessary

for thorough disinfection of instruments, surroundings, etc., were probably not observed, the channels for the introduction of the bacillus were, in all previous experiments, left unguarded; hence, they argue, it must have been this ubiquitous bacillus which induced the tubercle.

Further admitting, however, that innocuous substances may induce tubercle-like bodies, they claim that these bodies are not infectious, i.e., they are *false* tubercles.

All these objections would be very plausible if they were based upon actual observations and facts; but, unfortunately for the bacillus theory, they are not; they are *mere unfounded assumptions* [italics in original].[40]

Whether or not Formad was correct in his views, and in time they were shown to largely be incorrect, his arguments could be summarized as the following:

1. That the bacillus of Koch is a valuable diagnostic sign of tubercular disease.
2. That nothing is proved by its discovery for the etiology of tuberculosis.
3. That the too ready acceptance of the bacillus doctrine is not justifiable, and is likely to do more harm than good.
4. That neither phthisis nor any form of tuberculosis is contagious."[41]

The response from Koch's colleagues to Formad's arguments was rapid and pointed—even biting. That summer of 1884 Koch headed a German commission, first to Egypt, and then to India, investigating outbreaks of cholera in those two regions. Koch would subsequently identify the etiological agent, a vibrio, of that disease. Consequently he had temporarily ended his studies of the agent of tuberculosis. This did not mean others would be silent in light of Formad's allegations. "It is, perhaps, hardly fair to speak of Formad's deplorable failure to maintain his opposition to Koch by any reasonable arguments at the last annual session of the American medical association. Through imperfect counsel, the gentleman was induced to come before the meeting, and after announcing far and wide his intention to give results that would destroy the last vestige of strength to Koch's assertion in regard to the specific nature of the bacillus of tuberculosis, instead of doing this, proceeded to read a reprint of an article published by him last fall, announcing that his results would be published in the near future. This, in the present condition of all questions relating to micro-organisms in this country, seems to be almost inexcusable. These results have been promised for months, and at the time of writing have not yet appeared. It seems as if it were the bounden duty of all those honestly interested in the advancement of scientific knowledge to talk and publish less, and to work more. What is needed is the publication of the results of work carefully and conscientiously performed, together with the exact details of every step in every process by which those results were reached. In addition to this, we have a right to demand that all work of this kind shall be done by careful observers, in the presence of others equally well qualified for the observation,—not with and by half-trained students,—and that the very best appliances of modern research shall be employed in each and every observation made. In this way, and in this way only, can reliance be placed in observations recorded in work on micro-organisms; and it is the absence of work of this kind which gives so little force to the opponents of the specific nature of the bacillus of tuberculosis. At the same time, it is the presence of this very accuracy of the detailed account of every step in the process by which the results were reached, and of the completeness of the experiments and control experiments, that gives the convincing power to Koch's work. Nothing that can be for an instant compared with it for simplicity and directness of statement, or completion of detail, has yet been brought forth by his opponents. Until that is done, and it does not look probable at the present writing, his work must be accepted as conclusive; and measures should be taken to control to some extent the wide-spread destruction of this disease, as it is most certainly in our power to do."[42]

Formad died in 1892, ironically from a disease for which Robert Koch identified the etiological agent: cholera.

5

Training with Koch

As briefly addressed in Chapter 1, Koch began his courses in hygiene and bacteriology during the fall of 1885, following the move into his newly renovated Hygiene Laboratory on Klosterstrasse in Berlin. His training of visiting students, including some from the United States, actually began the previous year. As a result of his (likely, though still controversial) identification of the etiological agent of cholera early in 1884, the German government made arrangements with Koch, while still at the *Gesundheitsamt*, for the development of a laboratory course, the purpose of which was, first, to familiarize German physicians with the agent of the disease, and, second, the training of physicians in the growth and study of the organism. The course, divided into ten week portions, was to run from October 1, 1884, to the end of January 1885. Each group of trainees, primarily German physicians but also including some foreign visitors, would study for the ten day period, following which, another group would replace them in the laboratory. Physicians who were stationed in frontiers such as India in which the disease was endemic were required to enroll in the course. Among the first American trainees were Dr. George Lewis, a physician and practitioner of homeopathy, from Buffalo, New York,[1] and T. Mitchell Prudden, from Columbia University in New York. By the time in 1884 during which Koch's courses had been instituted, most of the innovated techniques for which he was subsequently known—the methodology to recognize specific species of bacteria and to produce pure cultures for their study, and application of the Abbe condenser and oil immersion procedure—had been developed and had become routine; the students in these courses were among the first to become trained in their use and widespread application. The success of the workshops and the growing international reputation of Koch resulted in a continuation of the training program in hygiene (bacteriology) for years, well beyond its initial purpose in familiarizing physicians with the cholera bacillus.

Both Lewis' and Prudden's descriptions, while obviously addressing their own situations and training, would nevertheless apply to the general experience encountered by any of the trainees enrolled in the course. The precise date during which Lewis participated in Koch's cholera course was vague, but likely either during December 1884, or in January of the following year. While Koch had described the likelihood that the "comma" bacillus he had identified in the intestines of cholera victims was almost certainly the etiological agent, the inability to test his hypothesis in the natural host for the organism—humans—meant there remained the question in the minds of some physicians as to whether this was indeed the source of the disease. Nevertheless, the working hypothesis was that Koch had indeed identified the correct agent, and that identification of the bacillus in discharges from victims of the disease had diagnostic value.

In order to carry out such identification, physicians should be familiar with culturing techniques. For example, "students" were expected to cultivate side-by-side, a variety of organisms with similar morphology—the Finkler-Prior bacillus, a biovar variety of *Vibrio cholera* now named *Vibrio proteus*, the typhus (typhoid in all likelihood) bacillus, probably *Salmonella*, and several micrococci. In some tests, a culture of mixed organisms was prepared, and students were expected to be able to differentiate them on different types of solid media (gelatin, agar-agar, blood serum and potatoes).[2]

The use of agar-agar, referred to as "Ceylon moss" by Lewis, was a relatively new innovation used by Koch as a solidifying agent. Now called simply agar, the substance is a seaweed extract which, unlike gelatin, has the advantage of being inert to liquefying, a characteristic to which Lewis alluded, "The fact that the agar-agar is not liquefied by even the advanced growth of the colony renders this substance very valuable as a breeding medium."[3] Koch's application of agar in developing his pure culture technique has been described in an earlier chapter. The idea of using agar as a hardening agent in place of gelatin may have originated with Angelina Fannie Hesse, the wife of Koch's associate, Walther Hesse. The history of background events has elements of apocrypha. According to the story, the Hesse's went on a picnic during a hot day when Walther noticed the jellies Fannie had brought remained solid even in the hot sun. When queried, she indicated that in place of gelatin she had used a hardening agent suggested to her by a Dutch neighbor from Java in the East Indies. It was suggested to Koch that he try replacing the gelatin with agar, a modification which proved successful. Loeffler later modified Koch's medium with the addition of peptone as a nutrient source.[4]

In a typical exercise, three sets of media are inoculated: one with fresh cholera "excrement," a second with filtered excrement, and a third with bacteria-free excrement to serve as a control. Only the first sample demonstrated colonies of growth of the "comma" bacillus, which Lewis went on to describe. Lewis also described the Koch method for growing the "comma" bacillus on sliced potato. "The potatoes should be as fresh as possible, not mealy or in any way discolored, and with few eyes. Those having bruises or scratches that have penetrated the surface should not be used. After carefully washing them and cutting out the eyes, they are to be placed in a five percent solution of sublimate [mercury chloride] for half an hour. At the expiration of this time they are to be thoroughly cooked in a steam-pot.... In cutting open the potatoes great care must be taken not to touch the cut surfaces with the fingers, nor should the same knife in any case be used twice. With cut surfaces up, the potatoes are placed in a bell-jar, lined with filter-paper, and saturated with sublimate solution. The inoculation should take place immediately after cutting the potatoes.... The contents of the platinum point should be spread over the greater part of the cut surface, then inoculated from the first potato into a second and so on.... Comma-bacilli flourish best at a temperature between 30° and 40° Centigrade."[5]

Once the bacteria had grown, methods developed by Koch were used to observe the organisms. As described by Lewis in the course: cells were mixed in a bouillon solution and a drop placed on a concave slide, "a peculiar kind of object-glass.... A little Vaseline is spread around the edges of this cavity to enable the cover-glass to rest firmly over it. With a sterilized platinum needle place a drop of the bouillon in the middle of the cover-glass over the cavity of the slide, taking care not to have it touch the sides. The vaseline keeps the air out and at the same time serves the purpose of Canada balsam or some other mounting medium.... They are now ready for examination with the Abbe artificial lighting apparatus and an oil-immersion objective. The appearance presented is that of a swarm of white particles in constant motion [essentially a hanging-drop technique]; the form is hardly discernible; now and then, however, their length is seen to be greater than their breadth. An almost infinite number can be noticed, but their violent movements prevent the characteristic 'comma' form from being detected. That is, to say the least, an unsatisfactory picture, but the only means of rendering it more real is to apply some artificial coloring substance such as [basic] fuchsin or methyl-aniline blue [a description which anticipates the acid-fast staining technique still in use 125 years later]...

"To give the dimensions of comma-bacillus would, indeed, be useless, because only a very poor idea could be derived from the extremely small numbers which would be necessary to represent its length, breadth and thickness. To compare it, however, with some other well-known bacillus, such as the 'tubercle,' will enable the reader to form at least some notion of its size, and at the same time admit of a comparison as to form and general appearance. The 'comma' bacillus is about three-fifths as long as the 'tubercle,' but much thicker and more bulky. A very evident curve, similar to that of a 'comma,' is noticed midway between the two extremities, hence its name."[6]

A more detailed portrayal of the work carried out by foreign visitors to Koch's Klosterstrasse laboratory was provided by Dr. Theophil Mitchell Prudden. During the spring of 1885, the secretary of the State Board of Health of Connecticut requested Prudden "to investigate the method of studying disease germs, particularly those causing Asiatic cholera, as employed in the laboratory of Dr. Robert Koch, in Berlin, and in such other laboratories as he might have occasion to visit."[7] Prudden subsequently spent two months traveling in Germany where he visited several laboratories and observed the bacteriological procedures carried out by Koch in Berlin, and Dr. Ferdinand Hueppe, in Weisbaden.

Prudden's report included a "backhanded" compliment of the state of bacteriological studies currently being carried out in the United States, before providing a description of that in Koch's laboratory. "In this [United States] country the pathological laboratories of some of the more prominent medical colleges have been, *usually at private expense* [italics added], more or less fully equipped with the necessary apparatus, and investigation and instruction are fairly under way. Under government auspices in Washington much excellent work is already in progress. But as the greatest advances in recent times have come from the labors of Dr. Koch in Berlin, or from those working under his direction or by his methods; and as his new laboratory in the Hygienic Institute is probably the most complete and perfect of any which exists, and as the procedures in most of the other modern laboratories are modeled after those here employed, it will best serve the purposes of the present paper, if the writer gives a general account of the course of study followed here, and the purposes which it is assigned to serve.

"It is assumed that the student who enters Dr. Koch's laboratory is familiar with the use of the microscope, with the general anatomy of the body, with the minute structure of its different parts as seen under the microscope, with the general methods of preparing diseased tissues for microscopical study, and with the appearance which the different parts of the body present in various diseases.

"The laboratory is a large well-lighted room with tables along the sides for work with the microscope, at which each student has his place before a window, with drawers and cupboards for keeping his apparatus. There are large tables in the centre of the room, supplied with gas and water, for the coarser manipulations, operation on animals, etc. Hoods and hot-air chambers are arranged at the sides of the room and in one corner a small space is partitioned off in which the bacteria which are being cultivated may be kept as much as may be free from dust, either at the ordinary or at an elevated temperature. Adjoining the general laboratory are laboratories for the assistants. Dr. Koch's private laboratory and study are separated from the others by a long hallway. Off from the general laboratory is a room for the janitor and his helpers, in which the apparatus is cleansed and in which is a cremating furnace into which the refuse from the bacterial growths, the bodies of animals which have served the purposes of experimentation and any infectious material, may be thrown and burned. Large photographic rooms are on the floor above, and also a loft in which smaller animals for experimental purposes are temporarily stored. The entire large building in which the laboratories are situated and formerly used for other purposes, will, when its reconstruction is completed, be entirely devoted to the purpose of an Hygienic Institute and will contain lecture-rooms, chemical laboratories, museums, etc.

"Each student is furnished by the institution with a set of the necessary apparatus which he is expected to return in good order at the end of the course, and is given a list of materials which will be used up in his work and which he may procure from the janitor. After cleansing and arranging his apparatus, he is given two or three well known forms of bacteria in the living condition to study. He is to learn all he can about them; their shape and size, whether they are movable or not when living, how they appear when growing, under what conditions they grow best, etc.; and finally with certain forms to see whether they are or are not disease-producing or pathogenic. In a word his task is to make out their life history, for himself, as completely as possible. He is aided in this work by Dr. Koch and his corps of well trained assistants."[8]

Prudden went on to describe, in some detail, the procedures carried out by the students, procedures reminiscent of those also described by Lewis (above), who had preceded Prudden in being trained by Koch (above). Many of these techniques are today second-nature to those enrolled in microbiology courses taught in colleges or professional schools. But it should be kept in mind such training was not the norm during the 1880s, when bacteriology was a relatively new field.

"The student is first taught the methods of staining them [bacteria] with the aniline dyes. But even when stained many of the bacteria look so much alike that it is difficult to tell them apart and moreover after staining they are always dead. So the next step is to plant them on some nutrient medium or soil on which they will grow. Boiled potatoes ... are cut in halves with knives sterilized by heat—being held in the fingers which have been freed from living germs by washing with corrosive sublimate [imagine the modern student being subjected to a similar procedure], and placed under sterilized bell-jars so that they may not be contaminated by the accidental falling upon them of bacteria from the air. Now by means of a platinum wire set in a glass handle, which has been sterilized by heating to redness, a tiny bit of the bacteria-containing material is conveyed to the cut surface of the potato and the latter is covered again and set away for a day or two in a warm place. Usually at the end of this time if all goes well, there will be a growth of the bacteria on the potato so large as to be quite visible to the naked eye. This growth, or 'colony' as it is called, which is made up of myriads of individual bacteria, the offspring of those planted, in many cases presents very characteristic ways of growing or special colors, etc., characters often by which particular species of bacteria may be distinguished from all others, even without the aid of the microscope...

"The next step is to make some transparent solid substance which shall be a suitable soil for bacterial growth. One of the most common and useful substances for this end is a ten percent solution of gelatin which is mixed with beef-tea, peptone, and a little common salt, and then made neutral or slightly alkaline by carbonate of soda. This mixture, carefully heated so as to destroy all bacteria which might be present in its ingredients, is filled into ordinary glass test-tubes which have been sterilized by a high temperature. These are filled about one-third full of the gelatin mixture and the opening is stopped by a plug of cotton batting. Through a long plug of cotton, bacteria cannot pass; the air can enter and leave the tube but all bacteria are caught by the fibres of the cotton. After the gelatin has become cool and solid, by means of a sterilized platinum wire, some of the bacteria are introduced into the gelatin, the cotton plug being removed for an instant for this purpose. Being transparent the gelatin permits us to see from the sides as well as from the surface the exact mode of growth of the particular form of bacteria introduced into the tube...

"But if we need to keep our bacteria at a higher temperature than that of an ordinary room, say at the temperature of the body, at which alone some forms will grow, the gelatin would melt and the bacteria would be scattered through it and the characteristic mode of growth of the masses or colonies would be lost. So for this purpose we use instead of gelatin, Agar-Agar, a material derived from a sea-weed, which in one per-cent solution forms a gelatinous solid transparent mass which may be heated to above the temperature of the body without fluidifying. To this are added, as to the gelatin, beef tea, peptone, etc....

"In all these methods of study it is of the utmost importance that we should be able to separate different species of bacteria from one another in the living condition, so that we may have growths or colonies which shall contain one species alone without admixture with any other. These are called 'pure cultures.' This is by no means an easy task, as will be appreciated when we consider how exceedingly minute the organisms are and how much danger there is that the bacteria floating everywhere invisibly in the air, may become mixed with those forms which we are studying. By a very simple device elaborated by Dr. Koch, we are nevertheless able at any time to separate one species from another with the utmost certainty, or from a mixture of many species to get into separate tubes pure cultures of each species by itself. This is accomplished by what is called the 'plate culture,' the details of which are as follows. Suppose we have a mixture, say a sample of impure drinking water, which contains four different species of bacteria which we wish to get into pure cultures in separate tubes, so that we may study them and their effects upon animals.

"We mix thoroughly a small amount of the bacteria-containing water with a much larger amount of the above described nutrient gelatin, rendered just fluid by heat. Then we pour this mixture out on to a glass plate which has been carefully sterilized by heat, so as to form a thin layer, which soon cools and becomes solid. The glass plate is now covered with a bell-jar to prevent the access to it of any bacteria which may be floating in the air and to prevent its drying, and set it away at the proper temperature. The individual bacteria which were scattered through the gelatin layer will presently commence to grow ... nothing is simpler than directly under the microscope, to take out on the tip of a sterilized platinum wire little bits from each one of the different forms of colonies, and transfer them to separate tubes of gelatin. Thus we secure 'pure cultures' of all the different forms of bacteria which were contained in the original mixture...

"There is still another feature of this method of working with the bacteria which is of the utmost importance. When we find bacteria in the body in connection with disease, the question always arises, do they actually cause this disease, or may it not be that the disease is produced by some other agency and simply furnishes favorable conditions for the growth of particular forms of bacteria, which may have come in from without and really have nothing to do with causing it? Still further, suppose in order to study the effects of the bacteria taken from a diseased, upon a healthy animal, we remove some of them, say on the point of a needle, and put them into a healthy animal, how can we be certain that we do not take with the bacteria some other unorganized material which may possibly itself be the real cause of the disease, and not the bacteria? We must be certain, in a word, that the bacteria which we have removed from a diseased animal are not mixed with anything else when we use them for inoculation. Now in order to attain this certainty, we do not usually transfer the material directly from the diseased to the healthy animal, but we transfer it to some of the above described culture media. When the bacteria have grown here, which they may in some cases do so rapidly as to have multiplied a thousand or ten thousand fold, even within a few hours, we remove the smallest possible quantity of the new growth—the descendants of the second generation from those taken from the diseased animal, and put it into a fresh portion of culture medium. This process may be repeated indefinitely, so that we may get the tenth, fiftieth, or the one hundredth generation. In this way, usually after from five to ten transplantations, we can assume, so enormous is the increase in number at each operation, that we finally have the species of bacterium which was removed from the diseased animal without any possible admixture of other material from the same source. If now, on introducing these remote descendants of the original bacteria into a healthy animal we can produce the disease, and if we find the same bacteria in the diseased parts of the inoculated animal, we have established the fact that it is this particular species of bacterium which causes the disease under consideration and nothing else.

"By the repetition of these various manipulations, the student in Dr. Koch's laboratory becomes practically acquainted with a considerable number of the better known forms of bacteria, carrying them through all the phases of growth, sketching and making notes of his observations. He learns to handle and experiment upon the bacteria causing the most virulent diseases—anthrax, glanders, tuberculosis, etc., without special danger of accidently communicating them to himself or to others, provided he works intelligently and carefully. He has the opportunity of making analyses of drinking water by which he determines the approximate number of living bacteria in different samples and studies the effects of filtration upon them. He may examine milk and other forms of food which frequently contain living bacteria. He furthermore has the opportunity of carrying on experiments upon the potency of a number of disinfecting agents under varying conditions. He also studies certain molds, which, like the bacteria, may cause well defined diseases in man and the lower animals. [Prudden is clearly extrapolating from the training which he received in Koch's laboratory, as he explained the applications of the procedures which he has learned.]

"As the end of the course approaches, when the worker has become practically familiar with the methods of research and the desirability of cautious manipulation, and has become acquainted with the varied characters of several species of bacteria, both the disease-producing and the harmless, work begins upon the bacterium causing Asiatic Cholera…

"So fully impressed was Dr. Koch with the virulence of the cholera bacillus, and so appalling would have been the calamity, should by any possible accident to his cultures, the bacteria have gained access to food or drinking water in Europe, that on his return from India after his discovery of the organism there and in Egypt, he destroyed all of his cultures and returned with only the records of his experiments and observations in the East. When the cholera broke out in Europe, however, in the following year, the source of infection being already there and the necessity for further experiments and studies urgently demanded for the public weal, pure cultures were made from the bodies of persons sick or dead of the disease in the Mediterranean ports and carefully carried to Berlin. Here investigations were continued, and under the order of the government, instruction was given, in ten day courses [see Lewis above], to classes of army surgeons, in the methods of recognizing the cholera bacillus, preventing its spread, disinfecting clothes, etc. But the most strict and unvarying precautions were taken against any possible escape of the bacteria from the single room in the laboratory to which studies on this organism were confined. Notwithstanding this, among the many men who did actual, practical work with the cholera bacillus in Berlin, in these courses, one contracted the disease, but happily recovered and did not spread the contagion. In his dejections the cholera bacilli were found in large numbers...

"The methods employed for studying the cholera bacillus in the laboratory are essentially the same as for other forms of bacteria, and have been sufficiently described in brief above.... Thus the student is furnished with the knowledge which will enable him to accomplish that which in the presence of a threatened invasion of the disease is of paramount and inestimable importance—namely, to recognize with certainty whether a given suspicious case is really Asiatic Cholera or not within a few hours. This done, an intelligent disinfection and isolation at the hands of the proper officials will, under all ordinary circumstances, suffice to stamp out the disease at once in countries to which it comes only by importation.

"Thus the course in the study of bacteria, of one month's duration, in Dr. Koch's laboratory, was brought to an end, and the writer cannot refrain from remarking that the calm, judicial mind of Dr. Koch—the master worker in this field—his marvelous skill and patience as an experimenter, his wide range of knowledge and his modest, unassuming presentation of his views are all calculated to inspire confidence in the results of his own work, to stimulate his students to personal exertion in this field, and lend certainty to the already widespread hope that ere long through the resources of science we shall be able to cope successfully with those most terrible and fatal enemies of the human race—the acute infectious diseases."[9]

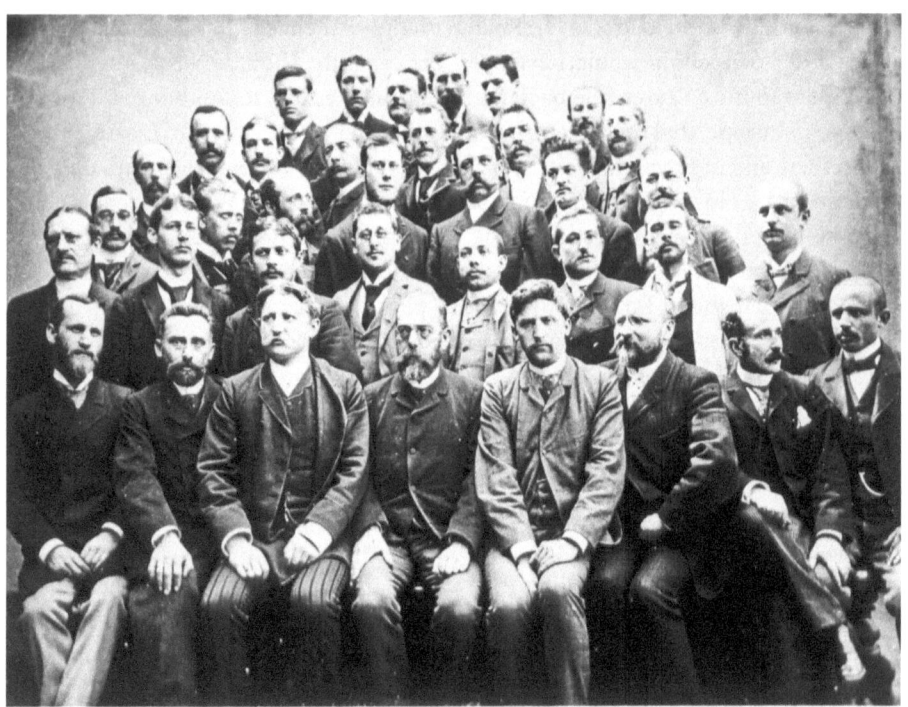

Bacteriology class taught by Robert Koch, Berlin, 1891. Beginning in the 1880s as a class to train physicians for the identification of the etiological agent of cholera, the course served as a magnet for American and other foreign students (National Library of Medicine).

Perhaps the most detailed description by an American student being trained in Koch's laboratory was that provided by Frederick Novy from the University of Michigan. Novy and his mentor at the University, Dr. Victor Vaughan, traveled to Germany during the summer of 1888, and were able to enroll in the course. Upon his return to Michigan, with plans to institute a similar course in the newly established Hygienic Laboratory on the university campus, Novy provided a detailed account of his (and Vaughan's experience) in Berlin. "The [Koch] Institute forms a constituent part of the University of Berlin, and possesses at its head, as director, Dr. Robert Koch, who has the able cooperation of his talented assistants, Drs. [Carl] Fraenkel, [Richard] Petri, [Bernhard] Proskauer and Kirchener. Before taking up the outline of work pursued in the laboratory, it will be well to say a few words concerning the building it occupies and the facilities for study which it affords.

"The present location of the Institute [Klosterstrasse 32–36] is in a large and spacious building, formerly occupied by an Industrial Academy which, upon the completion of the Polytechnicum at Charlottenburg, was transferred thither and its old quarters given up to the new department of hygiene, then but lately created. The building, which is three stories in height, consists essentially of two parts; the one occupied by a very complete and interesting Museum of Hygiene, and the other by the Laboratory proper. The latter is rectangular in form and surrounds an extensive open court. The first floor is occupied by the porter or concierge, and contains, moreover, the residence of the janitors as well as a number of neat and well kept animal rooms. The second story contains the large lecture room in which Dr. Koch is accustomed to deliver his lectures on hygiene, and a smaller room made use chiefly by the students engaged in the chemical laboratory, which is likewise situated upon this floor. The third floor contains the working rooms proper. There are here two large rooms for bacteriological work, each accommodating conveniently about twenty-five students, though a few more can be crowded in, if necessary. In addition to these two general laboratories, there are rooms for the use of the director and of his assistant, Dr. Fraenkel, as well as for special students engaged in advanced original work. Furthermore, there are contained here some well equipped rooms for photographing purposes, a splendid library and reading-room, and finally, though not the least in importance, a good lunch room. Owing to the fact that the building was originally erected for other purposes, it affords more room than is at present required by the Institute. As a consequence, fully one-third of the building is unoccupied…

"In order to meet the demand for instruction in the methods of bacteriological research, regular monthly courses are held throughout the year, except during the month of December when, owing to the short days [and loss of natural light], the regular work is discontinued. Of the remaining eleven courses which are annually held at the Institute, four are restricted to army surgeons, while the remaining seven are open freely to all comers without restriction of race, nationality or sex.

"This beginning course is presided over by Dr. Carl Fraenkel and his assistant, Dr. Kirchener, and constitutes one of the most prized courses offered among the many laboratories of Berlin. The maximum number of students that can enter one of these classes is about twenty-eight, and for anyone desiring to participate, it would be well to apply for a table some time beforehand.

"The daily work begins at about 9 o'clock in the morning with a lecture in which the day's work is outlined and the methods of manipulation are fully explained. The lecture over, the students betake themselves at once to their respective tables, and spurred on by the unusual interest of the subject, develop an enthusiasm for their work which is rarely seen elsewhere. Steadily and diligently each one looks after his own work, perchance endeavors to outdo his neighbors, but talks no more than is necessary. As twelve o'clock approaches, one by one suspend their work and withdraw to partake of lunch in the room set aside for that purpose. Here a substantial and cheap lunch, consisting of sandwiches of varied descriptions, eggs, as well as the inevitable beer, is provided. Each one helps himself to whatever he desires, and when finished, notes down the value of the articles consumed by him, in a book kept for that purpose. The account just entered upon with the janitor is settled upon completion of the course. As soon as the inner man is appeased, each student hastens to return to his table, where he remains until his day's work is completed, about four or five o'clock in the afternoon. Here, as in other laboratories one observes the traditional liberty of the German student in regard to smoking during working hours—a practice which at first sight would shock almost any of our American teachers. No attempt is made at the restriction of that habit, except that in the beginning the student is advised 'to smoke with caution and eat as little as possible whilst at work.'"[10]

"The first ten days, or so, are taken up with the study of the methods of manipulation and of the saprophytic or non-pathogenic micro-organisms. The remainder of the month is taken up with the study of the pathogenic germs, such as anthrax, tuberculosis, cholera, typhoid fever, erysipelas, etc. The methods of bacteriological examination of air, water, milk and soil are likewise given careful attention.

"The expense of such a monthly course will vary from twenty-five to forty dollars, according to the individual propensities of the student. Besides this expense, the student is expected to provide his own microscope, and it may be remarked here that the instrument employed by the students is, almost without exception, of Leitz manufacture. These instruments are much less expensive and almost as good as those of Zeiss. The 1–12th oil-immersion objective is employed exclusively in bacteriological work.

"In addition to this course, instruction is given in the Institute by Dr. Koch and by Dr. Petri, in the methods of inoculation and in original investigations."[11]

An entirely different perspective pertaining to Koch's laboratory was provided by Harry Luman Russell (1866–1954), then a graduate student in biology at the University of Wisconsin—in effect reversing the old axiom by making a "sow's ear from a silk purse." "We are in the 3rd story of an old and plaster building which would hardly be deemed worthy of warehouse purposes in America. Herr Koch has nothing directly to do with our work. He has just now something of more importance than the teaching of 'bugs.' Occasionally he passes through the laboratories and we see his general countenance. The deference with which he is spoken to by all is a surprise to an American. A German curtsy is something to be studied.... I expect it will be something to do before I shall be able to do the proper thing. The bow which is expected on all occasions begins at the hip joint and is a rigid inclination of the whole upper part of the body, at a considerable angle. The best way to practice it is to bind a crowbar from hip to lower spine.

"Dr. [Richard] Pfeiffer is first assistant and really has charge of all the laboratory work.... Dr. [Paul] Frosch, my overseer, is a genial good natured German. He is the only one of the assistants who can speak English to any extent."[12] As pointed out by Brock in his biography of Koch, Russell studied with Koch, or at least with his assistants, in 1890. The "something of more importance" which was occupying Koch at the time was the latter's work on tuberculin, mistakenly thought to serve as a treatment for tuberculosis. Certainly Russell's subsequent career benefitted from his work in Berlin. After leaving Koch's laboratory, he carried out further studies at the Pasteur Institute in Paris. Returning to the United States, Russell earned his Ph.D. at Johns Hopkins University in Baltimore in 1892. After spending one year on a fellowship at the University of Chicago, he joined the faculty at the University of Wisconsin, becoming a full professor in 1896. In 1903, Russell was appointed director of the Wisconsin State Hygienic Laboratory.

Russell's recollection of working with Koch's associates, albeit in 1890, rather than with the director himself was not inaccurate. Few students were so privileged to work directly with the director, particularly as the course progressed and Koch became involved in other areas of research. Prudden was among the few Americans to do so, as well as William Welch of Johns Hopkins and Harold Ernst from Harvard. Victor Vaughan, later the long-time dean of the medical school at the University of Michigan, along with his then student and colleague F.G. Novy, described in his memoirs the initial difficulty in simply meeting Koch, let alone enrolling in his course. But by the end of the 1880s and on into the next decade as the course evolved, an increasing proportion of foreign physicians, including Americans, were found in the Berlin laboratory. For example, in a course in bacteriology in 1891, the thirty-three students included ten Americans, as well as nine others from outside Germany.[13]

One does not wish to leave the reader with the false impression that Koch's laboratory was the sole training ground for American physicians interested in bacteriology during these final decades of the 19th century. Paul Ehrlich, an associate of Koch's at the latter's Berlin Institute during the 1890s and future Nobel laureate for his investigations into immunity, worked closely with several American physicians who spent time in his laboratory.

Edwin Klebs, whose work on germ theory was described in a previous chapter, and Paul Ernst, Director of the Pathological Institute in Heidelberg who, with Victor Babes, described the metachromatic granules seen in *Corynebacterium diphtheriae,* were among a growing number of German researchers who worked with American visitors. By the 1890s, however, a growing number of American universities, and even some medical schools, were incorporating bacteriology into their curricula. Many of their professors had received their initial training in Germany, and were now quite capable of passing on that methodology to the new generation of American researchers.

6

Theophil Mitchell Prudden

"Twenty-five years ago, pathological laboratories were rare in this country, and such as did exist were usually small corners in the deadhouse of some hospital which had more enlightened governors or more money than the rest. In the medical colleges, then largely proprietary, pathology was merged in the chair of the practice of medicine. The student could, if he were enterprising, witness an occasional autopsy, but beyond this his knowledge of this fundamental theme was derived from lectures, charts and books."[1]

Prudden was born in Middlebury, Connecticut, on July 7, 1849, the fourth son to Eliza Ann and George Peter Prudden. The father, an 1835 graduate of Yale College, was a Congregation clergyman and seventh-generation direct descendent of the Reverend Peter Prudden, among the founders of the New Haven colony.

Mitchell Prudden, the name he preferred, received his earliest schooling in his own home in New Haven where his father directed a private school. At age seventeen, in less than ideal health and unsure at the time as to whether he should endure the rigors of college, Prudden joined the business established by his brother Henry: "Bowditch and Prudden," a furniture manufacturing company. Starting with a salary of $5.00 a week for sweeping and dusting, Prudden within a year had worked his way up into bookkeeping. More important to his future, it was during this time he developed a greater interest in improving his education, particularly in the area of the physical sciences.

Prudden's fragile health during this period in his life resulted in living at home, while at the same time studying to fill the gaps in his education necessary for the goal of admittance to Yale College. A tutor helped him learn French, in addition to which Prudden attended lectures on the subjects of science and literature. In 1868, he entered Wesleyan Academy in Wilbraham, Massachusetts where, according to his own words, he "drifted along through the first term and then decided upon a long considered project to enter the

Sheffield Scientific School at Yale." While at the academy, he "engaged in his share of pranks ... while rather chummy with the boys and girls of his class."[2] Despite any hijinks, Prudden became sufficiently learned in Greek, Latin and mathematics for admission to Yale.

In 1869, Prudden enrolled in Yale College's Sheffield Scientific School, with a state fellowship covering the cost of his tuition. The original scientific school had been established in 1847, emphasizing science and engineering. During these first years of its existence, the scientific school at Yale was housed partially in the former president's house and partly in the building which formerly served as the chapel. In 1859, Joseph Sheffield, a New Haven lawyer, purchased the buildings for the medical school, had them enlarged, purchased the necessary equipment for a medical curriculum, and donated $50,000 for the endowment of the faculty for the school. The following year, in recognition of Sheffield's generosity, the name of the scientific school was changed to reflect its benefactor. Among its most famous alumni were physical chemist Josiah Gibbs and Lee de Forest, considered the "Father of Radio."[3] The school at the time of Prudden's admittance emphasized French, German and English, as well as physics, chemistry and mathematics. At the same time, what the Sheffield school did not offer were the subjects of zoology, botany, organic and physiological chemistry, scientific subjects necessary for Prudden's growing interest in medicine as a career.

Fortunately for Prudden, the early 1870s were a time of progressive ideas in the school. Prudden and a classmate, Thomas Hubbard Russell, who was also interested in a medical career, were able to convince the faculty to establish a "biological course in preparation for medicine."[4] The likelihood that it was on the initiative of Prudden and Russell that the course was established is supported by the description of the course in the Yale catalogue for 1870–71: "During one year the work of this course will be chiefly under the direction of the instructors in chemistry; during the second year, under that of the instructors in zoology and botany. In chemistry, especial attention will be given to the examination of urine and the testing of drugs and poisons; in zoology to comparative anatomy, reproduction, embryology, the laws of hereditary descent and human parasites; and in botany to a general knowledge of structural and physiological botany, and to medicinal, food-producing, and poisonous plants. The studies of the select course in physical geography, history, English literature, etc., are followed by these students."[5] In 1870, "these students" consisted of only Prudden and Russell.

Prudden graduated with a bachelor of arts degree in 1872, his thesis for graduation being "The Anatomy and Habits of the Larger Fiddler Crab," the work which he carried out for much of the late spring that year; the thesis was read during the graduation ceremony that June.[6] Prudden's experience was enhanced when he was asked to substitute for Professor William G. Mixter in the instruction of the freshman course in elementary chemistry in the Sheffield school during the several years the latter would be in Europe. In addition to paying Prudden a salary—$650.00 in addition to room rent—the time would allow him to enter the medical school at Yale.[7] Early visits from several faculty to Prudden's first classes, during which he professed to "much quaking," confirmed a wise choice had been made in filling Mixter's position; their confidence was further demonstrated when Prudden was appointed to serve as secretary at faculty meetings, the attendance in which made him initially feel "like a cat in a strange garret."[8]

Medical Training

Medical education at the Yale Medical School during the early 1870s reflected the largely cursory treatment of the subject common to most such schools in the country—a major reason some of the most highly qualified potential physicians preferred to train in Europe. A medical degree from Yale required a mere two years' worth of lectures; it was not until 1879 that the curriculum was increased to three years of study, with increased instruction in courses such as chemistry, histology, physiology and pathology. Students were expected to develop expertise in medicine through personal choices and interests.

During the spring of 1875, prior to graduating with his medical degree and on his own initiative, Prudden traveled to New York with the goal of enhancing his education. That spring, he attended lectures held at the College of Physicians and Surgeons at Columbia University, as well as participating in clinics directed by some of the leading physi-

Francis Delafield (1841–1915). A professor of pathology and practice of medicine in the College of Physicians and Surgeons at Columbia University, Delafield founded the first American laboratory of pathology. His *Handbook of Pathological Anatomy and Histology* (1885) was a standard text for many years in medical school curricula (librarything.com/pic/200381).

cians in the city. Among his contacts was Dr. Wesley Carpenter, a medical stenographer, who suggested to Prudden that he would benefit through the study of pathology with Dr. Francis Delafield, the recently appointed chair of pathology and practice of medicine at the College of Physicians and Surgeons. Delafield was well known for having developed a hematoxylin solution useful in staining cells, and the three months Prudden spent at his side were considered to be among the most important influences in his subsequent career.[9]

Following his graduation in 1875, Prudden, along with Thomas H. Russell, now a doctor, spent a year's internship at the New Haven Hospital, with six months in each of surgery and medical services. "Drs. [George Bronson] Farnam (1841–1886), [S. Henry] Bronson and Smith were the chiefs of the service at the time; Dr. Francis Bacon was the leading surgeon of New Haven. Dr. [William H.] Carmalt had just come. There was at this time no laboratory at the hospital for clinical tests and Prudden brought his New York experience to bear on a little urinary and other primitive analysis place in a tiny room at the west end of the basement in what was then the new wing of the hospital."[10] Farnum in particular seemed to take special interest in the new intern. When the former became incapacitated due to a rheumatic malady which ultimately proved fatal, and unable to continue in his capacity at the hospital, he also provided as a gift to Prudden, an expensive microscope he owned.

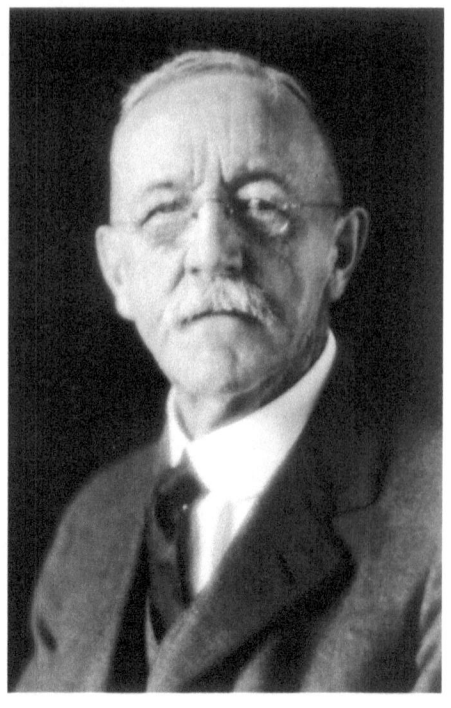

Theophil Mitchell Prudden (1849–1924). A professor of pathology in the College of Physicians and Surgeons at Columbia University, Prudden was among the first Americans to enroll in Robert Koch's bacteriology class. His 1885 report to the Connecticut State Board of Health on advances in bacteriology played a significant role in the improvement of health practices in that state (National Library of Medicine).

Upon completion of his internship, Prudden followed the path of many aspiring physicians and traveled to Germany, specifically Heidelberg, where he had the opportunity to further study pathology under the guidance of Dr. Julius Arnold (1835–1915), director of the Institute of Pathology, and who in 1879 provided the first diagrams of human chromosomes. Prudden's work with Arnold consisted of the study of changes involving living cartilage, portions of which resulted in Prudden being caught up in controversies between Arnold and other researchers on the subject. Upon completing his work with Arnold, Prudden visited other laboratories, including that of Salomon Stricker (1834–1898) in Vienna. "When most of us were serving our novitiate in pathology, the study of inflammation was largely limited to a bare description of visible phenomena and a cataloguing and classification of lesions … the more inquisitive among us were much exercised to find out whether it was the emigrated leukocytes or the fixed connective tissue cells which were most concerned in the formation of new cells. So earnest were the advocates of each of these views that the social amenities sometimes suffered. Thus it was my [Prudden's] hap to be banished from Stricker's laboratory in Vienna when it became known to that champion of the connective-tissue cells that I had been under the baleful influence of Cohnheim and Arnold."[11]

So what exactly was the work carried out by Prudden? As described by Hektoen in his biography, "The work deals with changes in living cartilage, a subject of special interest now in the day of vital staining and in vitro study of animal cells. He proves to have been endowed with a high grade of investigative workmanship. An effort was made to follow the effects of harmful agencies on living cells under otherwise normal environment. By a clever devise the transparent episternal cartilage of the frog was observed for hours under the microscope while connected with the body. The chromatin of the nucleus was recognized, variations in cell form and content were produced at will, and the important fact was noted that certain dye solutions do not color living cells but do color dead cells. 'But it seems to me particularly significant that it is possible to observe under the microscope, on living cartilage tissue, the process of contraction and the formation of vacuoles; and that it is possible thus to determine whether and under what conditions such changed cells return to the normal state or whether they undergo degeneration and die. The observations made with reference to the behavior of living and dead cartilage cells in response to dyes also seems to me [Prudden] noteworthy, because we thus learn that only the nuclei of the latter stain homogeneously. We are, therefore, in a position to distinguish whether cells are dead or living, and can thus exclude their participation in regenerative processes.'"[12] What distinguished Prudden's studies from those of others was his observation of living cells; previous works had involved interpretations of dead cells and tissues which had been fixed and stained.

Establishing a Career in Pathology

After two years in Europe, Prudden returned to New Haven with the thought of establishing a niche in the teaching and research of the subject of pathology; he had no real interest in following the common path of new physicians in developing a medical practice. After consultation with faculty members at several medical schools, he found there was little support in establishing a chair for the teaching of pathology; in general, the subject was subsumed within other areas of medicine. The only significant exceptions among those treating pathology as a unique discipline were in the medical school at Harvard, where Drs. John Barnard Swett Jackson, who previously had served as dean of the medical school, and Reginald Heber Fitz taught the subject.[13]

With few other options, Prudden opened an office for practice in a small clinic associated with the medical school at Yale, with the additional incentive of a lectureship in the medical school. During that first month, his first paying patient provided a two-dollar fee, which Prudden later had framed and hung in his laboratory; the remainder of the dozen patients he saw that month were non-paying.[14]

The perception of pathology as "merely" a sub-discipline of medicine began to change in the closing years of the 1870s. Two physicians practicing in New York were particularly prominent in motivating this change: Dr. Francis Delafield and Dr. Edward Gamaliel Janeway. Delafield was an 1860 graduate of Yale, earning his medical degree from the College of Physicians and Surgeons at Columbia University in 1863. After a brief appointment at Bellevue Hospital in 1874, he was appointed adjunct professor of pathology and practice of medicine in the College of Physicians and Surgeons the following year, a position he held for seven years, becoming a full professor in 1882. As noted above, Prudden spent three months in 1875 under the tutelage of Delafield. Edward Janeway (1841–1911) received his medical degree from the College of Physicians and Surgeons in 1864; in 1869 he received an appointment of professor of pathology and practical anatomy at Bellevue Hospital Medical College, where he remained for decades, even after its consolidation with New York University. Delafield, Janeway and others were particularly influential during these years in the investigation of the changes produced in the body as a result of disease—the immediate forerunner of modern pathology.

Prudden's opportunity in the new field came about shortly after he had established his practice in New Haven, a direct result of Delafield's long range view of the growing importance of pathology. The Alumni Association of the College of Physicians and Surgeons had established a fund of $10,000 in 1877, with the purpose of "advancing the standard of medicine." Delafield convinced the organization to use the money for development of a histological and pathological laboratory; in October 1878, Prudden was offered a position as director of that laboratory.[15]

Prudden was not Delafield's initial choice; the offer was apparently first presented to Dr. William Welch, a graduate of Yale College and at the time (October 1877) on the staff at Bellevue Medical College. Welch had been using a makeshift laboratory adjacent to the "dead house" in which he was carrying out pathological demonstrations for medical students enrolled at schools elsewhere in the city, and it was the popularity of these demonstrations that led the alumni to propose the generous funding. Welch was already acquainted with Prudden, and the two would subsequently have a long professional relationship. At the time, however, despite the opportunity to work in pathology, a field in which he had a growing interest, Welch felt his position at Bellevue would be more beneficial for his career, particularly if he could persuade Prudden to accept Delafield's offer in his stead. An additional benefit would be the close presence of a colleague likewise interested in developing the discipline of pathology. In a letter from Welch to Prudden that October 9th, the former outlined the position. "A few days ago Professor Delafield told me of the following scheme which the Twenty-Third Street Medical College has on foot. A laboratory for histology and pathology is to be established in connection with the college, by means of a fund given for the purpose by the alumni. It is to be taken hold of in an earnest way, for the laboratory is to hold the same relation to the college as the dissecting room does; that is, each student will be obliged during some part of his course to work there before he can take his degree. Dr. Delafield proposed that I should go in as his first assistant and have charge of the histological department, and assist him as much as necessary in the pathological part. The salary was to be five hundred dollars for the first year, and I believe more subsequently. I was naturally delighted with the offer and thought it to be just what I wanted, an opportunity to work in the direction where I had studied most. Upon speaking of the matter, before coming to a decision, with some of the professors at Bellevue, I find that they are reluctant to have me leave there, and even represent it as not the square thing for me to go at present. The latter motive especially has influenced me to stay, as I do not believe it pays to do anything unfair [particularly with those individuals who could have an impact on that career]. I feel as if I were relinquishing a great opportunity and do not see any equivalent for it at present at Bellevue, but as there is a feeling there that it would not be right for me to leave, I am going to stay and have so told Dr.

Delafield. He asked me if I knew anyone who would be competent for the position, saying there are a great many in New York who think they are, but few who really are.

"I immediately suggested your name and he at once seemed pleased, and deputed me to hunt you up by a letter and communicate the proposal to you. I really think the offer an advantageous one; in fact, presenting an opportunity better than any other I know for one with the tastes and resolution which you have formed. I do not know anyone who could do greater justice to the work there than yourself, and it seems to me to present great possibilities for the future. Personally, I should like to have you here in New York, for I fear I am going to rust out unless I have someone to talk with and help me on concerning the subject in which we are both interested."[16]

Prudden's first impulse was to politely decline the offer from Delafield, citing "pecuniary" circumstances. In a letter written the evening of the 16th, Prudden's reply stated "It is with great regret that after carefully considering the offer which you made me I find myself unable to accept it. I appreciate keenly the advantage it would be to me in my scientific career and the pleasure I should have in working with you. Pecuniary considerations alone compel me to decide thus. I am under such obligations in this respect that I think I should not be justified in assuming the risk which the transference of my residence to New York would involve.

"With many thanks for your kindness and deep regret at the necessity for this decision."[17] But once Prudden had a chance to sleep on his initial decision, coupled with "the spirit of adventure and the lead of a strong impulse of devotion to the advancement of science," he changed his mind. The following day, the 17th, Prudden sent his reply to Delafield: "I have decided to accept the position which you offered me. I should like to hear as soon as convenient how soon you would like me to come down."[18] Independent of the pecuniary needs, the $500.00 stipend was boosted by a curatorship of $250.00.

While the new laboratory was generously supported by the Alumni Association, expenses significantly exceeded the allotted funds, the deficit made up both directly by Delafield, and from student fees. In the immediate aftermath of the establishment of the laboratory, attendance being voluntary on the part of the students, relatively few participated in the studies. The numbers would increase with time and the growing reputation of the assistant. Prudden's description of the laboratory in its beginnings provides one explanation for the challenges he faced. "It was a narrow store on the ground floor, on Fourth Avenue, with a scanty strip of sky just visible through an iron grating, and with scarcely a feature adapting it to the needs of a microscopic laboratory, save that its walls kept out the wind and rain. An ice-cream store on one side and a harness shop on the other; the clatter of wagons and horse-cars and pedestrians sweeping endlessly along the street in front; the small boy peering curiously between the iron bars of the windows at the strange performances within, linked science to the busy world in a fashion truly cosmopolitan. The great brewery wagons rumbling heavily along the pavement set every microscope a-tremble; and the frequency with which microscopic observation must for this reason be suspended, while a severe strain upon the temper of the devotee to science, often left him free to muse upon the important role which beer plays in modern metropolitan life."[19] Prudden remained director of the laboratory until 1892, by which time the facilities were moved farther uptown to a "modern" building on West 59th Street.

Prudden, during these first months in New York, served as an assistant to Delafield in the autopsies the latter carried out at Roosevelt Hospital, founded several years earlier (and now known as Mt. Sinai Roosevelt Hospital). As recounted by Dr. William P. Northrup, president of the New York Pathological Society in 1888 and 1889 (having succeeded Prudden himself), "Granted that a college senior and a hospital house-physician are at the pinnacle of human pride and self-consciousness! Such a house-physician stood by the dissecting table at Roosevelt Hospital in 1878, while Dr. Delafield, the silent and dignified, made an autopsy on a medical case. At the foot of the table there appeared from an inner room a tall, pale, stiff figure in a black dissecting gown. A stranger stepping to a place in the front row seemingly assuming a place with the consent or tolerance of the operator! Who was this? Dr. [Henry] Heineman seemed to know him and bowed rather respectfully. 'This is the new assistant.' 'What has he to recommend him to assume so prominent a place in the front row where only house-physicians and professors dare to tread?' 'Who is he?' 'Why, he is so and so [Prudden],' and here followed a flow of encomium from Dr. Heineman which made some impression (not too much) on the house-physician. Long and motionless stood the stiff figure in the stringy, shapeless black gown and skull cap."[20]

Even though Prudden's scientific career was now settled in New York, and would continue to be for the remainder of his life, he did not yet completely sever his ties with Yale. For the first several years after accepting the position with Delafield, he continued to teach what was called "normal histology" at Yale, a course which dealt with general tissue and cell structure, and still closely linked with pathology. His first publication as a member of the College and Physicians and Surgeons was published at this time, *Notes on the Course in Normal Histology* (1879). Two years later a larger edition was published, *Manual of Practical Histology*, five editions for which were in print by 1893.[21]

Training in Koch's Laboratory

As described in greater detail in earlier chapters, the late 1870s and early 1880s represented an epochal period in the development of the germ theory of disease in general, and the study of bacteriology as its own discipline in particular. In March 1882, Koch reported the identification of the etiological agent of tuberculosis. As a result of this discovery, during this same period Koch established a hygienic laboratory, both to teach physicians methods for isolation and identification of the agent for diagnostic purposes, as well as a more general course, the purpose for which was to train future bacteriologists in that field. A description of that laboratory as observed (at a later time) by Frederick Novy and others, in particular Prudden, is also to be found in the previous chapter. Within a year after Koch reported his observations on the tuberculosis bacillus, Prudden published two articles on that same subject. In the meantime, Prudden arranged his own laboratory to allow for his own study of bacteriology. His laboratory, already barely large enough for several workers to be present at the same time, was further partitioned using glass sashes from a livery stable. It was said that a laboratory attendant standing at a table could touch the four walls at the same time.

In the first of these publications, in which Prudden described not only the significance of Koch's report, he also noted the importance of finding the same organisms in most, if not all, cases of the disease—in effect, repeating Koch's postulates. "In the prevailing furor, it is important to remember that even if all that is claimed for the new bacillus should be proven true, still the morphological basis upon which the present knowledge of tuberculosis rests has not been in the least disturbed, and that even the proof that this bacterium causes all the lesions of tuberculosis, would not explain either the peculiar reaction of the living organism against the parasite or the varied phenomena of the distribution of tubercle, heredity, variations in mode of attack, etc. While, however, a too ready acceptance of the new belief is to be deplored, it should not be forgotten that such a carefully conducted series of experiments as that by which Dr. Koch was led to his conclusions, is not to be met or shaken either by general skepticism or by reasoning based on analogy or more or less remote clinical data. It is only by actual experiments and observations, as minute, extended, and logical as his own, that Dr. Koch's conclusions are to be confirmed or disproved.

"The proof of the parasitic character of any infectious disease involves, first, the demonstration of the constant association of the parasite with the disease—this may be called the morphological part of the problem, and is often mistakenly regarded as the most important; second, the complete isolation of the parasite by cultivation; third, the production of the disease in a healthy animal by inoculation; fourth, and lastly—and this factor is, unfortunately, too generally ignored—it is necessary, in order to make the results of animal inoculation applicable to man, to prove that his organism will react in approximately the same way in the presence of the parasite as the animals experimented on.

"The present paper, which has almost exclusively to do with the first or morphological part of the problem, presents the record of the examination of a series of cases of tuberculosis with a view of determining to what extent, and in what way the tubercle bacillus was associated with the lesions in the material at the writer's disposal."[22] While there is little evidence that Prudden had direct knowledge of Koch's (or Henle's, for that matter) at this time, it is clear that he was following the concepts inherit in those hypotheses. In his analyses of over 100 patients diagnosed with numerous forms of tuberculosis, including acute military tuberculosis of the lungs, sputum in acute and chronic phthisis and tubercular lesions in various tissues, Prudden identified the tuberculosis bacillus in most. To account for those cases in which he was unable to observe the same bacillus, Prudden suggested the difficulty in staining, also noted previously by Koch himself, and the possibility that as the disease progressed, the numbers of organisms might be reduced.

In his second publication on the subject, Prudden addressed the problem that in some cases of the disease, including several of those examined personally, the bacilli are not readily observed. He presented several possible explanations for the apparent absence of the bacilli. "It is ... furthermore established, that in the great majority of phthisical cavities in the lungs, the contents and walls contain the bacilli in greater or lesser numbers; that the tuberculous areas and miliary tubercles in acute and chronic phthisis, many of them, contain bacilli; that in most cases of acute miliary tuberculosis the bacilli are present in many or most of the nodules. But it is equally true that in many of the miliary tubercles and cheesy areas, and in diffuse tubercle tissue in acute and chronic phthisis, and in some of the tubercles in acute miliary tuberculosis, the bacilli cannot be demonstrated by the technical procedures at present at our command...

"The popular conception of Koch's hypothesis would demand that the bacilli should be found in the peritoneal tubercles, particularly in those of presumably recent development. They could not, however, be found in any of the forms. But the writer [Prudden] is inclined to believe that the popular conception of Dr. Koch's hypothesis is not altogether correct. That the presence of the bacilli in each and every miliary tubercle, especially of younger form, must be demonstrable or the hypothesis is greatly weakened, is a notion founded in the misconception of the broad nature of his fundamental propositions. That tuberculosis is an infectious disease; that it can be communicated by the inoculation of the so-called bacillus tuberculosis, presumably freed from cultivations by all contaminating substances, and that this bacillus is the sole cause of the disease—these are the main features of his proposition. For Dr. Koch the criterion of a genuine tubercle lies in its infectious nature, and not in its anatomical character. Whether this criterion be accepted or not is at present a matter for individual decision, at any rate, it is a logical assumption as based on the data adduced by Dr. Koch. That the very frequent occurrence of the bacilli in the lesions of tuberculosis, in the human subject and in the victims of experimental inoculation, is a valuable confirmatory fact, there is no doubt, but so far as the writer is aware Dr. Koch nowhere states, nor does the establishment of his hypothesis require that the bacilli should be, or should have been bodily present in every tubercle.

"The fact that in cases of phthisis and miliary tuberculosis some of the tubercles do not, as judged by our present technical procedures, seem to contain bacilli, and that some apparently exceptional cases of tuberculosis do not reveal their presence anywhere in the body may be explained, it should be remembered, either, first, by the possibility that the parasites after inaugurating the morbid process may disappear from the seat of lesion or from the body; or, second, by the faulty nature of our demonstrating them; or, third, by the possibility that the bacilli may induce the growth of tubercle tissue in distant parts of the body by some product of their physiological activity at present entirely unknown to us; or finally, by the not improbably hypothesis that the morbid process which we call tuberculosis, may be induced by more than one agent...

"As the appearances and importance, from the diagnostic standpoint, of the tubercle bacillus become more and more familiar to the practicing physician, as they are unquestionably destined to do, it is very essential that it be clearly understood that its occurrence in sputa and other excreta in tuberculosis, however constant or practically valuable as a means of diagnosis, is not in itself a proof of the parasitic origin of the disease, nor does the search for it commit the observer in the least to the germ theory. For as far as all this goes it may be merely a harmless concomitant of tuberculosis and nothing more. When once it is proven beyond reasonable doubt to be one of the causes or the sole cause of tuberculosis in man then will arise questions in prophylaxis and therapeutics second in importance to none which can engage the attention of medical men.

"From the immediate practical standpoint, knowledge is most urgently needed on the subject of the occurrence of the bacilli in the sputa and other excreta in acute miliary tuberculosis, both in adults and children, and on their occurrence in cases of primary haemoptysis and in the incipient stages of various forms of phthisis, as well as in cases in which complete recovery has occurred or in which the disease has become latent."[23]

During the months following the appearance of his publications, Prudden planned on returning to Europe, with the goal of undergoing training with Koch himself. As he had worked with Julius Arnold during his previous time in Germany, making an excellent impression even as a largely inexperienced student at the time, he again called upon Arnold in hopes of arranging a meeting with Koch. However, in Arnold's reply, Prudden was informed that all positions in the course were at that time filled, though with the subsequent opening by Koch of the hygienic laboratory, space in a bacteriology laboratory would be available. In the meantime, Prudden might benefit by taking a portion of his time in Europe working in the laboratory of Dr. Ferdinand Hueppe, in Weisbaden, and an associate of Koch's.[24] In a fortunate juxtaposition, in May 1885 the Connecticut State Board of Health requested Prudden to present a report on the recent advances in bacteriology, and how they could best be applied in the improvement of health in the state: "to investigate the method of studying disease germs, particularly those causing Asiatic cholera, as employed in the laboratory of Dr. Robert Koch, in Berlin, and in such other laboratories as he might have occasion to visit, and further, to report to the Board the results of such observations."[25] Prudden's sojourn in Germany could provide the expertise to do exactly that. Some of the questions he presented, particularly in relation to practical applications of theoretical work, could be posed by the general public even 125 years later.

While the germ theory was quickly gaining credibility, an understanding of the concept was still not universal. As frequently stated in this and other chapters, bacteriology was a new field of science; physicians were more familiar with the "macro" as related to medicine, rather than the "micro." Therefore, among the reasons Prudden was asked by the Board of Health to visit European laboratories was to bring to the United States a greater understanding of both the evidence for germs as etiological agents of disease, and teaching the methodology for studying disease agents. Prudden began his report to the board by describing the current train of thought among European workers, such as Koch and his associates, in the field. "Everywhere in the air of inhabited regions, in the water and in the soil are myriads of tiny living organisms which belong among the simpler forms of plants, and which are commonly called bacteria. [The statement is in part a result of the work of Pasteur in refuting the idea of spontaneous generation, and its application by Joseph Lister in antisepsis.] They are very minute, requiring high powers of the microscope to make them visible. Some of them are capable of rapid multiplication, so that they may, under favorable conditions increase in number a thousand or a million-fold even in a few hours. Some of these organisms appear to be perfectly harmless, having no effect whatsoever, so far as is known, upon the health of animals and man. Others are of positive value in preserving a healthful sanitary condition of the water, soil and air, which they do by breaking down and feeding upon organic compounds which might prove deleterious to health. On the other hand, it has been definitely proven that a certain number of fatal diseases in man, and several in animals, are caused and caused alone by the entrance into the body of special forms of bacteria. These bacteria are often called 'disease germs,' and like the bacteria which are harmless to man and animals, are very minute. Thus the organism causing consumption, which is a little rod-like structure, is so minute that if placed end to end it would require from 4,000 to 6,000 of them to reach across the head of an ordinary sized pin. [Despite his inability to observe bacteria in all cases of tuberculosis—see his previously published two articles on the subject—he has acknowledged their role as the etiological agents of that disease.]…

"While it has been definitely proven that certain diseases in man, consumption, malignant pustule, erysipelas, Asiatic cholera, glanders, and certain forms of so-called blood poisoning, are due to bacteria and to them alone; there are several other diseases about which the proof is not yet so conclusive, but upon which investigations are yet in progress, which, there is good reason to believe, will ere long throw much light upon their nature; such diseases are, for example, typhoid fever, pneumonia, diphtheria, etc.

"The work then which is at present being done in laboratories which are devoted to the study of bacteria is of two kinds, first: the continued study of the life history of the bacteria, both those which are already proven to cause, or which there is reason to believe may cause illness, and those which are proven to be harmless; and second, the application of the knowledge already obtained to questions of the treatment of disease and of the preservation of public and private health. Work of this nature, whether applied to the first or second of these purposes, or, as is more frequently and naturally the cause to both at once, demands in the worker a considerable amount of special training in the use of the microscope, in the methods of some kinds of botanical study, and in the recognition of the changes which may be produced in the body by bacterial as well as other diseases."[26]

Prudden's detailed description of Koch's methods of study is presented in Chapter 5. A primary purpose of this report, of course, was not just such a description, as important as it might be in producing a guide towards the establishment of similar courses in the medical schools of the United States, but of providing recommendations for improvement of public health in both Connecticut, and in the United States as a whole. In summarizing the growing knowledge and potential applications which he observed, Prudden also ended his report with specific recommendations towards that end. "As we review this resumé of the modern methods of bacterial culture, we are impressed with the vast field for research which lies open to the scientific worker, and with the fact that our knowledge in this direction is still in its infancy. Its incalculable importance to the physical well-being of the race and the countless problems of general scientific interest which it suggests will insure the devotion of an abundance of capable investigators as soon as the means are furnished for the prosecution of the work by institutions of learning, by governments [using the German government in particular as such an example], or by private beneficence.

"At the present moment several questions of great importance present themselves to us. In the first place, of what practical advantage have the painstaking and expensive researches thus far been made to the human race, and what may we reasonably expect from their continuance in the future? It should be remembered here, as always when the practical utility of our knowledge is in question, that any and every addition to our knowledge of nature is of value to the human race, inasmuch as it enlarges its mental range and may throw light upon its origin and relationship to other forms of life. But in this particular case we are fortunately not thrown back upon the general utility of knowledge, for we can readily see how in very many ways the results of the few years of work upon the bacteria and related organisms have been of the greatest practical value. One of the most frequent questions of unthinking persons is, does all the knowledge of the bacteria which has been acquired enable you to *cure* [italics in original] any of the serious or fatal diseases of which you assert them to be the cause? To which we must answer at this date—November 30th, 1885—No. But this answer must be qualified. In the first place, the work has been going on in a systematic and scientific manner for but a very few years; second, the problems are among the most complex which any department of nature presents; third, the bacteria belong in an invisible and almost unknown realm, and our general knowledge of them must be built up as we go along, hand in hand with special knowledge which we are seeking in connection with the diseases of man. Long and tedious as are the investigations which must be made before we are certain in any single case that a particular form of bacteria causes a given disease, they are no means as extensive as are those which must be carried out before we are able to commence, upon a sound basis, the work of cure in individual cases...

"The practical results of the work thus far lie in another direction; not so much in the cure of persons already diseased—although the hope of this lies ever before the physician and the investigator—as in the *prevention* of the diseases or *prophylaxis*. Here the results have been positive and of incalculable worth, and bid fair to grow in importance with every day's advance in knowledge. We are no longer helpless in the face of a threatened invasion of Asiatic cholera; the studies of Dr. Koch and others have taught us characteristics of the bacteria causing the disease by which we may recognize it in the very first case which makes its appearance; and the studies upon disinfectants have taught us how to destroy in the most certain manner the source of the contagion. The diseases incident to surgical operations have lost many of their terrors since we have learned how to prevent the invasion of the bacteria which cause them. The dangers of prolonged intimate personal contact of well persons predisposed to the disease by inheritance or otherwise, with the victims of consumption, and the necessity for the destruction of certain excretions from these individuals, are points to which science has called attention, and by the heeding of which we may hope to do much towards checking the ravages of a bacterial disease which carries off nearly one-seventh of all who die. Glanders and anthrax are other diseases whose spread may be controlled by the application of knowledge already acquired. And the same principles of prevention which are efficient in the infectious diseases whose bacterial origin is already demonstrated, may be applied, with reasonable hope of success, to those which as yet are, by analogy alone believed to be due to similar causes.

"The duty of applying the knowledge already obtained upon this subject to the prevention of disease, belongs in part to the physician in his private and public practice, and in part to the national and local Boards of Health and their officers. So far as the physician's duties in this report are concerned, we need not discuss them here. A knowledge of the disease-producing bacteria and the methods of combating their ravages, is, or will soon become, a part of their professional furnishing at the hands of the medical schools. On the other hand, it may not be unprofitable to consider briefly the directions in which the States, through their Boards of Health, may render available and useful the results which bacteriological studies have thus far brought to light, and may contribute to the extension of our knowledge in this field. The work which must be done, and done with the authority which the sanction and support of the State can alone impart, is of several kinds. In the first place, in the presence of threatened epidemics such as Asiatic cholera, typhoid fever, diphtheria, etc., there should be in the employ of the State and located in some part of the State easy of access, some person vexed in the methods of modern bacteriology and familiar with the bacteria which are proven to cause disease, to whom might be entrusted the recognition of their nature at the earliest possible moment, the discovery of their source, and the enforcement of such measures as have been shown to be efficient in destroying the contagion. In the second place, the analysis of drinking water, either from wells or from more general sources of supply is no longer complete when its chemical composition has been determined, because a simple chemical analysis takes cognizance either not at all or only in the most general way of the presence of bacteria, upon whose existence or absence may depend entirely the salubrity or insalubrity of the water. The effects of the filtration system employed in the water supply of cities or of houses are to be judged with much greater accuracy by the determination of its effects upon the number of bacteria which the water contains—the so-called 'biological analysis'— than by the ordinary chemical methods. The writer does not mean to imply that the biological analysis is entirely to supersede the ordinary chemical analysis but rather that it should be practiced in connection with it.

"Furthermore, there is reason for believing that in many cases of poisoning from the use of impure foods such as milk, spoiled meat, sausages, etc., the source of difficulty lies, in many cases at least, in the presence in them of certain forms of bacteria whose existence can be revealed only by the bacterial analysis. Finally, an officer in the employ of the State for the above indicated purposes, should if possible be furnished with facilities for the prosecution of original researches on the relations of bacteria to disease, since in the imperfect condition of our knowledge important problems in this direction will arise at every turn.

"It should also be remembered that the bacterial diseases of animals, which in Europe have furnished problems of vast economic importance, are apparently becoming more and more frequent and important among us. So that the investigation of such disorders as swine plague, pleuro-pneumonia of cattle, glanders, etc., might well be associated with the duties above indicated for a duly authorized and competent officer in the employ of the State.

"An establishment somewhat similar in its general scope to the Agricultural Experimental Stations and under the direction of State Boards of Health, acting in concert with the local Boards, would form a suitable basis for the accomplishment of the desired end. Such an establishment sufficiently equipped for the performance of the most urgent duties need not, aside rom the salaries of the workers, involve great expense, since apparatus for bacteriological investigations is not in general very costly.... The expense which the carrying out of such a work would entail upon the State would at any rate be but trifling as compared with the possibilities of disaster which the invasion of a serious epidemic would bring with it, or the loss and danger which an impure water supply, or poisonous food would bring upon individuals or communities.... That the results accomplished are of vast importance may be seen by an examination of the work, for example, of the Imperial Health Bureau in Berlin, Germany.... The writer is certain that in order to fulfill his whole duty, in offering to the Connecticut State Board of Health this report, he could do no less than express his conviction of the urgent necessity for the establishment, even in a small way, of some such centre of research and control, as above indicated."[27]

One area of immediate impact which followed Prudden's return and subsequent publication of his recommendations, was the formation of a bacteriology department in the medical school at Yale. As was true at most university medical schools, at least in those which acknowledged the importance of the subject, bacteriology at Yale began as a department of hygiene, the primary function of which was water analysis for the State Board of Health. Indeed, at the time of Prudden's report, the new (1886) president of the college, Dr. Timothy Dwight V, Congregational minister and professor of sacred literature in the divinity school prior to his appointment, considered bacteriology "a passing phase of learning," interest in which would disappear in time. Events would soon prove Dwight to be near-sighted in his viewpoint.

The major concern of the hygiene department, as referred to above, was the quality of the streams and rivers in the state. In recent years, they had become increasingly polluted as human sewage combined with refuse from factories not only rendered the waters unpalatable—typhoid fever outbreaks were particular problems in the state—but the killing of fish created aesthetic problems as well, which could not be ignored. In response, the state legislature appropriated $5000.00 for the State Board of Health, the purpose of which was to investigate the cause and methods to address the increasing pollution.

The State Board of Health consulted Prudden for recommendations on how best to use the appropriation. Prudden's response was that the state should establish a bacteriology laboratory, with a paid bacteriologist in charge.[28]

Though it would be some years before Prudden's recommendations for establishment of a bacteriological laboratory in conjunction with a Board of Health would come to fruition, his report laid out what were likely the first such plans presented to any state board of this kind.

Bacteriological Legacy of Prudden

Prudden's training and early interests centered on pathology, more specifically on the changes which took place in tissues as a result of disease. Most of his major publications dealt with pathology, and, as stated earlier, his collaboration with Delafield produced the major medical work, *Handbook of Pathological Anatomy*, which went through numerous editions. By doing so, Prudden's studies ultimately served as a bridge between that discipline and scientific medicine, with a significant portion of the applications addressing an understanding between bacteria and public health. Largely self-taught in the newly emerging field of bacteriology, he was determined to increase his expertise in that area by studying with one of the most important leaders in that field: Robert Koch. In that end, he spent two months during 1885 in Germany, with much of that period learning methodology in the presence of the man himself. Koch's legacy, in turn, found an application in the training of new generations of bacteriologists, either by Prudden himself, or by his associates. Indeed, Prudden often thought of himself as primarily a teacher, in reference to his textbook, but as easily applicable to all of his teaching: "a slave to teaching and to keeping the breath of life in a textbook in pathology for successive generations of students and practitioners of medicine."[29]

As an example of Prudden's impact on bacteriology as a subject, in the same time period during which he received advanced training in Berlin, an associate in Prudden's laboratory, Dr. Timothy Matlack Cheesman, provided instruction in bacteriology, first for only a few students in 1885, and in 1887 before a larger audience of medical students in a course titled "Course in Pathology and Bacteriology." The format of the course was similar to that in which Prudden had been enrolled when he had undergone training in Koch's laboratory. Cheesman later became an important figure in the public health arena in New York, focusing on the safety of milk and water supplies, and was a charter member of the Society of American Bacteriologists, serving, in 1899, as their first secretary. Cheesman was one of—literally—hundreds of medical students, associates and personnel, who were ultimately influenced by Prudden over the course of the latter's career. As Dr. Edwin O. Jordan (1866–1936) later described his experience in Prudden's laboratory, "I spent the month of October 1888 in Dr. Prudden's laboratory. His energetic, genial personality dominated the whole place. Although my knowledge of bacteriology was exceedingly rudimentary, he gave freely of his time and advice. He told me briefly what to do, then turned me loose and after a few days, probably once a week, discussed results. It was a very stimulating and fruitful experience, and I have profited all my life from even that brief contact."[30] In 1892,

Jordan joined the faculty at the University of Chicago as an associate in the newly established Department of Anatomy. The subject of bacteriology became more prominent at that university during the following years, with Jordan receiving promotions to, first, an assistant professor in bacteriology (1895), and associate professor (1900), and a full professor in 1907. When a Department of Bacteriology was established in 1914, Jordan was appointed as its first chair.[31]

Nor were Prudden's publications entirely directed towards his peers in the field. Popular writings included "Our Ice-Supply and Its Dangers," published in *Popular Science Monthly* 32 (1888), 668; "Tuberculosis and Its Prevention," *Harper's Magazine* 88 (1894), 630, "To Live Past Three Score and Ten," *Harper's Weekly* 47 (1903), 934, as well as several later articles in *Harper's Magazine* dealing with his travels in the western mountains. Smaller booklets, *The Story of the Bacteria* (1890) and *Dust and its Dangers* (1890), also went through several printings.

Prudden's first publications dealing with the subject of bacteriology had been his observations of tuberculosis bacilli in patients diagnosed with that disease. Even with the widespread acceptance by the late 1880s of the role of these organisms as the etiological agents, methods of transmission—even the concept of contagion—had yet to be settled. Tuberculosis remained a significant problem in large cities such as New York. In May 1889, Commissioner of Health Dr. Joseph D. Bryant requested Prudden, in collaboration with Drs. Herman Biggs (1859–1923)

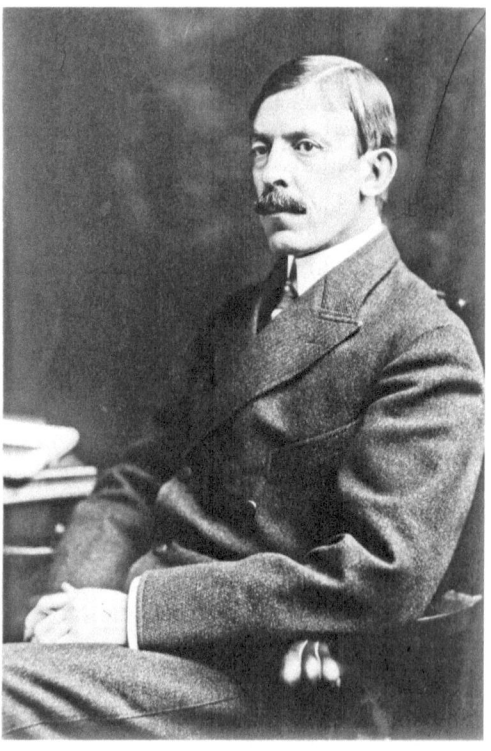

Hermann Biggs (1859–1923). In 1889, the New York City commissioner of health requested Biggs, Prudden and Alfred Loomis prepare a report addressing the spread and control of tuberculosis in the city. Biggs was appointed pathologist and director of the bacteriological laboratories in New York City in 1892, serving in that capacity until 1901 (National Library of Medicine).

and Alfred Loomis (1831–1895), pathologists associated with the department, to apply Koch's work with that disease, and address the continual presence of tuberculosis in New York.[32] Prudden was therefore instrumental in the first widespread campaign in that city, introduced with the goal of preventing the disease. While their report, the first such in the country on that subject, presented to the New York City Board of Health specifically addressed the problem in that city, its application was relevant nationwide. The report emphasized the contagious nature of the disease, that it is not directly inherited, and that prevention rests on preventing the spread from person to person.[33] Specific recommendations included "systematic surveillance, nursing follow-up of individual patients, public education, isolation of infectious patients, and free laboratory testing of sputum samples."[34] The New York City bacteriological laboratories, opened in 1892 with Biggs as its first director, were thought by him to have been the first such municipal laboratories established in the world. During the first ten months after some of the recommendations had been instituted (1892), approximately four thousand cases of the disease were reported, five hundred of which were confirmed by the laboratory.[35]

Prudden's bacteriological work in the 1880s extended into the study of diphtheria in children. His observations initially led Prudden to erroneously attribute that disease to streptococci, which had been found in large numbers in the throats of victims. With the identification of the actual diphtheria bacillus by Koch's associate Friedrich Loeffler, Prudden correctly recognized the role of the streptococci as the source secondary infections.

In 1892 Prudden was appointed professor of pathology in the College of Physicians and Surgeons, the position he held until his retirement due to declining health in 1909, at which time he became Professor Emeritus. Prudden died in his sleep from a coronary thrombosis in April 1924.

7

William Henry Welch

"Welch, who was making a collection of cultures to take back to the Hopkins, was not cast down when Koch refused to give him any cholera bacilli, for he had already obtained some from [Carl] Flügge. 'Dr. Prudden had them also,' he remembered; 'and I have often wondered whether Koch suspected us, for one evening when I had been looking at my cultures, Koch as he sat and talked with us remarked that it would be better a man had never been born if he introduced a disease germ into a region where it previously had not existed—suppose they escaped—supposed it could be traced to an accident in the laboratory—better that man had never been born!'

"Welch spent a sleepless night. At dawn he rose from the bed, unlocked his bureau, and took out the test tube in which was imprisoned the scourge of cholera. Having poured on a solution of bichloride of mercury to kill the germs, he hurried through the silent streets to drop them in the river. At last he reached a bridge; he put his hand into his pocket, but there the hand stopped. A figure with his hat over his eyes and his head down was approaching through the otherwise empty city. Welch stared innocently at the water, but when the footsteps had come so close that he could not resist looking up, he recognized the intruder; it was Prudden engaged on the same errand as his own. Each must have laughed, feeling both foolish and relieved; then both threw their cultures into the Spree. They expected, of course, to see the tubes sink immediately out of sight, instead of which they had the disquieting experience of observing them bobbing up and down as they floated slowly down the stream. The guilty pair hurried away just, it is said, as a large *Schutzman* [policeman] appeared on the scene. 'That,' Welch continued,' was long before there was any outbreak of Asiatic cholera in Berlin.'"[1]

Welch's anecdote originated with his second extended period in Europe, undertaken from September 1884 to August of the following year, with the purpose of developing expertise in the new field of bacteriology while studying with the avowed expert in the field at the time, Robert Koch. This was his second such trip to Germany and elsewhere in Europe, the first having taken place eight years earlier when, as a young medical intern, he took the opportunity to study pathology and physiology with experts in their respective fields, areas of study sorely lacking in an American education. In their own way, each trip would play a significant role in Welch's contributions to the beginnings of what would become one of the outstanding medical programs in the United States: The Johns Hopkins Medical School in Baltimore.

William Henry Welch was born April 8, 1850, in Norfolk, Connecticut, the only son and second child to William Wickham and Emeline Collin Welch. The younger William was born into a family with a long line of doctors; his grandfather, Benjamin Welch, and father, his father's four brothers, and four cousins were all physicians. Nor were these immediate family members the only members of the Welch ancestry to carry out public service. Benjamin's father and William Henry's great-grandfather, Hopestill Welch, had been a member of General Israel Putnam's army fighting with the British during the French and Indian War, and later served in the Continental Army under Benedict Arnold while the latter was still fighting the British; Hopestill Welch was among the few survivors of Arnold's ill-fated attack on the city of Quebec early in the war.

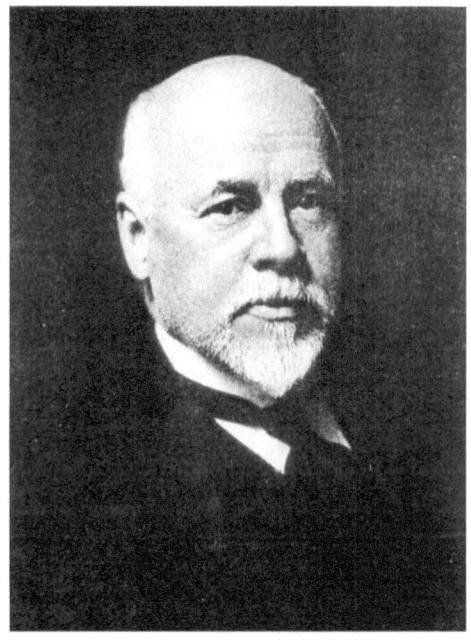

William Welch, both father and son, suffered a tragedy when, in October 1850, Emeline Welch, who had been in declining health for some time, died. The older child, also named Emeline and then three years-old, was sent to live with a nearby aunt and uncle, the Reverend Ira Pettibone; William Wickham's mother, Elizabeth, came to live with her son and grandson, helping to raise the latter during the frequent absences of the son when making his "rounds." William Wickham Welch would later remarry.

Welch's earliest formal education was at the day school run by two sisters, the Misses Margaret and

William Henry Welch (1850–1934). In 1884, Welch was appointed to the Johns Hopkins Medical School and Hospital, becoming dean of the School of Medicine in 1893. Welch helped train a generation of physicians and researchers in pathology, bacteriology and public health (National Library of Medicine).

Desiah Nettleton. In his old age, Welch looked back fondly on his early education. "Our life's as children centered around the family, the church, the Sunday school, the walks to the cemetery on Sunday afternoon, the school, the village green.... I was led to believe by my father, and I do not dispute it, that I owed everything in my start in life to my attendance at the Misses Nettleton's school, and I am sure that it was an excellent school of its kind."[2] Welch's education was enhanced by his fortune in being a part of a family which emphasized readings, including both classics and contemporary. "The educational advantages were good for that time and the intellectual and interests were not lacking. There was a small circulating library and as we grew in years there was much reading of books. It was a time when everyone was reading the same books, fewer in number but more intensely perused than today [1920s]. It might be Dickens, or Scott, or Harriet Beecher Stowe, or even Jane Eyre, Rutledge, or Beulah Dred or Wide, Wide World to say nothing of the Scottish Chiefs and Thaddeus of Warsaw. We exchanged books and we talked about them."[3] Not surprisingly, patriotism during the Civil War focused intensely on the Union; the children of Norfolk even formed a Zouave company which practiced drilling on the village green; whether William was a member of the "company" is unknown. Regardless, there is an element of irony here, coupled with Welch's familiarity with Stowe's *Uncle Tom's Cabin*. Later in life, Welch became friends with Dr. Victor Vaughan, dean of the University of Michigan Medical School, who was raised in Missouri in a family with a history of slave-holding.

In 1863, at the age of thirteen, Welch was enrolled in the Winchester Institute, a combination of a boarding school and military institute, advertised as maintaining "mild and parental discipline." Principal of the school was the Reverend Ira Pettibone, Welch's uncle and head of the family to which Welch's sister had been sent following their mother's death. Two of the instructors were Ira Welch Pettibone and Benjamin Welch Pettibone, family cousins. Welch's memories of the school were positive. Discipline was mild, and students had access to horses, picnics in the summer and sleigh rides in the winter.[4]

In 1866 Welch began his higher education with enrollment in Yale College. Education at Yale during his period was largely classical, with required courses in Latin and Greek, literature, moral philosophy and mathematics. During Welch's sophomore year French was added to the curriculum. The entire science curriculum consisted of a course in astronomy and one in geology. Upon graduating in 1870, Welch's ambition was to be a teacher of Greek, preferably at Yale, but if the opportunity did not present itself—and in fact it didn't—then he would teach at a secondary school. The best he was able to do was to serve as a tutor of German and Cicero in Norwich, New York, for a class of young women in a newly organized preparatory school. The school closed after one year, and almost by default, Welch returned to Norfolk, where his father was more than happy to have his son join him as a medical apprentice.

Career in Medicine

At the time he joined his father in 1871, Welch still had little interest in a medical career. It appears that while teaching in Norwich he had attended a chemistry lecture by a member of Columbia College's College of Physicians and Surgeons, Dr. Samuel St. John, which made little impression and certainly did not dissuade Welch in his preference for a career in the classics. By now, however, not only did his father encourage Welch to enter the medical profession, but both his sister and stepmother urged him to consider this step.

With few alternatives, Welch enrolled in the Sheffield Scientific School in New Haven in order to correct his deficiencies in science. As was presented in the previous chapter describing T. Mitchell Prudden's career, the Sheffield School possessed excellent laboratories, particularly in the field of chemistry. In 1872, Welch enrolled in the College of Physicians and Surgeons in New York.

Despite a faculty of dedicated and knowledgeable professors, the 1872 version of the medical school suffered many of the deficiencies common to such schools in the United States. There were few laboratories—classes were almost entirely lectures and memorization—and the curriculum consisted of two six month terms, with a third year in which the student served an apprenticeship. If the student passed a final examination, described by Welch as among the easiest examinations he ever took, he was now a doctor. Faculty were paid through student tuition—the University of Michigan Medical School was one of the few exceptions to this practice at the time—and consequently had little incentive to fail or remove underqualified students. In the words of Dr. Henry Jacob Bigelow, professor of surgery at Harvard University, "In an age of science, like the present, there is more danger that the average medical student will be drawn from what is practical, useful, and even essential, by the well-meant enthusiasm of the votaries of less applicable sciences, than that he will suffer from the want of knowledge of these.... The excellence of the practitioner depends far more upon good judgement than upon great learning.... We justly honor the patient and learned worker in the remote and exact sciences, but should not for that reason encourage the medical student to while away his time in the labyrinths of Chemistry and Physiology, when he ought to be learning the difference between hernia and hydrocele."[5]

Difficulties in medical training may have existed, but many of the faculty themselves had received excellent training, often through studies in Europe. Dr. Alonzo Clark, professor of pathology and medicine, had studied with the French physician Pierre Charles Alexandre Louis, among the most important early 19th century clinicians. As Welch later recalled, "He [Clark] was the one that brought that new French medicine to this country in his early days, and was greatly interested in pathological anatomy."[6]

Lectures were often supplemented by clinics, some of which were held at Bellevue Hospital. While not all medical students chose to attend these sessions, Welch found them particularly instructive. In particular, he enjoyed the clinic held by his neurology professor, Dr. Edward Seguin, on nervous disorders. One year, Sequin offered as a prize an expensive Varick microscope for the student who wrote the best essay on the course. Since the clinic was held on Saturday afternoons, at a time most students preferred to be elsewhere, Welch was awarded the microscope for his outstanding essay. Unfortunately, at the time Welch had not had any training in the subject of microscopy, and the instrument served more as an inspiration than could be put to a more practical use. More importantly, the clinic stimulated in Welch an interest in pathological anatomy. During this same period, Welch took advantage of the opportunity to meet and interact with another professor of the same subject, one who would play a significant role in his future career, and in Prudden's as well as we read in the previous chapter: Dr. Francis Delafield. Meanwhile, Welch received his medical degree from the College of Physicians and Surgeons in the spring of 1875.

Delafield had also studied with Louis in France—a common thread among many of those physicians who came of age in the earlier years of the century. Delafield was particularly interested in the dissection and study of cadavers, the subject of which Welch had in the recent year become fascinated. Delafield and his approach to the application of pathology had a strong appeal for Welch, and the feeling became mutual, as the professor likewise found Welch to be an able student. In the early summer of 1875, Delafield offered Welch an appointment as curator of the Wood Museum of Pathological Specimens, a position which Welch enthusiastically accepted. In a letter to his father, Welch described the position. "Yesterday Dr. Delafield asked me if I would not take his place as curator and pathologist at the hospital, for the summer. I accepted of course very gladly, but I fear I should not be able to do justice to the work. It involves my taking charge of the post mortem examinations two days in the week and recording in a book the pathological appearances. I understand pretty well the lesions visible to the naked eye, but I know nothing about the microscopical appearances. I am sorry I have not yet been able to study with the microscope, but I hope to find opportunity for it some time. It is very important and requires considerable training. It is the position which Dr. Delafield and Dr. Janeway have held as curators at the Bellevue Dead House that has given them their reputations as pathologists, and it is as such that they take rank among the first in the country."[7] Welch, of course, had not yet learned the use of the Varick microscope which he had won. Still, the experiences Welch encountered with Seguin in the clinic and his relationship with Delafield in the Dead House were primary factors in Welch's decision to choose pathological anatomy as his professional career.

Studies in Germany

Since Welch had little desire to establish a medical practice on the lines of that which his father carried out, his career choice of pathological anatomy immediately created a difficulty: During the 1870s few medical schools had established any department of pathology. In addition, if one wished to be appointed a professor at a medical school, the only realistic chance was to first having established a successful practice. The sole exception was the medical school to be associated with The Johns Hopkins University, then in the process of being established. What Welch lacked was the experience and expertise in certain medical disciplines, to say nothing of his lack of knowledge in the use of the microscope. Fortunately, he had made significant contacts during his years in school. Among them were Dr. James Wood, surgeon at Bellevue Hospital Medical College, and Dr. Abraham Jacobi, a Bellevue pediatrician, who both strongly advised Welch that a year or two studying in Germany could make up for some of these deficiencies. For example, at the time no medical school in the United States offered a course in microscopic anatomy (histology); German schools did. Convinced that the time abroad would significantly advance his career, and over the initial opposition of his father, on April 19, 1876, Welch sailed for Europe.

Welch's first destination was Strasbourg, a city which in effect straddled the border between eastern France and western Germany. In fact, until it had been annexed by Germany following the end of the Franco-Prussian War, it was located in the Alsace region of France (as it is today). In 1876 the intellectual life of the city was effectively German. In particular, this applied to the university, in which many of the most promising German students were now enrolled. The intent of the Germans, once they had annexed the region, was to create a university which would to be considered a model for such institutions; they largely succeeded, as many of the most outstanding professors and researchers were among the faculty. The medical school in particular was considered one of the best in Europe, which meant among the best in the world. To Welch's delight, the medical school included "laboratories for histology, pathology, physiological chemistry, superintended by the best teachers in Germany, viz., Waldeyer, von Recklinghausen, and Hoppe-Seyler."[8]

Dr. Friedrich Daniel von Recklinghausen (1833–1910) was considered by his contemporaries as among the most important teachers of pathology in Germany. Having studied and obtained his doctorate under Rudolf Virchow, arguably THE pathologist of his time, von Recklinghausen was the first to describe the eponymously named syndrome, also called neurofibromatosis as well as a variety of cell types and disorders. At the time of Welch's visit, von Recklinghausen was teaching a course in pathological histology, one which required some expertise in use of the microscope. Instead he settled for a demonstration course in gross pathology. The course was "unsurpassed," but not what he had wanted, and the speed at which von Recklinghausen spoke, in German, of course, made it difficult to follow.

Hoping to enroll in von Recklinghasen's course the following year, Welch enrolled in normal histology, taught by Dr. Heinrich Wilhelm von Waldeyer-Hartz (1836–1921), a course which included both lectures and laboratory. The laboratory component was largely self-taught, forcing Welch to become familiar with use of his microscope. "At first I made blundering work of it."[9] Welch was not Waldeyer's only American student; at least three, George Livingston Peabody, Landon Rives Longworth and A.J. Lanterman, had also worked with Waldeyer.

The third course in which Welch enrolled that summer was physiological chemistry, taught by Ernst Felix Hoppe-Seyler (1825–1895), chair of the Department of Biochemistry at the university, the only such department then in Germany, and also a former associate of Virchow. Unlike the other professors with whom Welch had studied while in Strasbourg, Hoppe-Seyler frequently made time for direct interaction with the students in the course. Physiological chemistry was a laboratory course; Welch spent his time developing useful expertise in quantitative and qualitative analyses.[10] In addition to the aforementioned courses, Welch also used his time—one cannot say "free" time, since there was little of that—to attend lectures by Ernst von Leyden (1832–1910) on the subject of heart disease.

Welch's preference now would have been for him to remain in Strasbourg in order to again attempt to enroll in von Recklinghausen's course. But still lacking in the experience the Strasbourg professor required, Welch found it necessary to go elsewhere in Germany. He decided the university in Leipzig, "the oldest and largest in Germany [with over 3,000 students]" would provide that opportunity. He arrived in that city, close to the center of the country, in August 1876, taking the opportunity to observe the university. "If you could visit the handsome and thoroughly equipped physiological, anatomical, pathological and chemical laboratories and see professors whose fame is already world wide, with their corps of assistants and students hard at work, you would realize how by concentration of labor and devotion to study Germany has outstripped other countries in the science of medicine. There is much less feverish energy and haste and consequent friction, far more repose here than with us in all departments of life. Men do not grow old so soon."[11]

Welch had originally chosen Leipzig in hopes of studying neurology with Dr. Johann Heubner, only to discover that Huebner was no longer teaching that subject, but had turned his interests to pediatrics. In place of Huebner's course, Welch joined the physiological laboratory of Dr. Carl Ludwig (1816–1895), director of the Physiological Institute at the university, and considered by Welch as one of the greatest living physiologists. Welch was not disappointed. He was assigned a project investigating the pathway of nerves in the heart, a natural choice given that Ludwig's research interests focused on functions of the circulatory system. His laboratory was particularly impressive, especially if compared with those back in the States. He described the atmosphere in a letter to his sister: "Ludwig is my ideal of a scientific man, accepting nothing upon authority, but putting every scientific

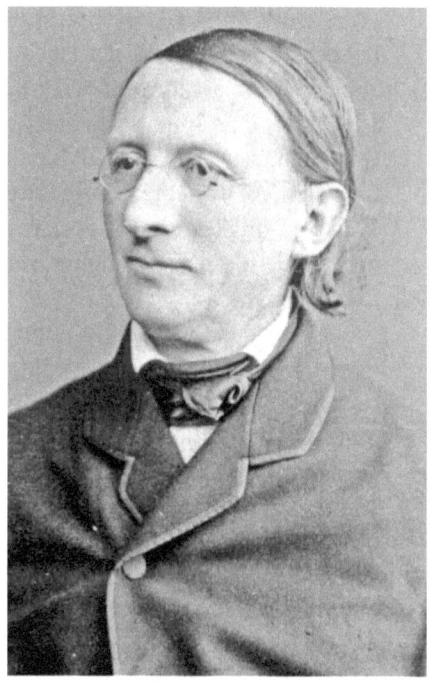

Carl Friedrich Wilhelm Ludwig. (1816–1895). He was a German physiologist and director of the Physiological Institute at the University of Leipzig. His work with William Welch on the physiology of the cardiac nervous system provided the latter with the opportunity to refine his microscopic techniques (National Library of Medicine).

theory to the severest test. His laboratory is a model of its kind.... Only those can work with him who are able to undertake original investigations, he receives no students simply for practice. Consequently the number is always small, and consists wholly of doctors. At the end of each year those whose work has resulted in making some contribution to science publish their results in a volume. These 'Contributions from the physiological laboratory in Leipsic' have probably added more to science than any similar work of the present day, and of course the credit is to be divided between Prof. Ludwig and his students. Prof. Ludwig, of course being interested that as many discoveries as possible should be made in his laboratory, gives to each individual's work a great deal of personal advice and supervision. The subject which he has given me to investigate is one which he personally worked up about thirty years ago viz. the microscopical study of the nerves and ganglion cells of the heart, and he thinks that I may be able to find out more than is yet known about the subject by employing new and improved methods."[12]

Welch's probing of nervous connections proved to be more successful than he had initially hoped; his observation of the nervous system connections had not been previously reported. For some reason, neither Ludwig nor Welch published the observation, and the work was later studied and described in a more complete version by a Frenchman, Dr. Louis-Antoine Ranvier.

Welch found the months spent with Ludwig well spent. "My work with Prof. Ludwig has been very profitable, especially in giving me an insight into the apparatus and methods of modern physiology, which is by far the most exact of any of the branches of medicine, this position of exactness having been obtained more through the effort of Prof. Ludwig than any living man.... I hope I have learned from Prof. Ludwig's precept and practice that most important lesson for a microscopist, as well as for any man of science, not to be satisfied with loose thinking and half proofs, not to speculate and theorize but to observe closely and carefully facts."[13]

Welch's microscopic and preparation techniques had been honed during these same months as a result of also having enrolled in Professor Ernst Wagner's course in microscopical anatomy. "My work this winter in Prof. Wagner's laboratory has been of a general nature, as I thought it best to obtain first a general view of the morbid anatomy of the different tissues and organs, before working upon any special subject.... I have acquired a knowledge of methods of preparing and mounting specimens so that I can carry on investigations hereafter wherever I have the material."[14] During this time in Leipzig, Welch also found the time to attend lectures presented by Rudolf Leukort (1822–1898) on comparative anatomy. Leukort's primary interests were in the field of parasitology—he had, for example, described the role of roundworms in the disease trichinosis—but he was also interested in organismal structure as it applied to classification. Leukort's influence on Welch extended to the latter embracing the controversial views of Charles Darwin.

The question for now, in Welch's mind, was where he should next proceed for continuing his studies. At the time, a year earlier, of his decision to travel to Europe, his initial inclination had been to study with Rudolf Virchow, considered the father of modern pathology, in Berlin. Instead, Ludwig convinced Welch he would benefit more by studying with Julius Cohnheim at the University of Breslau. Accepting Ludwig's advice, Welch traveled to Breslau in April 1877.

At the time of Welch's arrival in Breslau, Cohnheim was interested in the pathology of oedema, more specifically, the underlying process by which excess fluid from the blood built up in tissue, resulting in swelling; it was this project to which Welch was assigned. In a letter to his father, written soon after joining Cohnheim's laboratory, Welch described the difference he perceived between Ernst Wagner and Cohnheim.

"Prof. Cohnheim and Prof. Wagner are in some respects the antipodes of each other. Wagner has perhaps a greater array of facts at his disposal ... has gone deeper into the microscopic details of a pathological change, but while Wagner is often satisfied with the possession of a bare fact, Cohnheim's interest centers on the explanation of the fact. It is not enough for him to know that congestion of the kidney follows heart disease or that hypertrophy of the heart follows contraction of the kidney, or that atheroma [buildup of plaque] occurs in old age, he is constantly inquiring why does it occur under these circumstances. The result is that Cohnheim has taken for his

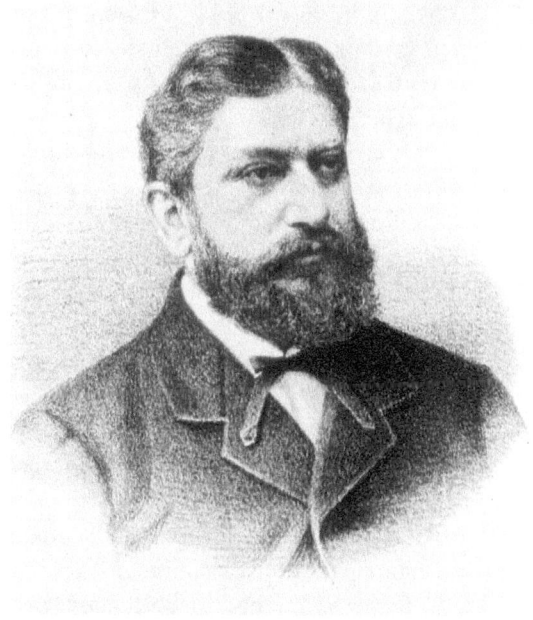

Julius Friedrich Cohnheim (1839–1884). In 1877 he was professor of pathological anatomy at the University of Breslau, where William Welch received his early training in pathology (National Library of Medicine).

especial studies such common subjects such as inflammation, dropsy, embolism and through his investigations these have become perhaps the only subjects in pathology in which our knowledge approaches in exactness what is known concerning a physical or chemical process."[15]

The underlying cause for the accumulation of fluid in body tissues—oedema—was well understood by then. Any form of blockage or constriction of the veins could restrict fluid flow, resulting in a backup of fluid in the tissue. The question which Cohnheim was attempting to address, and the project to which Welch was assigned, was why fluid buildup occurred in the lungs when the heart began to fail. The pathway of blood circulation was well known; the left ventricle pumps the blood through the body, which then returns to the right side of the heart, from which the right ventricle pumps the blood to the lungs. From there, blood returns again to the left side of the heart. Welch suspected that a backup of fluid would take place if the pumping of the left ventricle was inefficient.

Welch's testing of this hypothesis was elegant in its simplicity. Upon opening the chest of an animal, and squeezing the left ventricle, in effect paralyzing it, fluid would build up in the lungs. His idea was confirmed when various methods were used to reduce the pumping efficiency of the left ventricle, the same results were observed. The work was subsequently published.[16]

It was while Welch was working in Cohnheim's laboratory that he had his first opportunity to meet Robert Koch. As described in an earlier chapter, in 1876 Koch had demonstrated to Cohnheim, Ferdinand Cohn and others, the life cycle of the anthrax bacillus, including the spore stage. In 1877, likely in June of that year, Koch again came to the university in Breslau to demonstrate his anthrax work to the English physiologist Burdon-Sanderson. When Koch appeared in Cohnheim's laboratory, he and Welch were introduced. This, of course, was before Koch had made his identification of the tuberculosis bacillus, and, while well known in the microbial community, was not the world-renowned figure he would later become. Welch would only later realize the significance of what he had observed.

In his defense, at this time in his professional career Welch had no particular interest in the discipline of bacteriology. He had come to Breslau to study the newer methods of pathology; Cohnheim himself had little interest in bacteriology at the time, ironic in that several of his colleagues—Cohn, Carl Weigert and others, including Edwin Klebs whom Welch met in a visit to Prague[17]—played important roles in the early development of that field.

Welch was one of Cohnheim's first non–German students, and the first American to join his laboratory. That, and the recognition that Welch had significant potential in research, resulted in Cohnheim including Welch in activities outside of the laboratory. For example, Welch described a picnic to which Cohnheim had presented an invitation. It also provided an opportunity for Welch to observe the social strata of 19th century Germany. "The party consisted of five professors with their wives and a very moderate supply of unmarried young ladies and three young doctors including myself. The professors were all quite young and very sociable. Much as I admire German science, I must admit that American ladies are more agreeable and understand how to entertain better than German ladies. My experience is not very great but I rarely see a German professor and his wife without wondering how the professor came to marry her; the wife seems almost always to be inferior to the husband. She is generally well educated but seems to lack that tact and conversational talent which I imagine exists nowhere in a higher degree than in America. I was introduced to a young lady last evening who began the conversation, 'Oh, you are from America. I think English is such an ugly language,' which was not a very soothing way of opening an acquaintance.... I am very glad to see something of the social side of German life, but am not so infatuated with is as to care to change my residence from America here. So far as art and music and science are concerned we are very far behind the Germans, farther than is generally believed in America, but as regards the social amenities of life the Germans could take a lesson from us."[18]

"We are very far behind the Germans." A description of the average day in the laboratory provided a ready explanation. Welch's friend Carl Salomonsen and colleague in Cohnheim's laboratory described the typical session: In addition to carrying out experiments, students routinely attended lectures and demonstrations, including those in clinical laboratories. "The day began very early, with breakfast in the many 'gardens,' which were divided into beer, coffee and milk gardens. They arrived at work by 7:00 AM and worked the entire day, returning to the laboratory after dinner and staying until 7:00 or 8:00 PM."[19] Students were also urged to participate in presentations carried out by the medical societies associated with the university. In addition to the opportunity to meet many of the most important figures in medicine on a personal basis, both professionally and on an informal basis, Welch was exposed to the extensive experimental research being carried out in these fields, something not readily found in American medical schools of the time.

If given a choice once he would return to the United States, Welch would have chosen positions at either Bellevue Hospital Medical College, or at the College of Physicians and Surgeons, where he could once again interact with Delafield. Neither school had a position into which he could step. It appeared the only real option would be to open a practice, a default position in Welch's mind, but at least a means to earn a living. In hopes of filling any gaps in his knowledge of clinical medicine, Welch next traveled to Vienna, then considered the center of knowledge in that field.

Welch arrived in Vienna in October 1877, where he would spend the next six weeks. Welch was disappointed in what he found there. The city was expensive, particularly for someone living on a modest budget. He enrolled in courses dealing with dermatology, taught by Ferdinand von Hebra, neurology, taught by Theodor Meynert, and courses in a variety of other subjects. But in general, Welch felt the courses were being taught by young men with no significant reputations in their respective fields, and whose interests seemed focused primarily on making money. In attempting to make contacts useful for his future, Welch attempted to meet with Salomon Stricker (as had Prudden as well, described in the previous chapter), but when Stricker heard Welch had spent time with Cohnheim, a rival, he refused to invite him into his laboratory. Welch had more success when meeting with the embryologist Leopold Schenck, spending most of his visit in his laboratory, and having the opportunity to meet Prudden for the first time. "He [Prudden] is a very good fellow and I think an excellent microscopist and pathologist. I do not think he has anything to look forward to in America more than I have in a pathological line."[20]

With the experience he had gained during his nearly two year period of study, particularly in the field of normal histology, Welch returned to Strasbourg where he was then able to join von Recklinghausen's laboratory. He was assigned a project involving the source of "pus" which accumulated as a result of irritation in the cornea in the eye of a frog—whether from an external source (Cohnheim's view), or through multiplication of fixed cells (Virchow's view). The question was solved in a rather elegant manner. After exposing the eye to an irritant, Welch transplanted the cornea into the aqueous humor of another animal, where he observed the infiltration of external cells into the cornea, supporting Cohnheim's hypothesis.

Welch spent a month in Strasbourg, following which he traveled to Paris for a week or so of sightseeing—the Louvre and Versailles—and even attended a lecture by the pathologist Louis-Antoine Ranvier. One thing Welch did not do while in Paris, was to make an effort to visit the laboratory of Louis Pasteur. Nor did he refer to Pasteur, by then among the most prominent scientists in Europe, and a national figure in France, in any letters to his family. The reason may be related to the general perspective of bacteriology in 1877. As pointed out by the Flexners in their biography of Welch,[21] Pasteur by this time was moving into the study of infectious diseases, ultimately developing vaccines against both anthrax and rabies. Still, it is perhaps unfair to criticize Welch for lack of recognition of the role played by micro-organisms and disease. While physicians were increasingly accepting of the germ theory by 1877, this belief was not by any means universal. Even among those who acknowledged that some diseases were infectious, the question remained as to which diseases. For example, Carl Weigert accepted the etiological role of bacteria in some illnesses, but remained uncertain in others: "*Ich meine, dass für einige Fälle (Rekurrens und Milzbrand) die Einwirkung der Bakterien mit der für wissenschaftliche Untersuchungen für eine Reihe anderer Fälle wahrscheinlich, für sehr viele aber noch gar nicht sicher anzunehmen ist.* (I believe that in some cases (recurrent fever and anthrax) the action of bacteria has been proved with such certainty as is attainable for scientific investigations, that in a series of other cases this action can be assumed as probably but that in a great many cases it cannot yet be assumed with any certainty.)"[22] Whether other illnesses in addition to relapsing fever and anthrax were infectious was undecided. Cohnheim himself, albeit initially an early skeptic of germ theory despite being an admirer of Koch, expressed similar uncertainty: "*Für die ganze, so hochwichtige Gruppe der Infectionskrankheiten ist jetzt ja das Contagium animatum der Früheren Autoren keine Hypothese mehr, und mit vollem Recht fordert heute die Wissenschaft von dem Pathologen, dass er bei jeder Infectionskrankheit die pärasitaren Organismen auffinde, welchen sie ihre Entstehung verdankt...* (For the whole very important group of infectious diseases, the *Contagium animatum* of earlier authors is at present no longer a hypothesis and science today quite rightly demands of the pathologist that in each infectious disease he find the parasitic organisms to which it owes its origin. The only point where unity has not yet been reached is the question as to how far the territory of infectious disease should be staked: there are authors who attribute an infectious character even to the malignant tumors, and there other others who do not hesitate to refer every so-called cold, every catarrh, to an infection.)"[23]

After a brief stay in London, Welch returned to the United States in February 1878, hoping to obtain a research position at the College of Physicians and Surgeons. His contact, Delafield, was able to offer a position as unpaid lecturer, with the possibility of a research laboratory if space could be found anywhere; nothing could be found. Welch's backup choice was a position at the lesser Bellevue Hospital Medical College, a place at which his former classmate Dr. Frederick Dennis, a wealthy member of New York society— Dennis' father was president of the New Jersey Railroad and Transportation Company—and member of the medical college, had considerable influence. After significant negotiations, Welch was offered a laboratory, consisting of three rooms with kitchen tables for work space and little else. There were no microscopes, instruments or specimens available for teaching. A letter to his sister expressed his frustration. "I have been trying to get the laboratory in order so as to organize a class this summer, but the material was so scanty that I should have given up the idea of starting anything there this summer, unless those who wish to have their students work there were not so urgent to have me begin. I can get as many students as there are places for, but I can not make much of a success of the affair at present. I seem to be thrown entirely upon my own resources for equipping the laboratory and do not think that I can accomplish much.

"I some times feel rather blue when I look ahead and see that I am not going to be able to realize my aspirations in life. I may be able to make a support in New York, and even if I should succeed in accordance with the hopes of my friends, it would not be the kind of success which I should like. I am not going to have any opportunity for carrying out as I would like the studies and investigations for which I have a taste. There is no opportunity in this country, and it seems improbable that there ever will be. I can quiz students, I can teach microscopy; and pathology, and perhaps get some practice and make a living after a while, but that is all patchwork and the drudgery of life and what hundreds do."[24]

The college finally provided $25 towards the purchase of equipment, and Welch was able to obtain six antique microscopes, slides and stains. For specimens, Welch personally captured frogs from marshes in New York. With such meagre resources, Welch started in 1879, the first laboratory course in pathology at an American medical school. His salary consisted of the fees paid by the six students who had been enrolled in the course.

During the following years at Bellevue, Welch was increasingly recognized as a young physician with significant potential. He was offered a partnership with Dr. Henry Goldthwaite in helping prepare medical students for examinations.[25] The quality of many of these students for medicine was questionable, but the position paid adequately. More important for his future career was a position as assistant to Dr. Austin Flint, professor of the practice of medicine at Bellevue, and considered one of the most important members of the medical school; his text, *Flint's Practice of Medicine for the Practitioners and Students of Medicine,* was a required resource for students in that field. As Flint's assistant, Welch not only helped him with preparation of lectures and professional presentations, in addition to an uncredited editing of Flint's text, but he—Welch—also had the opportunity to participate in pathological examinations. Within months after his joining Bellevue, the quality and importance of Welch's work came to the attention of Welch's mentor Francis Delafield at the College of Physicians and Surgeons. When Delafield obtained funding from the alumni for establishing a similar pathological laboratory, he offered the position of head of the laboratory to Welch. Though this would have been exactly the position Welch had wanted upon his return from Europe, his obligations to Bellevue, no doubt including pressure from Flint to remain, resulted in turning down the position. As related in the previous chapter, Welch recommended the position be offered to Prudden, who accepted. The result of Prudden's hiring was the second such pathological laboratory to be established in an American medical school.

A New Position and Training with Koch

Welch spent six years in New York, conducting autopsies—he and Dennis were demonstrators of anatomy—writing and developing a small practice. He was offered a full professorship in clinical medicine by Flint, turning the offer down in hopes of fulfilling his goal in becoming a research pathologist. Meanwhile, he, and Prudden, had arguably single-handedly instituted a German model of pedagogy into a staid medical educational system. As noted by Fleming in his biography, the medical system had until then in the United States functioned in a more or less seniority system—a Congressional inflexibility, in Fleming's words.[26] Still, with the meager support Welch received, he remained limited in his ability to carry out any form of creative research. Only a single piece of experimental work was carried out. Dr. Samuel Meltzer, a physiologist among the faculty, asked Welch for permission to use his equipment to test the result of shaking red blood cells with various chemically inert abrasive materials; the result was the disappearance of the corpuscles. Facilities were limited, and Meltzer and Welch even had to

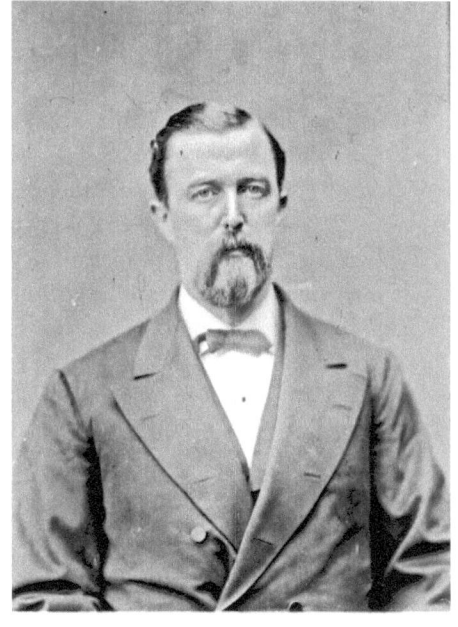

John Shaw Billings (1838–1913). Billings helped design the buildings for the newly established Johns Hopkins Hospital and served with the committees involved in the recruitment of faculty. William Welch was among those new faculty (National Library of Medicine).

borrow a mechanical mixer for the experiments. The experiment was hardly groundbreaking, but did result in a publication.[27]

What of Welch's dream of a professional career in pathology? During the mid-1880s, there were few medical schools in the United States worthy of the name; one was the medical school associated with Johns Hopkins University. The university had its origins with the fortune, some $7 million, donated by Johns Hopkins, philanthropist and director of the Baltimore and Ohio Railroad, upon his death in 1873. Half of the donation was for establishment of the hospital and associated medical school. In February 1876, the university officially opened, with Daniel Coit Gilman, then president of the University of California, as first president. Gilman, in turn, selected John Shaw Billings (1838–1913), who had already made Welch's acquaintance in 1877 while traveling in Europe, to design the hospital and medical school. Billings' professional career included the merger of two seemingly unique fields: medicine and library science. During the Civil War, Billings had been medical inspector for the Army of the Potomac, subsequently becoming head of the Library of the Surgeon-General's Office—later renamed the Army Medical Library—the position he held at the time of Gilman's selection. Gilman and Billings together made the decision to design the medical program using the European model, with a strong emphasis on research.

In the process of recruiting faculty for the new medical school in Baltimore, specifically the position of professor of pathology, Billings renewed his acquaintance with Welch in February 1884, appearing in the amphitheater during an autopsy demonstration carried out by the latter. Inquired as to which area of research would he find of interest, assuming adequate facilities and funding, Welch indicated he would wish to study the cause and pathology associated with dysentery. After some further conversation, Billings left. Billings' visit was not by accident. Gilman, in searching for a pathologist for the medical school, had first contacted the physiologist Dr. Willy Kühne, who indicated to Gilman that the person who might provide a better perspective was Cohnheim; Cohnheim, in turn, and literally on his deathbed at the time, recommended Welch for the position.

Billings was duly impressed with Welch, writing to Gilman: "I saw Dr. Welch, had a long talk with him, heard him lecture and saw him directing work in his laboratory. He is 33 years old, unmarried [and would remain so throughout his life], of good personal address, modest, quiet, and a gentleman in every sense so far as I can judge. He is a good lecturer, an excellent laboratory teacher, and has a keen desire for an opportunity to make original investigations, being activated I think by the true scientific spirit. He has written little under his own name. He has been trying to make some original investigations in the causes and pathology of Dysentery but has very little time as he has to make his living by students and Doctors fees and must give them the first place. Upon the whole I think he is the best man in this country for the Hopkins. He has not the reputation yet which is possessed by [Emil] Ponfick or [Johannes] Orth or Weigert or several other Germans who are probably available—but I think he will develop well."[28]

Gilman was clearly satisfied with Billings' evaluation, and early in March invited Welch to come to Baltimore for a face-to-face interview. There he met with a committee consisting of Gilman, two members of the board of trustees, and two members of the Philosophical Faculty of the university: Dr. Ira Remsen, a chemist, and H. Newell Martin, a biologist. Prior to the interview, Welch had injured his heel, and Gilman happened to notice he was wearing only one shoe. Unfazed, Gilman's only comment was "Wait a moment, Dr. Welch. The Johns Hopkins does not regard eccentricity as a sign of intelligence."[29]

An offer for an appointment as professor of pathology was tendered to Welch on March 15, with a starting salary of $4000. He would also have a laboratory as well as two assistants. Along with the tenured offer, President Gilman enclosed a personal note, indicating the offer was "hearty, unanimous and earnest.... You must come."[30]

The medical school had yet to be completely organized at the time of the offer—March 1884—and would not be for another two years. If Welch accepted the offer, and in the moment it was not a certainty, his appointment would be the first to the medical faculty. Among his responsibilities would be to not only play a major part in organizing the new school, or more appropriately a faculty of medicine as he described it to his father, but Welch would also be immersed in the politics of the program, and to help in the recruiting of additional faculty. The conflict felt by Welch was expressed in letters to his father and sister. To his father, Welch wrote, "I have not yet given a definite answer to the proposal, nor have I had time to speak about it to anyone. The main attraction at the Johns Hopkins for me is the opportunity it gives me for investigation. It is undoubtedly the best opportunity in this country, with the exception that pathological material can not be abundant there, and certainly before the hospital is organized will be very scanty. I had much rather live in New York than in Baltimore, and from some points of view I am fortunately situated here. The field for teaching is vastly greater here, and perhaps I have been as successful as a teacher as in anything. I do not think that I should better myself peculiarly by going to Baltimore. I did not learn definitely what the salary is to be ... but I think probably at first about $3000. [It was to be $4000.]

"But with all the pleasant associations and acquaintances in New York, and not withstanding the wide circle which I reach in teaching and in my pathological work, I do not feel as if I was accomplishing what I want to do. My energies are split up in too many different directions and are likely to be so long as I remain here. In Baltimore everything would be quieter, more academic; I should be expected to give myself up mostly to original work, to renounce practice altogether. I should be equipped with everything which I want in the way of a laboratory. If I accept the offer I should expect to go abroad this summer and to remain a year preparing myself for the work, taking up especially cultivation of bacteria, comparative and experimental pathology, the fields which it is desired to cultivate especially in Baltimore."[31]

To his sister, the conflicted Welch wrote, "since the aim is to make the university a center for research, [he would be largely relieved of] the drudgery of teaching.... The choice seems to be between an academic, scholar's life with a chance to contribute somewhat to science, and the busy, restless, withal enticing life in New York. I have had a taste of the pleasures and comforts of New York life and they are not easy to relinquish. One who has lived here does not care to live elsewhere. But I suppose that I shall abandon Mammon and go to Baltimore. Still I have not come to a positive decision. I dread the interviews with [Frederic] Dennis and Dr. Flint."[32]

His colleague Frederic Dennis certainly did not make the decision easy. In hopes of countering any offer from Baltimore, Dennis was able to convince the industrialist Andrew Carnegie to provide funding of $50,000 for construction of a pathological laboratory at Bellevue, while the trustees of the school appropriated $45,000 for purchase of a site in the city.[33] Others as well—not least of whom was his father—attempted to convince Welch that going to Baltimore would be a mistake. In response, Welch laid down conditions necessary to keep him in New York, expectations which were largely unrealistic: a substantial salary ($4000), and money to pay an assistant, the money to come from Bellevue, and not earnings in a practice or student fees. The specifics were not met—not that Welch would have remained anyway—and on March 31 he accepted the offer of a professorship in the nascent medical college in Baltimore, Johns Hopkins.

By 1884 recognition of bacteriology as a unique science, central to the study of medicine, had changed significantly. During the six years Welch had spent in New York, the germ theory, if still perhaps not universally accepted, had still become well established. Either Koch, or his associates, had identified the etiological agents for illnesses such as tuberculosis, cholera, typhoid fever and diphtheria. His associate (and superior) at Bellevue, Austin Flint, described as "an enthusiastic bacterian," had upon the report of Koch's identification of the tuberculosis agent, "come bounding up the stairs in Welch's house, crying 'I knew it, I knew it.'"[34]

Among the first students at Bellevue Welch was able to inspire with this discovery was Hermann Biggs (1859–1923), later a bacteriologist and subsequent professor of pathological anatomy at Bellevue, who played a significant role in the development of public health programs in New York. "He [Welch] showed us methods of staining sputum and demonstrating the tubercle bacillus. I can now see quite clearly the steam rising from the dish of carbol-fuchsin in the sand-bath containing the sputum while he talked."[35]

Despite his enthusiasm with Koch's discovery, Welch was well aware of his shortcomings in the field of bacteriology. He was certainly cognizant of its growing importance in the years since he had been in Europe. But the few resources he had available at Bellevue, barely enough to cover his work in pathology, allowed no flexibility to apply significant effort, or money for equipment and supplies, in the newer field. Welch looked on this lack of experience as, in fact, a blessing in disguise. As he later wrote after gaining that experience with Koch, "I am glad that I did not attempt to dabble at the subject in New York, for I might have made as melancholy a failure of my cultivations and experiments as [Henry] Formad. The methods can be learned only by personal observation in a laboratory."[36]

The solution for Welch was to study with the master himself: Koch. In September 1884 Welch embarked on his second trip to Europe, with the goal of meeting with Koch in Berlin, and obtaining a seat in his laboratory. He was to be initially disappointed. Koch met with Welch, but informed him that the laboratory was not set up for instruction, and in any event, since the laboratory belonged to the war department, Welch would need permission from the German minister of war. It is unclear how this would substantially differ from the training Koch would provide to physicians, albeit German physicians, during this period, or even the training Prudden would receive in the future. It is likely Welch was simply premature in his expectations.

There was an option. Koch's former student Wilhelm Frobenius had developed a course in bacteriology in Munich, the first such public course in that subject to be established; Welch enrolled in Frobenius' second course in November. In the meantime, he sent a letter to President Gilman at Hopkins, requesting that Gilman use his connections to provide an opportunity for Welch to meet with the American Minister in Germany (possibly John Kasson), hoping the latter would intercede with the war ministry on behalf of Welch.

The ultimate goal of Welch's second trip to Europe, to study bacteriology with Koch, was to prove successful. However, it came about only after months of laboratory studies elsewhere in Germany; though frustrating at times, these "side" adventures not only provided Welch with needed experience, they also allowed for the opportunity to make important contacts in related medical fields.

In November 1884, Welch enrolled in the course taught by Frobenius at the University of Munich. To say Frobenius had been a student of Koch's would be a stretch. Though a physician, he learned his bacteriology primarily through three brief visits he had made to Koch's laboratory, and would spend much of his professional career as a medical missionary to German colonies. His teaching methods consisted largely of reading from notes he had taken while working with Koch, and expecting his own students—including Welch—to simply learn by rote. This extended even to holding a test tube in a manner identical to that by Koch. The professor, Welch later wrote, "had rather a narrow horizon."[37]

While in Munich, Welch took advantage of the proximity of other laboratories. The pathological laboratory of Professor Otto Bollinger, in fact the site in which Frobenius' course was being taught, allowed Welch to observe autopsies. The nearby veterinary laboratory of Theodor Kitt provided a means to compare animal diseases with their human counterparts, particularly tuberculosis. Welch also spent time in the hygienic laboratory of Max von Pettenkofer, who despite his dispute with the germ theory of disease, developed sanitary reforms which allowed the control of gastrointestinal infections such as cholera and typhoid fever.

Welch spent two months in Munich, and after travels to Vienna, Budapest and Prague where he visited a number of laboratories, he arrived at the Physiological Institute run by Carl Ludwig at the University of Leipzig. In the years since Welch had studied with Julius Cohnheim in Breslau, Cohnheim had joined the faculty in Leipzig. Cohnheim had died in August 1884, and his assistant, Carl Weigert, had taken over many of Cohnheim's duties. Weigert had hoped for a professorship, but had been denied—Welch believed this was because he was Jewish, though Cohnheim himself had been. Regardless of the reason, Weigert provided instruction to Welch on the techniques used in staining bacteria. Welch also took the time to visit with Cohnheim's widow, who related to Welch how impressed her husband had been during his time in the laboratory.

Welch's earlier work with Cohnheim had focused on the buildup of fluid in the lungs which resulted from weakening of the left ventricle in the heart. Taking advantage of Welch's experience in that subject, Ludwig assigned to him a related question: whether vasomotor nerves which control dilation of arteries elsewhere in the body may also regulate that of the pulmonary arteries; Welch was unable to provide a definitive answer, but his methodology in addressing the problem significantly impressed Ludwig. Welch described his daily routine in working with Ludwig in a letter written to his step-mother. "One day is about the same as another. After my coffee at half past eight I go to Professor Ludwig's lecture from nine to ten, then work in the laboratory until one, then go to a rather frugal but substantial dinner and then renew my laboratory work until five when the laboratory closes. I usually then attend a lecture on logic to fill up the hour from five to six. The subject is presented in an entirely new and very interesting manner. In the evening I sometimes go to the theatre or make a call on some American or German friend, rarely the latter as one must be very intimate to call in the evening in Germany, or visit a café and read the newspapers."[38]

Welch's goal of working with Koch took a step forward in February 1885 when he received a letter from Gilman which had been signed by Frederick Frelinghuysen, Secretary of State under President Chester Arthur. In the letter, Frelinghuysen requested that the American Minister intercede with Germany's war ministry to allow Welch to work in Koch's laboratory. Though Koch was now more amenable to Koch joining his laboratory, the timing was not perfect. He had just received an appointment as professor of hygiene at the University of Berlin—ironically eliminating the need for permission from the war minister previously necessary for Welch's acceptance—and Welch was now welcome to enroll in the course to be taught by Koch, but the three current available positions had already been filled.

Once again Welch returned to Leipzig, though first taking the time to visit Göttingen to enroll in the bacteriology course taught by Karl Flügge, another of Koch's former students. Though some of the material was similar to that to which he had been exposed months earlier in Frobenius' course, Welch found Flügge to be, by far, the better instructor. Not only did Flügge's laboratory include some of the world's most important bacteriologists, providing important contacts for the future, the less formal approach shown by Flügge included invitations to dinner at the professor's home.

Welch planned to join Koch in June, assuming the laboratory was ready. It was not, and in the interim Welch traveled to England to purchase equipment for the laboratory at Hopkins. His visit included more than simply shopping, as Welch had the opportunity to visit Cambridge University, now being received "with almost embarrassing" hospitality. At a dinner held at Trinity College, Welch also had an opportunity to meet Prince Albert Victor, Duke of Clarence, Queen Victoria's grandson and second in line to the throne.[39]

Welch returned to Germany in June, bypassing Paris (and Louis Pasteur) and visiting more laboratories in Strasbourg, Heidelberg and Frankfurt, before arriving back in Leipzig. Welch was finally able to enroll in Koch's course in July.

During the previous months, as Welch awaited the opportunity to work directly with Koch, he had studied in courses taught by two of Koch's former students: Frobenius and Flügge. As related earlier, the methodology employed by Frobenius was largely that which had been taught by Koch himself. Certainly the experience was important for Welch, and there was the further opportunity to develop professional contacts. As a consequence and it is important to not overplay the significance, much of what he learned from Koch was a repetition of that which had already been covered. But Welch recognized that training in any field, not merely in medicine, involves more than simply learning the material. Those early years also involve meeting the outstanding figures in the field, or, as Welch put it, students should "not tie themselves down by attempting research in a single laboratory.... You must get into contact with the great teachers. Then you will have an impression of the men and their work which you will never forget, and every time you read their writings you will remember. Everything will be much more vivid to you."[40] The same advice is as valid today as it was during the 19th century. Graduate students at universities are urged to complete their training elsewhere when possible, allowing for greater perspectives and a wider range of thought when dealing with a problem.

The Robert Koch that Welch encountered on a daily basis was nearly unrecognizable to those who remembered him in later years. "He was in every way most approachable and affable—indeed in those days he was one of the most simple-minded, unaffected men imaginable. It was a rare opportunity! About once every two weeks he would come and sit with a small group of us about a little table at a restaurant and would join us in refreshment. Indeed, you cannot imagine anyone more approachable in every way. He was not very talkative, but he told a story well and he had a good deal of dry wit and humor. It is said, it is true, that later, in consequence of unfortunate experiences [tuberculin episode? Personal issues?], he became somewhat unapproachable and suspicious of others, but I confess I am very much surprised at this, for I found him unchanged when he came to this country, and only a year before he died when I was in Berlin I spent an hour with him in his laboratory and he was most cordial in his reception.... He was a man, I think, of a singularly attractive and agreeable personality, though I cannot claim having had any real intimacy with him."[41]

That July, Welch was able to renew his acquaintance with another student in the course, T. Mitchell Prudden. Having completed training in the methodology of bacteriology, and planning on offering such courses on their own following their return to America, Prudden and Welch, particularly the latter, had been collecting bacterial specimens to be used in their own laboratories. Of particular interest were cultures of cholera. Koch might have been a logical source. Koch had isolated cultures during his period in India in 1883 when he identified the etiological agent. But fearful of the consequence if the organisms gained access to food or water back in Germany, Koch destroyed his isolates before returning. An outbreak of cholera in France, however, made his concern moot, and recognizing the need for possessing such cultures to be used as a training tool for physicians, Koch obtained samples from an autopsy in Toulon, sequestered the bacteria in a tube in his pocket, and returned to Germany. The cultures were secured in his laboratory, and access was only allowed on the basis of need.

Welch had hoped to include the cholera bacilli among the organisms he would carry back to Hopkins, but Koch, it appears, refused his request. Unbeknownst to him, however, Welch had already obtained a culture from Flügge (as did Prudden, from an unnamed source). The result was the anecdote related at the beginning of this chapter, when both Welch and Prudden destroyed their cultures.

Welch spent the month of July enrolled in Koch's bacteriology course. No detailed account is available describing the specifics of his time spent there, but his experience likely mirrors that provided by Prudden in the latter's report to the Connecticut Board of Health. (See Chapter 5.) Students learned how media was prepared, as well as procedures for growing, observing and identifying bacteria.

After a brief visit at the University of Copenhagen with his previous acquaintance from Breslau Carl Salomonsen, Welch returned to New York in August 1885, bringing with him equipment for his new laboratory, and a level of experience which he had lacked during his previous visit in Europe.

Welch's Legacy

Welch's laboratory at Hopkins, a two-story building originally planned for use as a dead house, though not completed, was at least ready for occupancy the beginning of November. In February, Welch presented the first of nine public lectures on the subject of bacteriology, the first such in this country. Indeed, Welch and Prudden were the only such instructors in bacteriology in the United States at the time. The subjects ranged from the early history of the subject, and the relation of putrefaction to disease, classification and methods of cultivation in the laboratory, characteristics of infectious disease and methods of transmission, the role of specific bacteria as etiological agents of disease, and diagnosis of disease, to immunity and treatment, at least as far as was understood in the 1880s.[42] When some of his cultures died, Welch was forced to briefly return to Germany, where Koch's assistants replaced the cultures Welch planned on using. That October, Welch began formal instruction in pathology, the subject with which he had been most familiar, and his primary choice as a professor at Hopkins. Among the twenty-six medical students in the laboratory over the following seven months was army physician and future Army Surgeon-General George Sternberg, sometimes considered the first specialist in bacteriology in the United States. Among the studies in pathology Welch himself carried out during his first decade at Johns Hopkins were characteristics of glomerulonephritis in patients with Bright's Disease, a non-description condition of kidney failure often fatal at the time, the pathology of fever, the structure of thrombi, and hemorrhagic infarction (blockage) in the intestine.[43]

During this same period, Welch also directed work in the area of bacteriology with many of his students and assistants. These included studies on hog cholera, the role of the pneumococcus in lobar pneumonia, and with Alexander Abbott and Simon Flexner, the etiology and pathology of diphtheria. Perhaps Welch's most important investigation during this first decade involved the gas producing bacillus, initially known as *Bacillus aerogenes capsulatus* (though a capsule is implied, it was not consistently observed).

In July 1892, Welch, and his student and colleague George Nuttall (1862–1937), identified a gas-producing bacillus throughout the tissues of the heart, liver and kidneys, and in the blood of a man who had suffered a fatal aneurysm.[44] The bacilli which they isolated from the tissue did not appear initially pathogenic when inoculated into rabbits, but upon death of the host Welch and Nuttall observed the formation of gas bubbles. Their conclusion was that the origin of the gas was not from the atmosphere, but was a product of the bacteria themselves.[45] The organism was determined to be anaerobic as it would not grow on media exposed to the air. Welch's contributions to the story of the organism, later named *Clostridium welchii* in his honor, consisted of reviews of cases of infection provided by his colleagues at Johns Hopkins, Drs. William Osler, William Halsted and Howard Kelly. In part, the importance of the discovery, in the view of Flexner, was the establishment of the field of pneumopathology.[46]

Though Welch considered himself more of a pathologist, or even a physiologist, his own work in integrating bacteriology into those medical subjects, and his influence on the students who followed, played a significant role in the future adoption of bacteriology as a science on its own in the United States. Among his numerous professional accomplishments, in 1893, Welch was appointed as the first Dean of Medicine, serving until 1898. He was a charter member of the Society of American Bacteriologists—now the American Society for Microbiology—founded in 1899, and in 1901 served as its second president. He served as president of the American Association for the Advancement of Science from 1906 to 1907, and of the National Academy of Sciences from 1913 to 1916. Ironically, given his strong interest in the subject, Welch's view of bacteriology often was as an adjunct to the medical sciences. In his summary of Welch and his relationship to the development of bacteriology in the United States, Barnett Cohen related two anecdotes which would seem to suggest a conflicted viewpoint on the part of Welch. Simon Flexner, Welch's assistant and biographer, was not permitted by Welch to take the regular course in bacteriology. Later, Welch advised a medical student interested in bacteriology, that he would be better off emphasizing medical training. Cohen's explanation was that at the time, bacteriology was an applied science, with little in the way of pure scientific knowledge. The subject was often subsumed within departments of hygiene or pathology. That would of course change at first in the medical area as the role of microbes in disease became a research area on its own, and in a more general sense in the view of bacteria as prototype cells for the study of areas such as metabolism.

During World War I, Welch was a member of the United States Medical Corps. He remained active in administrative duties at Hopkins nearly until the time of his death, serving as a member of the Advisory Board at the Institute for Biological Research, and as the first director of the Institute of the History of Medicine. Welch succumbed to prostate cancer in April 1934.

8

Edward Oram Shakespeare

Edward Shakespeare spent only a brief period with Robert Koch, primarily to develop expertise in isolating and identifying the cholera bacillus while studying the disease in Europe and Asia. Nevertheless, Shakespeare's extensive contributions to the field of public health were significantly influenced by Koch.

Shakespeare was born in Dover, Delaware, on May 19, 1846, the son of William McIntire Shakespeare and Catherine Haman Shakespeare. Through his father's lineage, Shakespeare traced his ancestry to Edmund Shakespeare, brother of the 16th century English bard.[1] Through his mother, Shakespeare was a descendent of the Barons of Crevefuer and Cathan. Following his 1867 graduation from Dickinson College in Carlisle, Pennsylvania, Shakespeare enrolled in the University of Pennsylvania Medical School, graduating in 1869. The next years were spent practicing medicine in his hometown of Dover, specializing in ophthalmology, until 1874, when he was appointed lecturer in operative ophthalmic surgery at the University of Pennsylvania. In addition to lecturing on the subject, his work included practicing eye surgery and refraction at Philadelphia General Hospital. While there, Shakespeare developed a more advanced ophthalmoscope and ophthalmometer, with which he could study not only diseases of the eye, but their physiology as well. He published his work in *The American Journal of Medical Sciences*.[2]

As recounted in Chapter 2, in March 1882, Robert Koch reported his identification of the tuberculosis bacillus. While most heralded the discovery as a vital component in the fight against a disease Sir William Osler referred to as "Captain of the Men of Death," some remained skeptical. In the United States, one of the more vocal opponents of Koch's interpretation was Dr. Henry Formad, a notable Philadelphia physician and pathologist (see Chapter 4). Formad was born in Russia in 1847. He came to the United States in 1875, at which time he enrolled in the University of Pennsylvania Medical School, graduating two years later. He maintained a practice for a short period of time before becoming involved in medical research. His initial work involved the study of the contagious nature of diphtheria, which included traveling to Michigan during 1881 and 1882 to investigate an outbreak in that state. The following year, he was appointed Demonstrated of Morbid Anatomy and Pathological Histology, and Lecturer on Experimental Pathology at the University of Pennsylvania. In 1884 he was also appointed as a Coroner's physician in the city of Philadelphia. It was during this period that Formad became most involved with the topic of tuberculosis.

Formad's perception of that disease was that there existed an inherited predisposition affecting the susceptible tissues. "A simple inflammation resulting from any cause can produce tuberculosis." (See below.) In support of this argument, Formad used examples of experiments in which a large variety of irritants, including powdered glass, were capable of inducing the disease.[3]

Formad continued to express his views at meetings and in the medical journals of the time, largely without significant efforts among his peers to dispute his interpretations. Finally in late 1883 and in 1884, Shakespeare— perhaps reminiscent of Thomas Huxley as Charles Darwin's "bulldog"— responded in defense of Koch's discovery in a series of arguments which came to be called the "Philadelphia debate."[4] Formad: "Today, while the bacillus is acknowledged as a common morphological concomitant of tubercle, pathogenetic properties are denied it, on account of a want of sufficient confirmation of the evidence. Tuberculosis may arise from other causes. The bacillus may be one of the causes, conditionally, but it is not THE cause. The question of predisposition stands in the way of the bacillus theory. Furthermore, I will try to show that *tuberculosis is not a contagious disease* [italics in original]. Koch and others who believe in the contagiousness of tuberculosis disregard, as a rule, the negative evidence. Tuberculosis cannot be produced in some animals, nor in some persons, although every individual is liable to acquire syphilis, smallpox, and other contagious diseases. A special predisposition and a special individual are required. In such an individual a simple inflammation, resulting from any cause whatever, can produce tuberculosis, although bacilli act more readily than other irritants. Tubercle is primarily a simple granulation tissue of inflammatory origin. Phthisis is a local tuberculous inflammation of the lung, which may manifest itself in various ways. Lesions representing the different forms of phthisis, and their transition from one form to another, are often seen in the same lung. Virchow insists that nothing should be considered tubercular unless it shows true tubercle nodules, and hence he does not recognize cheesy pneumonia as tubercular, although he does not object to the term 'phthisis' for this lesion. But if we consider the presence of the bacilli of Koch as the differentiating point between what is tubercular and what is not, we find that catarrhal and cheesy pneumonia *are the most tubercular of all* [italics in original], because they contain, as a rule, more bacilli."⁵

Shakespeare's criticism of Formad's recent arguments, both the current as well as several previously published, was summarized by the editor. "Dr. Formad opposes Koch's theory of tuberculosis by the claim that there is no necessity for the action of a specific agent in the production of tuberculosis; that scrofulous animals have an anatomical peculiarity—that is, a narrowing of connective tissue lymph spaces; that the inflammatory process in such animals, from any exciting cause, is necessarily tubercular. To support this view, Dr. Formad exhibited sections showing cellular hyperplasia of the connective tissue, but no section capable of demonstrating lymph spaces—not one silver nor gold preparation.

"Even admitting Formad's hypothesis, it only explains predisposition; the exciting cause of tuberculosis is a different question. The claim of Koch is not that the tubercle bacillus excites tuberculosis under any and all circumstances, but that a suitable soil and favorable conditions are also essential."⁶

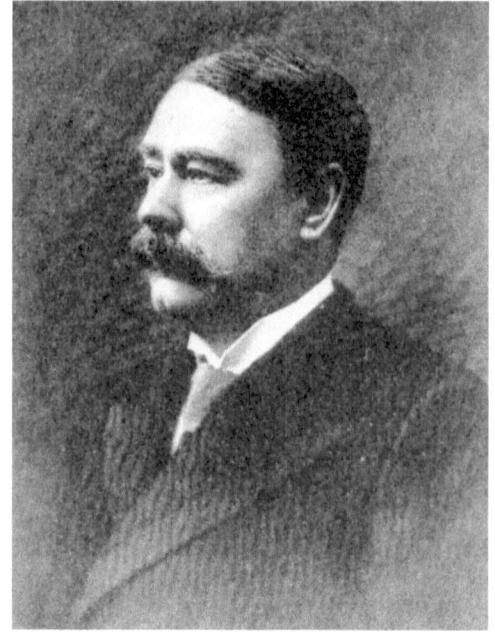

Edward Oram Shakespeare (1846-1900). Shakespeare, a descendent of the Bard's brother, was considered one of the world's foremost experts on cholera when he was sent by President Grover Cleveland in 1885 to investigate an outbreak in Europe. His "Philadelphia debates" with Dr. Henry Formad in 1883 and 1884 addressed the question of the etiological basis of tuberculosis (Historical Medical Library, The College of Physicians of Philadelphia).

The "Philadelphia debates" between Formad and Shakespeare continued throughout the year, both in addresses before the Philadelphia Medical Society, and published in medical journals, each refuting the other's statements. The (sometimes) nasty tone of the debate can be summarized using excerpts originating with the protagonists. In June 1884, Formad wrote, "There is ... in Dr. Shakespeare's remarks ... a statement of importance, and of such character that I cannot leave it unchallenged. It may be due to some mistake of the stenographer, perhaps. [Could this represent we what today call a snide comment of sorts?] I am quoted by Dr. Shakespeare as having made the declaration that 'Koch had so far modified his views that he now admitted that neither the form, size and aspect of the tubercle bacillus, nor its want of individual motion, nor its peculiar behavior towards staining fluids distinguished it from any other bacilli.'

"This would be, evidently, a misrepresentation of Koch's view upon this point, and I am *not* [italics in original] guilty of it. What I ever said or published on this point was this: 'Dr. Koch kindly demonstrated to me a number of specimens of bacilli, and, in particular, the appearance of these bacteria exhibiting under low amplification the peculiar S-like figure in the growths in masses. Koch seems now to lay more stress upon this low-power appearance and upon the pathogenetic properties of the *Bacillus tuberculosis* as a distinguishing feature from other bacilli than upon the color test. During the conversation, he admitted that some other bacilli may also yield the same micro-chemical reaction as the tubercle bacilli, but insisted that the latter bacilli can not be stained brown. The failure of the tubercle bacilli to take the brown stain, he said, was the reason that they can not be well photographed (blue and red-stained objects not being suitable for photographing).'"[7]

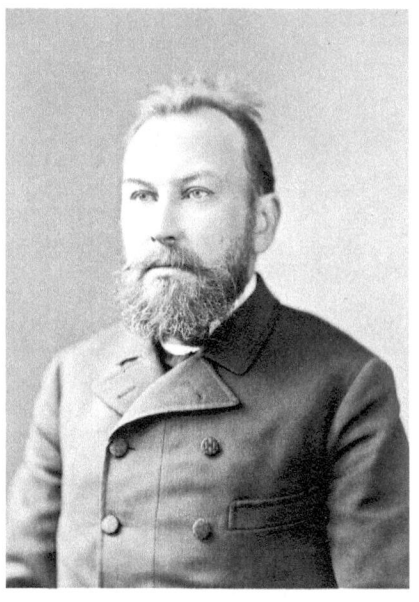

Henry Formad (1847–1892). He was a faculty member in pathology at the University of Pennsylvania and coroner's physician for the city of Philadelphia during the 1880s. Formad's opposition to Koch's identification of the tuberculosis bacillus led to a series of "Philadelphia debates" with Edward Shakespeare in 1883 and 1884 (University Archives and Records Center, University of Pennsylvania).

Shakespeare shortly afterwards responded to Formad's comments in a like (sarcastic) manner.

> In the [*New York Medical Journal*] of June 28th appears a quite characteristic letter from Dr. Formad, written from the Pathological Laboratory of the University of Pennsylvania. In that letter are certain disclaimers and denials of responsibility for misrepresentation of Koch's present views and animus, with which he was charged during the ... discussion before the Philadelphia Medical Society.

It is to be remarked that it is a little odd that these disclaimers and denials have been addressed to the readers of the *Journal* rather than to the members of the society before whom his address was delivered. Perhaps, however, those who heard Dr. Formad as he delivered his address, seeing him only occasionally refer to the notes at his side, and also heard at the close of the debate a most positive reiteration of the statements which had been criticized by Dr. Shakespeare, can readily appreciate the reasons which may have caused the author of the letter [i.e., Formad] to address a denial to the readers of the *Journal* rather than to themselves. If, after mature reflection, aided no doubt by the recent appearance of the second volume of the *Mittheilungen aus dem kaiserlichen Gesundheitsamte* [*Communications from the Imperial Health Office*], in which Koch has declared his present views concerning the tubercle bacillus, Dr. Formad has found it necessary to retract what he said before his audience in Philadelphia in misrepresentation of those views, it would have been manly, honorable, and praiseworthy for him to do so in a straightforward manner. But he has preferred to deny his words, and to address his denial to those who did not hear them. Probably those few of the readers of the *Journal* who did hear the author's words, and have also read the printed article, will not only be struck with the vast difference between some of the oral and the printed statements, but will also be surprised at the declaration that the quotation given in his letter contains *all* [italics in original] that he has ever spoken upon that point. The remarks which Dr. Shakespeare made before the Philadelphia society during the debate were in criticism of statements *orally addressed to the ears* [italics in original] of that body, and not in criticism of what had been for the most part rewritten and prepared for publication many weeks after the address was delivered. But, unfortunately for the author of the letter, there is sufficient basis, even in the greatly modified and tempered language which he quotes as his own, upon which to ground a charge of misrepresentation.

The charge which the author of the letter denies and to which, in his own language, he pleads 'not guilty,' is substantially reported by the recorder as follows:

2. The author had further announced that Koch had so far modified his views that he now admitted that neither the form, size, and aspect of the tubercle bacillus, nor its want of individual motion, nor its peculiar behavior toward staining-fluids, distinguished it from many other bacilli.

The language quoted by our author [Formad] as his genuine and only utterance, and which he thinks to justify his denial, comprises the following sentences: 'Koch seems now to lay more stress upon this low-power appearance (the S-shape of the culture colonies), and upon the pathogenic properties of the bacillus tuberculosis, as a distinguishing feature from other bacilli, than upon the color test. During the conversation he admitted that some other bacilli may also yield the same micro-chemical reaction as the tubercle bacilli, but insisted that the latter can not be stained brown...

Speaking of the peculiar action of Ehrlich's special staining method upon the tubercle bacilli and their surroundings, Koch says: 'But in the differentiation of the tubercle bacillus this peculiarity (staining the tubercle bacilli a color in contrast to that of their surroundings) renders still further assistance, for not alone do the connective-tissue constituents assume the contrast color, but all other bacteria at present known to me, except the lepra bacillus [a member of the same genus as the tubercle bacillus], ... likewise stain by Ehrlich's coloring method in contrast to the tubercle bacilli.... Recently I [Koch] have tested Ehrlich's method of staining upon numerous substances containing bacteria ... but have never found bacteria which gave the same color-reaction as the tubercle bacilli. I must therefore regard all assertions concerning the occurrence of bacteria which may have been found in sputum ... and stained like the tubercle bacilli, as erroneous and dependent upon a faulty application of the method of staining.[8]

"It is by no means our intention to enter upon an exhaustive criticism of those papers. Neither does time nor inclination serve for such a task, for, judging from the abundance of material presented, it might prove almost interminable. Yet the position which their author occupies in this country as the demonstrator of pathology and lecturer in experimental pathology in one of the greatest of our medical schools would seem to entitle him to speak with authority upon the subject of which he writes, and would also seem to enable him to exert no little influence in the development of public opinion concerning those matters. Moreover, he claims to be a leader among the few who, from the standpoint of personal observation and experiment, have denounced Koch's claims for the agency of the tubercle bacillus in the etiology of tuberculosis." In this particular article, Shakespeare continued, on a point by point basis, to refute the arguments Formad had previously presented in print and before the Medical Society, concluding with a question as to the reliability of the author on the question. "Indeed, as to the authority of our author, if we are to judge a man by his utterances, it may justly be said there is ample ground if he possesses really any definite notions as to what a genuine tubercle is or appears to be.... Justification of this doubt would seem also at the same time to warrant a suspicion that he is, in addition, still far at sea and greatly befogged in his knowledge of the nature of tuberculosis and pulmonary phthisis, in spite of those 'long years of research he has almost exclusively devoted to this subject.'"[9] In any argument it is immensely helpful when the individual is correct. In time, Koch, and of course Shakespeare, were proven correct in their assertion as to the etiological agent of tuberculosis. Formad continued to remain skeptical, even in the face of overwhelming evidence.

In 1885, a typhoid epidemic broke out in Plymouth, Pennsylvania, killing 100 residents. Labor strife, particularly associated with a large number of Eastern European immigrants hired to work in the mines, and living in overcrowded and often unsanitary housing, exacerbated the problem. That year, Shakespeare and Dr. Morris French, Surgeon to the Philadelphia Police Department, were commissioned by the mayor of Philadelphia, William Smith, to investigate the cause of the outbreak. The Pennsylvania State Board of Health also requested a report. After conferring with Dr. Lewis Taylor, a local Wilkes Barre physician who provided a history of the outbreak, as well as a map of the area, Shakespeare determined the source was a local dairy farmer with the disease, whose contaminated feces entered the town's temporary water supply, a creek which flowed from the nearby mountain. The house was located approximately eighty feet from the creek, and feces was somehow allowed to contaminate the nearby ground.[10] In February, an early thaw allowed the waste to enter the creek. "The town ... is supplied [nine months a year] from a mountain stream, and in periods of drought the water is pumped direct into the mains from the Susquehanna River. About March 20 [1885] last the mountain supply became to a large extent suspended owing to severe frost, and the water company had to pump direct from the river into the lower streets of the town, whilst the upper streets were still supplied from the reservoirs of the mountain stream. A thaw, followed by rain, ensued on March 26th, when the river supply was abandoned. During the brief period in which the river water had been resorted to, the surface of the Susquehanna was deeply frozen, and its volume was otherwise diminished. About two miles above the Plymouth pumping-station the sewage of 30,000 people of Wilkes-Barre found its way into the stream, and was rapidly swept by the mouth of the Plymouth mains; garbage and mine refuse also had access to the river. On April 10th the epidemic commenced, some fifty cases occurring daily up to April 20th. At first sight the relation of the foul river water to the disease seemed evident; but this turned out not to be the case. One part of Plymouth, supplied exclusively from the Susquehanna and a few wells, entirely escaped—except, indeed, a few cases amongst persons who had drunk the mountain water; and in other parts of the town the amount of disease was distinctly related to the extent to which the latter water had been used. Indeed, it was the mountain water itself that, as the result of the investigation showed came prominently under suspicion. The mountain stream has four reservoirs, all of which were frozen and all but empty at the date in question. The stream is a small one, and at one point a dwelling is situated about eighty feet from its bed. In this dwelling a case of typhoid fever, which lasted from January to March, had occurred; and the excreta had been regularly deposited in the ground towards the stream. Until the thaw and rain referred to, the mass of typhoid excreta was frozen; but when the frost abated, the long accumulation of infectious refuse was suddenly swept by the rain into the lower reservoir, and within fifteen days an epidemic resulted, which, amongst 8000 people, caused 1200 attacks of typhoid fever, and 100 deaths. We have here another of the proofs, which have so often come to us [in England] from America, to the effect that the infection of typhoid fever is not destroyed by freezing, and that the process of freezing only affects it in so far as it holds it in store until it has opportunity of gaining access to the human system. When held in ice, its potency is found to be in no way diminished when that ice is melted by being mixed with drinks, or otherwise used for human consumption.... Another point of interest is indicated in the report: mere filth, such as was contained in the sewage-befouled river, is often quite powerless to produce typhoid fever, whereas a comparatively small proportion of the excreta of a typhoid patient is potent for widespread mischief."[11]

The report subsequently submitted by French and Shakespeare provided additional lessons for public health agencies:

> First. For the production of the specific infectious disease known as typhoid fever, whether individuals or communities are considered, there are required the presence and action of one specific cause, which, elaborated in the intestinal canal of one or more patients suffering with that disease, must be transmitted in an active state to those susceptible. This specific cause being absent, typhoid fever can not and does not occur. [This statement was a response to the belief, noted in the report, by some public health officials that typhoid fever is the result of decomposition of organic matter.]
>
> Second. Epidemics of typhoid fever are a reproach to the communities which they afflict. They are absolutely preventable and controllable, and, from the standpoint of modern experience, neglect to employ proper means to those ends should be regarded as inexcusable.
>
> Third. It is the bounden duty of the physician in attendance upon any case of typhoid fever, wherever it may be located, to cause each and every evacuation from the bowels to be *immediately and effectually disinfected* [italics in original], and it is of paramount importance also that the danger of infection of the healthy should be further guarded against by the adoption of efficient means for the destruction of any infectious agent which may exist in the water or in the food.[12]

The outcome of the report did have some positive effect. Better methods of water treatment, including development of a sand filter method for removing contaminants, were ultimately implemented.[13] In part the result of his expertise in investigating infectious disease, Shakespeare's reputation also grew beyond the region of eastern Pennsylvania.

Early in 1884, Robert Koch reported the identification of the etiological agent of cholera, a comma-shaped bacillus eventually named *Vibrio cholerae*.[14] World-wide pandemics of the disease during the 19th century often originated in India, and had become endemic throughout much of the world. By the early 1880s, the germ theory of disease had been accepted by most of his contemporaries. Koch's report on the agent was not universally accepted, primarily because of the difficulty in

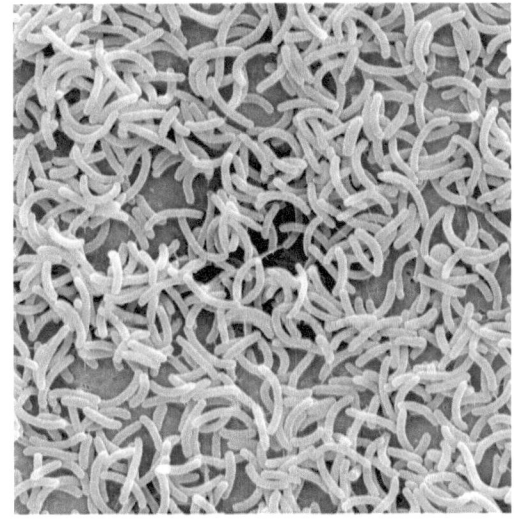

Shown here is *Vibrio cholerae*, often referred to as the "comma bacillus," the etiological agent of cholera. Isolated by Koch in 1884, the difficulty of finding a non-human test animal resulted in skepticism by some as to whether this was truly the cause of that disease (courtesy Louisa Howard, Dartmouth College).

finding a suitable (non-human) test subject in which to reproduce the disease. However his identification was subsequently proven to be correct.

During the early 1880s, subsequent to Koch's identification of the cholera bacillus, outbreaks of the disease were taking place in much of Europe. In response, President Grover Cleveland, using the guidelines of a Congressional act to investigate potential epidemic disease which might threaten the United States, in 1884 authorized Shakespeare to travel to Spain, the purpose of which was to investigate a cholera outbreak which was taking place, and to investigate the "causes, progress, and proper prevention and cure" of the disease, making a full report to Congress upon his return:

Executive Order
By the President of the United States of America

Whereas, by the provision of the act of Congress entitled "An act making appropriations for sundry civil expenses of the Government for the fiscal year ending June 30, 1886, and for other purposes," approved March 30, 1885, for the suppression of epidemic diseases, the President of the United States is authorized, in case of threatened or actual epidemic of cholera or yellow fever, to use certain appropriated sums made immediately available, "in aid of State and local boards or otherwise, in his discretion, in preventing and suppressing the spread of the same, for maintaining a quarantine and maritime inspection at points of danger"; and

Whereas there is imminent danger of a recurrence of a cholera epidemic in Europe which may be brought to our shores unless adequate measures of international or local quarantine inspections are taken in season; which measures of preventive inspection are proper subjects to be considered and to the end that their efficiency in diverse countries may be secured:

Now, therefore, in virtue of the discretionary power conferred upon me by the aforesaid act of Congress. I designate and appoint E.O. Shakespeare, M.D., of Pennsylvania, as a representative of the Government of the United States, to proceed, under the direction of the Secretary of State, to Spain and other such countries of Europe where the cholera exists, and make investigation of the causes, progress and proper prevention and cure of the said disease, in order that a full report may be made to Congress during the next ensuing session; and I direct that the necessary expenses of travel and sojourn of the said E.O. Shakespeare in proceeding from Washington to Spain and elsewhere in Europe as he may find it absolutely necessary to go in pursuit of the desired information and in returning to Washington at the conclusion of his labors, be adjusted and paid from the appropriation and available under the aforesaid act of March 3, 1885, upon his statement of account approved by the Secretary of State.

Done at the city of Washington this first day of October, in the year of our Lord one thousand, eight hundred and eighty-five, and of the Independence of the United States the one hundred and tenth.

Grover Cleveland[15]

It would not be the "ensuing" session of Congress to which Shakespeare made his report. Rather, it was a full five years before the task of writing was completed, resulting in Shakespeare becoming one of the world's authorities concerning cholera. His report also acknowledged the role played by Koch in developing the expertise he needed:

I was directed by his excellency the President, during the early part of the autumn 1885, to proceed to Europe and prosecute in the various countries which were then experiencing the ravages o the disease, or had recently suffered from them, such investigations into the cause, prevention, and cure of Asiatic cholera as my judgement would suggest.

Upon my arrival in Europe pursuant to this commission I found that cholera was rapidly vanishing from that continent, for the season at least, and I learned that the field for most active observation was then in Palermo, the principle city of the island of Sicily.

After equipping myself with a traveling laboratory, purchased in Berlin, and familiarizing myself in that city with the characteristics of the so-called "comma bacillus of Koch," through the courtesy of Dr. Robert Koch, professor of hygiene at the University of Berlin, and Dr. Georg Gaffky, director of the Pathological Laboratory of the Imperial Board of Health at Berlin, whose kindness I take this public opportunity to gratefully acknowledge, I went at once to Palermo, where a severe epidemic of cholera was raging, and began my work of investigation and experiment.[16]

Shakespeare spent the next year traveling, first to Spain in January 1886, and then to India in June of that year. He spent two months in the latter country, a great deal of the time suffering from the diseases associated with the poor sanitation conditions there, before returning to the United States in August. The result was a report comprising nearly 900 pages, including photographs, tables and figures illustrating the extent of the epidemic crisis in those regions of Europe, including France and Italy, and in Asia. Contributors to material in the report included active researchers throughout Europe and Asia, including Koch himself, who provided additional information about the cholera bacillus and its characteristics. Some even described their work on developing a vaccine.[17] The four years following Shakespeare's return were spent collating the enormous quantity of material and developing the report in its final form.

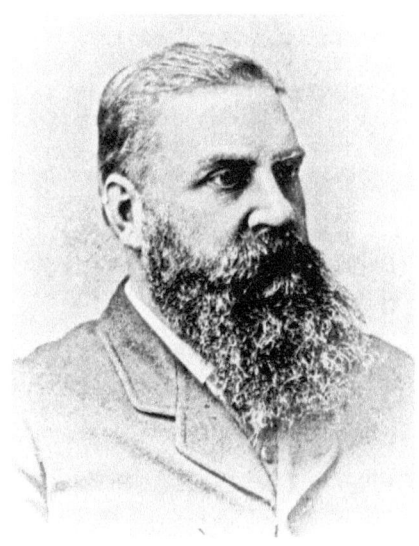

Heneage Gibbes (1837–1912). He was a British pathologist who, during his tenure at the University of Michigan (1888–1895), attempted to discredit the germ theory of disease. As a member of the 1884 British cholera commission with Dr. Emanuel Klein which traveled to India to examine Koch's identification of the etiological agent, Gibbes disputed Koch's conclusions. A portion of the report produced by Edward Shakespeare addressed some of Gibbes' arguments (National Library of Medicine).

Even in the face of growing evidence linking Koch's bacillus to cholera, not everyone remained convinced. To his credit, Shakespeare included some of the arguments presented by some of the skeptics. Among the contributors were Emanual Klein and Heneage Gibbes, both included with the cholera commission sent by the British government to investigate the outbreak in Calcutta, India in 1884. Each remained skeptical of Koch's conclusions, but the tone of their discussion, found in Shakespeare's report, was decidedly neutral.[18] "The nature and origin of cholera have until recently been subjects about which a great many speculations and theories have been forwarded, in all of which the fundamental fact, viz, the demonstration and actual isolation of the cholera virus, was absolutely wanted."

> The large number of observations made concerning the spread of cholera in India and the different visitations of cholera of Great Britain, the continent of Europe, and the Mediterranean has yielded a number of facts, which have brought the different observers, as it were, under three well-defined flags:
>
> 1. According to some, cholera in its causation depends on no definite 'entity,' but is due to certain atmospheric and telluric [terrestrial] conditions. Where these conditions prevail, as in Bengal, or where by some unknown change they obtain, as in the epidemics in Europe, cases of cholera occur. These cases stand in no causal relation to each other, but occur, like ague [malaria] or intermittent fever, independently of one another, but are dependent on a common cause of soil and atmospheric state. This theory, then, does not admit cholera into the rank of infectious diseases, and it is hardly necessary to say that in Europe this theory has no great number of followers, since, with few exceptions, almost all medical authorities are opposed to it.
>
> 2. Other authorities maintain that, in the history of all the visitations by cholera of Europe and the Mediterranean countries, the character and course of every epidemic point clearly and unmistakably to the fact that cholera is dependent to a great measure on human intercourse, that each epidemic has had its origin from a country where cholera cases had previously occurred, and that when once imported is liable to and generally does spread to larger and larger areas; that if the first cases are isolated and sanitary precautions are taken the plague remains limited. This theory further says that cholera, being communicable, belongs to the group of infectious disease. i.e., diseases in which a virus, having had access to the body of a person, therein multiplies to an enormous extent, and thereby causes the disease; that the morbid products in the case of cholera—the vomits and evacuations—are charged with this new brood of virus, and that the smallest quantity of this is capable to start the malady in a new individual.
>
> The upholders of this theory, viz, that cholera is a communicable disease, group themselves into two distinct classes, (a) those that maintain that cholera is a contagious disease, i.e., directly communicable from person to person, and (b) those that do not admit of direct contagion, but say that the substances voided by the patient in the vomits and evacuations are harmless while fresh and do not as yet contain the actual virus, but acquire this power only after they have undergone certain changes, these changes being dependent in a certain measure on the medium into which the cholera dejects pass, not every medium being suitable for producing this change; having undergone this change, this substance assumes the character of the cholera virus; i.e., finding access to the human body, either through the air we breathe, or food, or water, produces cholera. [Klein and Gibbes refer to these advocates as the contagionists.]
>
> 3. There is a third group of observers, headed by [Max] v. Pettenkofer, who, as is well-known, is justly concerned to be the greatest living authority on cholera. v. Pettenkofer is

a localist, with this distinction, that, judging from his earliest and latest writings, he does not admit of the evacuations of a cholera patient containing the virus at all either potentially or actually, but considers the product of an organism altogether extraneous to the body of a patient. This product is a kind of ferment, created by that organism only under certain favorable, seasonal, and local conditions...

If it could be demonstrated with the same accuracy and to the same degree as has been done for some of the infectious diseases—notably splenic fever [anthrax], tuberculosis, glanders, swine fever, erysipelas, etc.—that the virus is a living entity, capable of multiplication within the infected body and thereby causing the disease; that the products of the disease are charged with the same living entities; that these organisms are capable of starting the malady when introduced into a new individual, then the whole problem might be said to be practically solved.

To have achieved this demonstration is claimed by Mr. Robert Koch, sent out in 1883 by the German government to investigate the outbreak of cholera in Egypt and to study cholera in Calcutta. Koch has published in full his observations and conclusions in the 'Berliner Klin Woch,' 1884, No. 31. In the periodical reports sent to his Government from Egypt and India, and still more in the above publication, the views of Koch on the nature and cause of cholera have been expressed with so much precision and definiteness, and Koch being justly considered a great authority on questions concerning the relation of micro-organisms to infectious diseases, it is not to be wondered at that a great section of the general and medical public take it for granted that the whole problem of the nature and cause of cholera is definitely and satisfactorily solved.

Now what are the observations and conclusions of Koch? Koch failed to discover in the blood and other tissues of patients dead of cholera of anything that could identified as infective particles. He failed to find any kind of micro-organisms, and he therefore looked to the alimentary canal, which, as is well known, is the seat of grave disturbances. In the intestine he found this: In some cases the lower portion of the ileum [also spelled ilium below] ... was of a dark brown color, owing to hemorrhage into the mucous membrane, which in some instances amounted to necrotic and diphtheritic changes.... The contents of the intestine were, more or less, a fluid, like rice water, in which were suspended the characteristic flakes, i.e., masses of detached epithelium cells held together by mucous...

In acute typical cases of cholera the rice-water stools showed the comma bacilli in greater numbers the fresher the stools. Koch found this condition to be characteristic of cholera; he saw it in Egypt, in Calcutta, and more recently in Toulon, and not finding the bacilli in any other disease except cholera, he is led to attribute to them an important relation to cholera. Seeing that the more typical and fresher the case, the more pronounced the presence of the comma bacilli is, seeing that in the most typical and acute cases the mucous membrane of the intestine is so crowded with the comma bacilli that it represents, as it were, a pure cultivation of them, he concludes that these bacilli are the true cause of the disease.

To explain the manner in which these comma bacilli produce the disease, he assumes that a chemical ferment is elaborated by the comma bacilli, analogous to the septic or putrid ferment produced by putrefactive bacteria; this ferment, while at the same time killing and detaching the epithelium, is being absorbed into the general system, and then sets up all the symptoms constituting cholera. The more acute a case the greater the number of the comma bacilli in the intestine, and consequently the greater the quantity of this chemical ferment produced. This—the presence of large numbers of comma bacilli in the mucous membrane— is a point, the verification of which being obviously of central importance, Koch has been able to ascertain hold good in a large number of cases, for he found that the more acute the case the more conspicuously was the mucous membrane of the ilium a pure cultivation, and also the more affected the mucous membrane, the more numerous were the comma bacilli...

The comma bacilli are then, according to Koch, the producers of the cholera poison, and the intensity of the disease is independent [sic] in a direct ratio on the number of comma bacilli present in the mucous membrane of the ilium. A very necessary conclusion from these statements is this, viz, is that the rice-water stools, and particularly the mucous flakes suspended in the clear fluid (being charged with the comma bacilli) are the vehicles of the virus, and the minutest quantity of these materials finding entrance into the small intestine of a person multiply in the mucous membrane, and produce the chemical ferment acting as the cholera poison, the more rapid the multiplication of the comma bacilli, the greater their numbers and the more acute and intense the disease; as long as their number is limited, the amount of the ferment is too small to produce any other symptom except diarrhea, but as their number increases, the amount of ferment increases, and a general infection of the system with all the typical symptoms ensues...

These views of Koch, it is evident, favor in an eminent way the theory of contagiousness, inasmuch as the comma bacilli directly derived from the fresh evacuations are considered as the contagium vivium. Particles of these evacuations, linen and clothing soiled with them, provided these particles remain in a damp state, water, food, and other articles contaminated with comma bacilli can, under this view, directly convey the disease, if they find access to the alimentary canal, particularly to the small intestine. There exists a great many *a priori* in accepting this view of Koch. Foremost is the well-known fact, observed over and over again, that direct contagion does not exist at all, or is of the greatest variety; the attendants of the cholera patient, the persons living in the same room, physicians and nurses, persons occupied in handling and removing the evacuations of a cholera patient, are, according to almost all accounts, particularly exempt; if the comma bacilli were in reality the contagium, then it is impossible to understand why direct contagium should not be a very common thing.... Again, it is well established by the researches of Pettenkofer and others, that between the introduction of the cholera virus into a new locality and the outbreak of disease in the form of an epidemic, there is always a considerable lapse of time: according to Pettenkofer the cholera matter introduced into a locality must, before becoming active virus, pass a certain stage of development in the soil, this soil must be at the same time of a definite character, and only after having undergone these changes and having had access to the system of persons can produce the disease...[19]

Another great difficulty in accepting the theory of Koch is this: The comma bacilli can not, according to Koch, exist in acid media, and therefore when introduced into the stomach, this mode of infection being, according to Koch, the general one, they could not pass unscathed into the small intestine (the ilium being their true breeding ground).[20]

Klein and Gibbes were correct in stating *Vibrio cholerae* is sensitive to acid. For this reason, its selection and growth in the modern laboratory is carried out on the selective medium TCBS (Thiosulfate-citrate-bile salts-sucrose) agar, at a slightly alkaline pH. Its ability to survive stomach acid is likely due to the slight buffering capacity of the food or water in which it is found. The large quantity of cholera bacillus in contaminated water likely contributes to survival of sufficient numbers entering the small intestine.

Koch was also correct in suggesting the production of a ferment as the immediate cause of the symptoms of cholera: vomiting and diarrhea. The existence of the primary virulence factor, now known as cholera toxin, was conclusively proven in 1959.[21]

Shakespeare's firm conclusion was that Koch was correct in his identification of the comma bacillus as the etiological agent of the disease. He concluded his report with a summary of the agent, its method of transmission, and methods for treatment. And though the specific toxin involved in the disease would not be recognized for nearly 75 years, he acknowledged Koch's belief in its existence. "Cholera infectiosa has, as a specific exciting cause, a specific infecting agent, which enters the person attacked by way of the stomach.

"This agent is in all probability a vegetable parasite—namely, the comma bacillus of Koch. In the process of development and growth of this parasite, both within and without the human body, a specific poison or *ptomaine*—a chemical alkaloid possessing specific chemical and physiological properties— is produced; the primary action in the human system is upon the mucous membrane of the intestinal canal, chiefly the small intestine, and the ultimate result is the desquamation and destruction of the epithelial elements."[22]

His report also contained specific recommendations for controlling an outbreak, the most obvious among numerous requirements being: "(a) speedy isolation and isolation of the sick; their proper treatment; absolute and rapid destruction of the infectious agent of the disease, not only in the dejecta and the vomit, but also in clothing, bedding, and in or upon whatever else it finds a resting place. (b) The convalescents should remain isolated from the healthy so long as their stools possibly contain any of the infecting agent, say for ten to fourteen days after the commencement of the attack… (c) The dead should be well wrapped in a cloth thoroughly saturated in a solution of corrosive sublimate… (d) Those handling the sick or the dead should be careful to disinfect their hands and soiled clothing at once, and especially before touching articles of food, drinking, or culinary vessels."[23]

As a result of his thorough and painstaking report, Shakespeare would be regarded as the country's leading expert on cholera. His "great work" work was cited by the American Medical Association: "The valuable cyclopedic 'Report on Cholera in Europe and India,' by Dr. E.O. Shakespeare, who was appointed by President Cleveland, October 1, 1885, and who on November 17, 1890, transmitted his great work to Secretary Blaine, after having given five years of travel and study to its preparation, 'all voluntary and without pay for personal service.' Perhaps there is no other instance of an individual holding the high appointment of Commissioner from our National government, acting in so patriotic and liberal in manner, and furnishing an example so worthy of imitation by men of means and culture. Well may the medical profession take an honest pride in such a worthy colleague."[24] Shakespeare returned to Philadelphia a hero. When cholera appeared in the European emigrant ports of Hamburg and LeHavre in August 1892, the Philadelphia health authorities feared the outbreak would subsequently be brought to the city. In 1873, the American Steamship Line, originally formed as the American Steamship Company of Philadelphia, had begun a regular passenger service between that city and European cities. By the early 1890s, over 1100 passenger ships, carrying over 17,000 passengers arrived annually at the port of Philadelphia, any of whom, in the minds of the city health authorities, might be carrying infectious disease.[25] In response, Shakespeare was appointed Port Physician by Pennsylvania Governor Robert Pattison.[26] The concern was to prove unfounded, however, as the few suspected cases turned out to be only minor intestinal illnesses.

Following the outbreak of the Spanish-American War in 1898, epidemics of typhoid fever spread through many of the army camps in the southeastern United States. Shakespeare and Drs. Walter Reed and Victor Vaughan, were appointed to a commission tasked with investigating the outbreaks, and providing recommendations for control and elimination; each of the members received an appointment as officer, with Shakespeare as Major and Brigade Surgeon in the United States Volunteer Army:

> War Department
> Adjutant-General's Office,
> Washington, August 18, 1898
>
> Special Orders No. 194
>
> A board of medical officers, to consist of Maj. Walter Reed, surgeon, U.S. Army; Maj. Victor C. Vaughan, division surgeon, U.S. Volunteers, and Maj. Edward O. Shakespeare, brigade surgeon, U.S. Volunteers, is appointed to meet in this city at the earliest date practicable for the purpose of making an investigation into the cause of the extensive prevalence of typhoid fever in the various military camps within the limits of the United States, under such instructions as it may receive from the Surgeon-General of the Army [Dr. George Sternberg]. The board will call the attention of the proper commanding officers to any unsanitary conditions which may exist at the camps visited by it, and will make recommendations with a view to their proper correction. The report of the board will be forwarded to the Surgeon-General as soon as practicable after the completion of the investigation contemplated.
>
> Such journeys as may be required under the above order are necessary for the public service.
>
> By order of the Secretary of War:
>
> H.C. Corbin, Adjutant-General[27]

Between August 20 and September 30, the Typhoid Board visited camps throughout the region, producing a "landmark study" of the sanitary conditions which allowed for the outbreak. Their final report, published in 1904, contained fifty-seven specific determinations, focusing primarily on improper handling and disposition of fecal excretions.[28] Recommendations from the Board were subsequently instituted, and typhoid fever ceased to be a significant problem within American army camps during World War I. Tragically, the untimely deaths of both Reed and Shakespeare left it to Vaughan to complete and submit the final report. Despite his relatively young age, Shakespeare developed symptoms of heart disease which became more apparent with time. On June 1, 1900, he died suddenly from a heart attack in a Philadelphia hotel room. Shakespeare's expertise in bacteriology, demonstrated by his application of Koch's studies on the subjects of tuberculosis and cholera, moved him to the forefront of American physicians involved in those areas.

9

Harold Clarence Ernst

"While Dr. Ernst possessed the true spirit of investigation and the abilities of a great investigator, his temperament ... left him constantly engaged in efforts to accomplish work of immediate utility."[1]

H.C. Ernst was born July 31, 1856, in Cincinnati, Ohio, the third of three sons of Andrew Henry Ernst, who came to the United States in 1804 from Hanover, a region in what is now Germany, and Sarah Otis Ernst, born in Massachusetts, and an early suffragette. Harold's oldest brother, Oswald Herbert Ernst (1842–1926), had a long military career, serving as an engineer with General William Tecumseh Sherman during the Civil War, and later as superintendent of the United States Military Academy at West Point. A second brother, George Alexander Otis Ernst (1850–1912), was a lawyer and member of the finance commission in Boston.

Their father, Andrew, died during Harold's childhood, and he and his mother returned to her birthplace in New England, where Harold attended secondary school. Ernst was graduated from Harvard College in 1876. But it was not solely his academic performance for which he was remembered. Legend has it that Ernst was equally famous as a pitcher on the Harvard baseball team, and also played an instrumental role in development of the catcher's mit. "The popular tale begins in 1875 with a late season game between arch-rivals Harvard and Yale. Somewhere in the early innings, Harvard pitcher Harold Ernst came to bat. As the first pitch approached he jumped back, startled by the extreme new swerving movement on the ball as it crossed the plate. Ernst struck out on three pitches. The rest of the Harvard lineup also seemed to be swinging at air. Ernst watched Yale pitcher Charles Avery's throwing motion very closely for the rest of the day. Yale went on to easily defeat Harvard for the sixth time in their last seven meetings. After the game, Ernst knew that to be one of the best he would have to learn the delivery of this tantalizing pitch. In the off-season he went about teaching himself how to throw what we now call the curve ball. The effects of Ernst's offseason work were immediate. On opening day in 1876, throwing as many curves as his elbow could stand, Ernst no-hit the powerhouse Lowell, Massachusetts club. He led Harvard to a 25–12 record that season and established himself as one the pioneers of pitching."[2] Centerfielder on the team was James Tyng, who alternated positions with catcher Harry Thatcher whenever the latter's hands (and face) grew sore from attempting to catch Ernst's pitch. When Thatcher graduated, team captain Frederick W. Thayer (Class of 1878) asked Tyng to become the regular catcher. He agreed, but only if Thayer could devise some form of facial protection. Thayer developed a modified fencer's wire mask which served to provide a measure of protection.[3] It appears there was some attention among professional teams for Ernst's services, though he never expressed any interest in signing with them.

Ernst received his medical degree from Harvard Medical School in 1880, and a Master of Arts (A.M.) in 1884. During these years he became interested in the new field of bacteriology, and while developing a medical practice, published several papers during 1883 and 1884 on the subject of tuberculosis, observations of which included his own work. Ernst's conclusions mirrored those of Koch, who had observed the bacillus the year before. "1. A staff-shaped micro-organism exists in all forms of the tuberculous process, and its presence has been demonstrated in them. 2. It is more abundant in the rapid than in the slow form of the process. 3. Its specific nature as to the cause of tuberculosis has been claimed by Koch on the ground of his observations. 4. Its specific character has not been successfully refuted by trustwor-

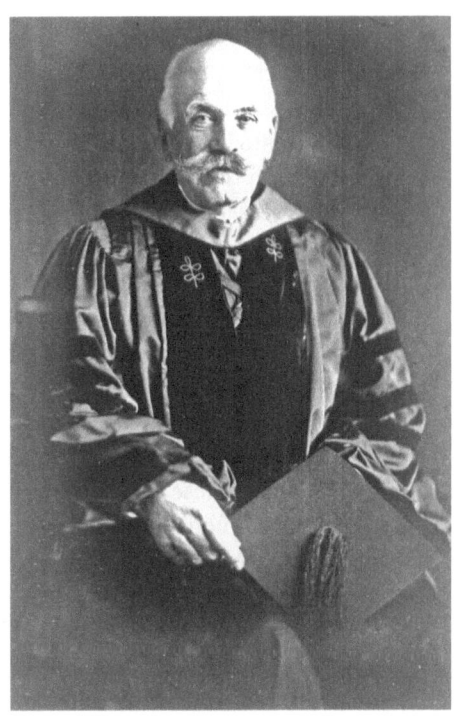

Harold Clarence Ernst (1856–1922). In 1885, Ernst, William Welch and T. Mitchell Prudden enrolled in Koch's bacteriology course, the first Americans to study with Koch in that capacity. Despite minimal cooperation from the Harvard administration in the beginning of his tenure at that institution, Ernst eventually developed the bacteriology laboratory incorporated into the medical program (National Library of Medicine).

thy observations. 5. Its value as diagnostic evidence of tuberculosis is very great, although its absence cannot be considered as excluding the existence of that process."[4]

It was one thing for Ernst to summarize Koch's work with the tuberculosis bacillus. But if he were to develop and teach a course in bacteriology for medical students—a goal of Ernst's—then it would be necessary to learn firsthand the laboratory methodology for the subject. With the lack of suitable facilities in the United States, the only alternative for Ernst would be to travel to Europe, preferably to Koch's laboratory, and participate in the instruction of the subject. During the summer and fall of 1885, Ernst traveled to Europe where he, along with Welch and Prudden, became the first Americans to enroll in Koch's course. Returning in November, he was appointed as an Assistant in Bacteriology. His lectures on the subject were the first in the United States presented to students in a medical school.

The reception by faculty for Ernst's course was decidedly mixed. There were some who lent him support: most notably physiologist Henry Bowditch, the dean of the medical school, but most faculty were opposed to adding bacteriology to the medical school curriculum. Prevented from obtaining laboratory space at Harvard, Ernst was forced to use a small room belonging to the Warren Museum in a local school. It was only in 1888, that laboratory work in bacteriology was added to the instruction for medical students.

Promotion for Ernst soon followed. In 1889, he was promoted to Instructor, in 1891 to Assistant Professor, and in 1895 he became professor of bacteriology. During these years he continued to maintain a practice, while at the same time conducting and publishing research on a wide range of topics in bacteriology. When Koch announced his use of tuberculin as a "cure" for tuberculosis in 1890, Ernst made a second trip to Berlin that year to gather information about the treatment. Upon his return in the fall of that year, Ernst proceeded with treatment of a small number of patients. His results were presented twice, once before members of the medical profession, and a second time before the Harvard Medical School in January 1891. Ernst's visit with Koch was acknowledged in his introduction by Dr. C.H. Porter for the first lecture: "A member of the staff of this hospital, by laborious work in the laboratory of Professor Koch of Berlin, by painstaking research in his own laboratory at the Harvard Medical School, has made himself an authority in bacteriology. Recently he has had exceptional opportunities, both by personal interviews with Professor Koch himself, and personal observation by himself at various Berlin clinics for acquiring a knowledge of the action of 'Parataloid,' which is the name given to the fluid by Professor Koch, which he claims is of service in the treatment of tuberculosis."[5] In the beginning of his presentation, Ernst acknowledged the experimental nature of the treatment, while at the same time expressing full confidence in Koch's expertise. "I have had the honor of sharing in the introduction of this treatment in Boston; and the first patient upon whom it was tried in this city, is still under my care at the Massachusetts General Hospital in Dr. [George] Tarbell's service and by reason of his courtesy. The number under treatment is for the present limited, because when we look at the matter soberly, we must all acknowledge that this is a great clinical experiment, and the impressiveness of the stage through which we are passing is one which will grow greater as time goes by. We, as medical practitioners, are doing a thing which has never been known in the history of medicine. We are, at the suggestion of one man, employing a material of whose composition we are still ignorant. And we are doing this in perfect faith, and feeling we are justified in its course, because this material, and the suggestion of its employment, comes from one of the greatest medical minds the world has ever produced. This one fact of the general acceptance of Koch's parataloid, and its employment against tuberculosis by the medical profession, says more than any one individual can find words to express, of the greatness of character of this man, who has been, to my mind, for a number of years, one of the most impressive characters that has ever crossed the medical stage. He is the one man in scientific medicine who thus far has never made a mistake. Going back some twenty years to the time of the Franco-Prussian War, through which he served as an assistant-surgeon, passing from that period to a struggle for a practice in an obscure north German town, without money, influence, or friends, he stands today at the pinnacle of the medical profession; and we all look to him for further developments in the line of his previous researches. He is practically the one man by whom the possibility of research in bacteriology has been laid open to us by the development of methods which enable the average man to carry out something in the line of work in which he himself is engaged. This does not enter a claim for his absolute precedence in bacteriology, for there were others before him, Pasteur, of course. Among them; but it is owing to the introduction of his methods that we have reached our present point."[6]

The obvious question here which should be addressed, was what exactly was this parataloid which Koch had developed, and which Ernst among others was testing? Ernst's description was primarily what the treatment *was not*, not what its actual composition might have been. "Probably what it is not, is the thing which has been impressed upon you that it is. In the first place this material is distinctly not a vaccine. It bears not the slightest resemblance to one, and it is very easy to see why, if you recall what a vaccine really is. A vaccine requires for its effect and action something in the nature of vitality—

an organism. There must be something present capable of reproduction. It must have some vitality, and the best example is the 'vaccine [sic] virus,' which we see employed daily as a preventive against smallpox. A vaccine has distinctly the power of reproduction, if a minute amount is introduced into an abrased part, and a local reaction of a marked degree is set up; this does not occur in our experiments with parataloid, therefore this material is distinctly not a vaccine...[7]

"Having shown that Koch's material is neither an attenuated virus nor vaccine, what else can it be?... Nutrient gelatin is somewhat of an amber color, and the method of planting the bacteria in the tube is by means of a platinum wire which has been sunk into a glass rod at one end and is free at the other. The free end is dipped into material containing the organism, and then immediately plunged directly through the centre of the nutrient material. The result of such a procedure is a visible line through the centre of the gelatin. If this is kept under observation for a short time, depending upon the time necessary for the development of the colony of bacteria, there is observed a gradual thickening of this line on both sides, and occasionally an elevation above the gelatin; then the further spreading of this colony of bacteria ceases, and does not go on any more at any time. For a long time it was difficult to explain why that occurred, but the knowledge which has come to us of late years furnishes a perfect explanation of why the colony does not grow farther out, and why its vitality is not destroyed. The bacteria take from the nutrient gelatin certain elements necessary for their development. They leave, therefore, the nutrient gelatin in a state of partial chemical decomposition, and these unstable chemical elements come together and form new chemical compounds, all of which occurs directly along the outlines of the colony.... A great characteristic is that they [i.e., new chemical compounds] are inhibitory to the development of bacteria, and each variety of bacterium produces in a given nutrient material a special alkaloid or ptomaine, which is inhibitory to its further growth, but does not destroy its vitality. This, it seems to me, furnishes a very perfect explanation of what Koch's material must be, if the explanation of what goes on within the body after its use is correct.... This material, it seems to me, can be nothing else than the ptomaines produced by the development of the bacteria of tuberculosis in some medium which permits of this alkaloid being separated out of the nutrient material after the bacteria of tuberculosis have produced it."[8]

The reality was, parataloid, or as it was more frequently termed, tuberculin, simply did not work. Ernst was forced to acknowledge that even in Koch's hand it was ineffective, though using the caveat of advanced cases. "I am sorry to say that a large amount of the clinical material which is being collected in Berlin will be more or less unsatisfactory in helping us to determine this particular question [of the efficacy in pulmonary tuberculosis]. The reason is that in the hospitals there they are overwhelmed by the number of applicants for admission for treatment; and in the excitement attendant there have been a number of cases accepted, which will tend to throw discredit upon Koch's material, because they are in too advanced stages for treatment with any hope of recovery."[9]

Koch's parataloid was an extract prepared from the tuberculosis bacillus. Its composition was not initially revealed, not because of some dark secret, but likely because Koch had no means to patent the material. It was only after other physicians observed a lack of efficacy in its use as a treatment that it, and Koch as well for a time, fell into disrepute.

In addition to his work with tuberculosis, Ernst's professional career included research on topics as diverse as diphtheria, in which he helped develop the first anti-toxin for use in Boston, rabies and immunology. He was among the first to develop a method to sterilize milk for infant feeding. His research also included the subject of whether milk from tuberculous cattle was capable of transmitting the disease to humans. He found that even when udders appeared normal, milk from tuberculous cattle could produce the disease when fed to pigs. The obvious conclusion was that milk from diseased animals was not safe for humans.[10] "The virus may be present in the milk while yet the closest examination fails to reveal the tuberculosis of the udder."[11]

In 1896, Ernst founded the *Journal of the Boston Society of Medical Sciences,* which continues as *The Journal of Medical Research.* He served as editor of the journal until his death. His endeavors for the acceptance of bacteriology as a distinct discipline were highlighted by President Emeritus of Harvard Charles Eliot, following Ernst's death. "I was cognizant of all the circumstances which attended his long struggles for proper treatment of the subject of bacteriology in the program of studies at the medical school, including the slowness of his own promotion. These difficulties were due not only to the failure of several important members of the Medical Faculty to realize the importance of the science, but also to the slowness of the medical profession in general to recognize the important service which bacteriological examinations could render in the practice of both medicine and surgery. I admired the dignity and courage which Dr. Ernst met all the rebukes and obstacles, and finally succeeded in obtaining proper recognition for his subject and himself."[12] Ernst died September 7, 1922.

10

Victor Vaughan and Frederick Novy

> "Bacteriology was taught to medical students at the University of Michigan probably before the subject was seriously presented in any other medical school in the United States. This caused concern to the Professor of Pathology who had no faith in the infectious theory of disease. In fact, the Professor of Pathology suggested to the University administration that Vaughan and Novy be relieved of their posts. After some consideration a new Professor of Pathology was appointed!"[1]

The professional careers of Vaughan and Novy were so interconnected, that it is only appropriate to consider the two scientists together in describing their respective vocations, as well as the influence that the time spent in Koch's laboratory had on each. Vaughan and Novy came from two very different backgrounds. Their connection originated in the late 1880s, beginning when Novy was a student of Vaughan's. After earning a doctorate in chemistry in 1890, and his medical degree the following year, Novy became a professional associate of Vaughan's, the same year the latter was appointed dean of the medical school; for years, the two carried out collaborations on numerous projects in the area of hygiene. Vaughan's professional interests were largely in the area of physiological chemistry, Novy's in the newly emerging field of bacteriology. Together they played what could be described as a symbiotic role in establishing the bacteriology program in the medical school at the University of Michigan.

Victor Clarence Vaughan (1851–1929)

> "Working in Dr. Victor Vaughan's laboratories, directed by him, in personal contact with him and his students, was more than a mere scientific experience of great value. The influence of that remarkable personality cannot be calculated. The busiest man on the campus, yet never hurried, lecturing at the College of Arts, as well as in the Medical School, looking into the face of each student present till each felt the personal appeal, he also attended to a considerable private practice, yet that equanimity was never disturbed. AND WHAT HE TAUGHT—indeli-

ble and incomparable. Such a man! If only our children could always have even one such fine figure to steer by."²

Victor Vaughan was born near Mt. Airy, Missouri into a family of considerably mixed ethnic heritage. Vaughan's paternal side was of Welsh ancestry. Vaughan's grandfather, Sampson Vaughan, after serving in the Napoleonic Wars—a service implied in Victor Vaughan's autobiography—arrived in America with his new wife, Mary Jones, on their honeymoon. Purchasing a small farm near present-day Durham, North Carolina, Sampson Vaughan earned a living growing and selling tobacco. Their son, Victor's father, John Vaughan, chose instead to be trained as a cabinetmaker. Desiring to see the western United States, John enlisted in the quartermaster department of the army, later taking part in the reconstruction of Fort Laramie (Wyoming) and Fort Kearny (both ca. 1846–1849) in the present state of Nebraska. Following his discharge, and a marriage to Adeline Dameron, Vaughan settled in Mt. Airy, Missouri, located near the central portion of the state. It was in Grandmother Eliza Dameron's house east of Mt. Airy, that Victor Vaughan was born October 27, 1851.³

Vaughan's maternal side was of French Huguenot ancestry. Though family tradition traced his ancestry as far back as the 11th century in Burgundy, accurate information begins about the year 1650, with the birth of one Bartholomew Du Puy. When Du Puy was thirty-five years old, the Edict of Nantes, published in 1598 by Henry IV, which granted religious tolerance to the Protestant subjects in France, was revoked. Du Puy and his new bride, Susanne Lavillon, fled first to Germany, and subsequently to England. In 1699,

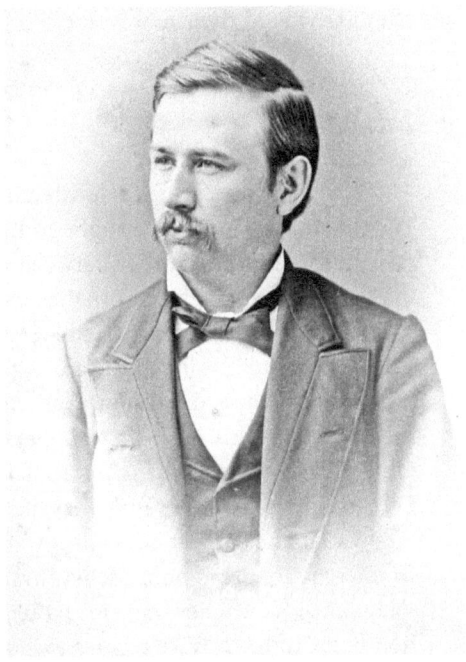

Victor Clarence Vaughan (1851–1929). Longtime dean of the medical school at the University of Michigan (1891–1921), Vaughan instituted many of the changes which modernized the medical program at the school. Along with Drs. Walter Reed and Edward Shakespeare, Vaughan was a member of the commission which investigated outbreaks of typhoid fever in army camps during the Spanish-American War (Victor Vaughan file, Bentley Historical Library, University of Michigan).

Du Puy and his family immigrated to America, settling in Virginia in a region north of Richmond. The family remained in this region north of the James River for several generations. Vaughan's great-great grandfather, Joseph Dameron, served with the colonial army during the revolution, and was wounded during the Battle of Guilford Court House in 1781. The family prospered during these years; some became slave holders. Joseph's son, George Ball Dameron, a "well-to-do farmer," married Mary Moore, and served as a deacon in the Methodist Church. Their son, William Moore Dameron, Victor Vaughan's grandfather, married his cousin, Eliza Dameron. Along with five children, four brothers, and slaves, William and Eliza Dameron moved to Missouri in 1829. Their daughter Adeline, Victor's mother, was born shortly after arriving at their new home.[4]

Education

The Vaughan farm was located in what was then still frontier. The Civil War, beginning in 1861, brought additional challenges. Missouri was a slave state, located on the border between the North and South, and subjected to the horrendous slaughter from the guerrilla warfare carried out by both sides. Two of the more infamous Confederate raiders, "Bloody" Bill Anderson and William Quantrill—including among the members of his fighters, Frank and Jesse James—carried out some of their most vicious actions in that region of the country. In his memoir, Vaughan described an 1864 (uninvited) visit of Quantrill to their home, shortly before his raiders slaughtered unarmed Union soldiers in Centralia, Missouri.[5]

Vaughan's earliest education was typical of that for young boys on the frontier: a mixture of home-schooling and some formal schoolhouse learning. Vaughan's first teacher was a local physician, Dr. William Watts, with instruction likely in his private residence, but who shortly afterwards moved away. A more formal schoolhouse, with the fancy name of Hazel Hill Academy, was constructed to provide a broader education for the local youth, and it was here that Vaughan received more comprehensive opportunities for study. With one exception, all Vaughan's teachers were women. Vaughan was also fortunate in having an extensive library present in his home, readings provided by his mother.

Vaughan's education continued beyond secondary school. After turning sixteen, Vaughan enrolled in Central College, a Methodist school founded in 1854 and located in Fayette, Missouri. Now known as Central Methodist University, the school still exists over 150 years later. Admittedly still too immature to devote the necessary time for learning, Vaughan withdrew after one semester. Vaughan was not forgotten. In 1910, forty-three years later, he was awarded an honorary degree by the school.

A year later, Vaughan enrolled at a Baptist school, Mount Pleasant College, in nearby Huntsville. The president and owner of the college was a former Confederate soldier, the Reverend James Terrill. The best Terrill himself could provide for Vaughan, was a rudimentary training in Latin, so limited that Vaughan himself was forced to study the subject sufficiently enough to serve as the instructor shortly afterwards. This is not to imply the instruction at Mount Pleasant was second-rate. During the early years of the schools development, Terrill significantly enlarged both the main building, as well as the campus as a whole, while at the same time attracting some of the best teachers in the state. Unfortunately, the war had left most of the region impoverished, and unable to properly maintain the infrastructure, or pay the teachers a salary commensurate with their abilities, the school subsequently lost much of its initial prestige.[6]

The more important long-term impact of Vaughan's training at Mount Pleasant was in the subject of chemistry. Vaughan's interest in chemistry began with what could be considered a fortuitous accident. Vaughan came upon a locked room located in the college's main building, and upon obtaining permission to open the door, discovered a treasure-trove of chemical supplies and equipment. The materials had likely been purchased prior to the war, and had remained unused since then. Three walls were lined with glass cabinets containing a large quantity of apparatus for use in chemistry experiments, as well as pure chemicals in bottles which had never been opened—even the paper wraps were intact. Using several editions of early chemistry books as texts—primarily [George] *Barker's Chemistry (a Textbook of Elementary Chemistry)* (1870)—Vaughan taught himself enough of the subject that he was able to teach a chemistry course at the school, while at the same time establishing his own laboratory. His acquisition of a first edition of *Qualitative Analysis*, authored by Drs. Albert Prescott and Silas Douglas from the University of Michigan, not only provided an additional source for his interests in chemistry, but would play an important role in his future career. Vaughan was graduated in 1872, but continued to teach both Latin and chemistry at Mount Pleasant for another two years.

Vaughan briefly continuing his teaching after leaving Mount Pleasant, this time at Hardin College in Mexico, Missouri, a school associated with the Missionary Baptist Church of Missouri, and established for the education of young women. But in order to continue his own education, Vaughan was forced to look beyond the immediate area of his home. There were six "so-called" colleges located within a fifty mile radius of the Vaughan farm, but none offered anything but rudimentary learning. Vaughan was also handicapped as a member of a family which had been Confederate sympathizers during the war. In these years immediately following the conflict, a ban had been established by the Union "occupiers," that only those instructors who had taken an oath to support the Union would be allowed to teach at most of the state's public schools; neither Vaughan nor his family had done so.

Vaughan's choices were schools beyond the borders of Missouri. His initial interest was the University of Virginia. Unfortunately, the school had not yet recovered from the devastation of the war. Ivy League schools such as Harvard, Yale, Dartmouth or Princeton were ruled out, either because of the lack of scientific programs, or for religious differences. One school stood out in Vaughan's mind: the University of Michigan.

The choice to come to Ann Arbor in 1874 was not inevitable, but several factors entered into Vaughan's decision. First, the school was already well-known for its teaching in the classics as well as in math and science. In astronomy, James Craig Watson had reported the discovery of well over a dozen asteroids. Alexander Winchell, professor of geology and serving as well as the state geologist, was well-known for having generated controversies with his personal arguments in support of evolution, rather than adhering to literal Biblical interpretation. The most important factor in Vaughan's decision, however, was the presence of an excellent chemistry program, considered among the best in the world. Among the chemistry professors at the university were Prescott, then a professor of organic chemistry, but shortly to be appointed dean of the college of pharmacy, and Douglas, who in addition to his position in chemistry, had just completed a tenure as mayor of Ann Arbor.

The goal of enrolling in the university was laudable, but first Vaughan had to be accepted into the graduate program. His bachelor's degree from Mount Pleasant was considered insufficient by itself for admission into the program. However, the president of the University, Dr. James Angell, provided a compromise. In personal interviews with three members of the faculty, Vaughan would have to demonstrate competency, not only in chemistry, but in geology and biology as well. Prescott was chosen to conduct the chemistry interview, which Vaughan passed easily. The interview for the subject of biology was conducted by Professor Mark Harrington, a multi-talented member of the faculty with appointments in botany and zoology, as well as in astronomy. The interview did not go well, with Harrington reportedly telling Vaughan, "I suppose you know as much about biology as our freshman do."[7] Professor Eugene Hilgard, briefly serving as professor of mineralogy, and considered among the founders of what is now called soil science, was the third member of the faculty chosen to quiz Vaughan. Fortunately for Vaughan, Hilgard was in California, and would not return for several weeks. Vaughan put the time to good use, studying the subject sufficiently enough to at least acquire a minimal level of expertise. The interview with Hilgard was impressive enough that the professor hired Vaughan to be his assistant the following year. When Hilgard accepted an appointment at the University of California, Berkeley in 1875, he offered Vaughan the opportunity to accompany him; Vaughan declined the offer. Vaughan received his Master of Science degree in June 1875, with his thesis entitled "The Separation of Arsenic and Antimony."[8]

Vaughan remained at the university for continuation of his doctoral work, graduating in 1876 with two theses: "The Osteology and Mycology of the Domestic Fowl," and a second thesis which was a continuation of his work on the separation of antimony from other minerals.[9] That year he was also admitted to the program in medicine.

During these early months of 1876, Vaughan received his first teaching appointment, as an instructor in physiological chemistry. What under other circumstances might have been a rare honor, was in this instance the result of an unfortunate "scandal" and controversy in the department. Professor Silas Douglas, one of the authors of the aforementioned text on qualitative analysis utilized by Vaughan at Mount Pleasant, had been a major figure in the original effort to fund the construction of a laboratory building devoted completely to the teaching of chemistry. The original building was completed in 1855, and Douglas continued in his role as an instructor in chemistry. During this period (1875), another member of the faculty, Dr. Preston Rose, who had been teaching toxicology and urinalysis to the medical students, was appointed assistant professor of physiological chemistry.

According to the bylaws of the university, "Each student should be furnished with apparatus and chemicals at their cost price, or according to the price list of a New York dealer, and only such chemicals as shall actually be used shall be charged, and the amount thus received by the professor of chemistry shall constitute a fund in his hands for the purchase of apparatus and chemicals for laboratory use, which amount shall be properly accounted for at the close of the year."[10] Douglas was then director of the laboratory. Rose was the instructor in physiological chemistry, receiving in cash the funds for purchase of materials. The rule was seemingly clear. Students paid a fee, approximately $10, for use of reagents and equipment, the funds for which went to the university. (When this author was enrolled in The Pennsylvania State University a century later, the laboratory fee for chemistry was still $10.) Left over money was given to Douglas, who would initial a receipt.

The controversy began when it was discovered that, between 1866 and 1875, the sum of $831.10 was unaccounted for—the confusion actually involved several thousand dollars; Rose was accused of having stolen the money. The primary reason for the accusation lay in the informality of the accounting methods. Card vouchers served as receipts, and no accountants were involved in keeping track of the money. Rose eventually paid the university a portion of the alleged missing amount, mortgaging his house to do so. In December 1875, Rose was suspended from the university, and Vaughan was appointed in his place. Six years later, the State Supreme Court placed the blame on both parties for their informal accounting methods.

Member of the Faculty

In June 1877, Vaughan was appointed to the "position of instructor in medicinal chemistry and lecturer on physiology."[11] His teaching duties included the subjects of histology and physiological chemistry. Nine months later, in March 1878, Vaughan received his medical degree, one of sixty-five students which included six women. He received an additional appointment as lecturer on medicinal chemistry in June 1879. The promotions continued. The following year, Vaughan was appointed assistant professor of physiological chemistry (also referred to as medicinal chemistry). The appointment provided the opportunity in 1881 to teach a course called Sanitary Science, considered to be the "unofficial" start of bacteriology at the university. The course consisted of twelve topics, one of which included topics such as "ferments and germs; physiological ferments, and fermentation; disease germs; filth diseases; antiseptics and disinfectants and their use; quarantine, vaccination, etc."[12] The course would be taught by Vaughan for the remainder of the decade. In June 1883, Vaughan received another promotion, becoming a full professor of physiological chemistry, as well as the additional title of associate professor of therapeutics and *Materia Medica*.

That same year (1883) marked the beginning of Vaughan's evolution in the field of public health and hygiene. The Michigan State Board of Health had been established in 1873, with Dr. Henry Baker as its primary founder and first secretary. Baker had been the driving force in the establishment of the Board, with significant experience in the area of sanitation from having served as a regimental surgeon during the Civil War. Following the war, Baker returned to his home in Michigan, where he became an advocate for the establishment of a board of health. The danger of contagious disease was a significant problem—understanding the role of "germs" was still premature during the late 1860s—but there were other health concerns as well among the populace. Illuminating oil was routinely used for lighting, and explosions were not uncommon. The use of the poison arsenic as an ingredient in pigment for wallpaper was likewise a health concern. Baker's initial attempts to establish a board in 1870 were initially unsuccessful. However, Baker was able to convince several physicians, most notably Dr. Ira Bartholomew, of the need for such a board. In 1872, Bartholomew was elected to the Michigan State Legislature, and, through his efforts, establishment of a State Board of Health was signed into law on July 30, 1873, making Michigan the fifth such state to establish such a board.[13]

In 1883, Vaughan was appointed to the Board of Health by the Michigan governor, Josiah Begole, ultimately serving as a member of the board for thirty-five years. The first concept of a state hygienic laboratory was brought before the members by Vaughan in January 1884. Dr. John H. Kellogg, superintendent of the Battle Creek [Michigan] Sanitarium and a member of the Board, had brought a request for "using a part of its appropriations for making special investigations" of designated unsanitary conditions such as those which existed in the State Reform School.[14] Vaughan, Kellogg and Dr. Henry Baker had been appointed to examine sanitary conditions at the school and in its surroundings. However, no laboratory yet existed in Michigan capable of carrying out such investigations. In support of the idea, Vaughan "spoke of the need for a fully equipped sanitary laboratory at the university." While the Board of Health took no immediate action towards creation of a physical laboratory, a resolution was passed designating that "a sum not exceeding three hundred dollars be appropriated to pay for results of original investigations in sanitary subjects, provided such results be presented to and accepted by this Board. [It was further resolved] that this Board desires to encourage special investigations into sanitary conditions at localities, with special reference to water supply, ventilation of public buildings, and the origin of epidemics."[15]

It was not long before the issue of public health was brought before the Board. Between August 1883 and August 1884, outbreaks of violent illness were reported in several regions of Michigan. The first report came from Oxford, then a rural area north of Detroit. The local health officer, Dr. E.P. Wilder, reported that during August 1883, over a dozen persons were reported ill with an intestinal ailment. Wilder suspected the source of the illness was cheese which had been eaten by the victims. The food had originated with the Eagle Cheese Company, located in Lyon, Ohio. Additional cases of food poisoning were subsequently reported in Barry and Hillsdale Counties. By the time the outbreak ended the following August 1884, some 212 persons had suffered from the same illness. In an early epidemiological study in which a comparison was made between those in individual households who became ill, and those who had not become ill, and the foods each had eaten, it was determined that the source of the illness was the cheese. Even within the same family, only those who had eaten this particular cheese became ill. The source was ultimately traced to one cheese manufacturer, the Old Original Fairield Factory located in Fruitridge, Michigan.[16] In hopes of determining the specific contamination, samples from the contaminated cheese were analyzed by Vaughan and his assistant, Dr. Charles Pengra, in Vaughan's university laboratory.

Vaughan found obvious evidence for the presence of toxins as the immediate cause of the illness, perhaps associated with the extensive bacterial contamination also found in the samples. In his final report on the subject, published the following year, Vaughan described his isolation and testing of the contaminant he found in the cheese. After extracting the material in alcohol, and allowing it to dry, he observed a "fatty mass," which upon tasting—self-experimentation being common during the time—resulted in a dryness in his mouth and a constriction of his throat. Vaughan further purified the mass, the result being a "needle-shaped" crystal which, when he placed a small quantity on his tongue, produced the symptoms of nausea previously described by the victims who had eaten the contaminated cheese. Vaughan termed the toxic agent "tyrotoxicon."[17] Vaughan correctly believed the presence of the toxin was the result of unsanitary practices carried out by the farmer in the collection and storage of the milk. This was the mid–1880s, a time when the germ theory of disease was just undergoing widespread acceptance by the physicians of the period. Vaughan correctly attributed the source of the toxin to be the result of bacterial contamination of the milk. "As the putrefactive changes in the milk are due to the growth of minute organisms, the introduction of these organisms into the milk may hasten its putrefaction, and, consequently, the formation of the ptomaine [poison]. The germs may be present in portions of milk which adhere to the sides of vessels which are not cleansed as often or as thoroughly as they should be. I would suggest that cheese manufacturers thoroughly inspect the cans in which milk is brought to them. When cows are kept in filthy stalls, the milk is likely to undergo speedy putrefaction."[18]

Chemical analysis of the tyrotoxicon resulted in the beginning of a long collaboration between two rising "stars" in the department: Vaughan and Frederick Novy. Working together, they determined tyrotoxicon was identical to a salt of the toxic material diazobenzol, and was likely produced as a result of bacterial putrefaction. When a small quantity of the substance was fed to a cat—research using live animals was common during the period—the animal developed symptoms identical to those exhibited by humans in the outbreak. Vaughan attempted to identify the micro-organism at fault. "We are conducting some experiments with the hope of ascertaining the nature of the micro-organism which produces this poison, but are not ready yet to make any definite report on this point. We will only say that it seems to be a germ which develops best in the absence of air [an anaerobe] or with only a limited supply of air. We have inoculated two samples of milk with the same material, leaving one sample open to the air and placing the other in a stoppered bottle, and after a few days found the poison in the stoppered bottle but not in the open beaker, though this may be explained by supposing that decomposition goes on more readily in the open jar and the poison does not accumulate. Fresh oysters, inoculated with poisonous material and left in an open beaker, become poisonous, and the same was true of some thick custard. Though here, again, the upper layers of the oysters or custard may have prevented free access of air to the underlying portions."[19] The collaboration between Vaughan and Novy, originating with the subject of tyrotoxicon, also resulted in the joint publication of their work in a book, *Ptomaines and Leucomaines*, the first in a long series by these authors on that general subject.

The methodology for precise identification of bacterial species had not yet been developed in the 1880s. Consequently, Vaughan and Novy could not determine exactly which bacteria were responsible for the toxicity in the milk beyond the likelihood that it was an anaerobe. From the vantage point of 125 years, we can say the toxin was a likely nitrogen compound by-product produced as a result of butyric acid fermentation, a process carried out by several species of anaerobic bacteria. Vaughan, in fact, suspected some of the decomposition of the cheese might have been due to butyric acid. The investigation did result in a positive outcome. Recommendations that proper sanitation measures were to be instituted were carried out. These included what today would seem to be obvious: proper cleaning of hands by the food handlers, better maintenance and cleaning of stalls, sterilization of food receptacles, and refrigeration of milk when stored or transported. Outbreaks of milk-borne illnesses became less common.

Vaughan's investigation of the milk-borne poisonings produced an additional benefit for the state: the establishment of a sanitation laboratory. Another request was presented to the Board of Health in October 1886. This time it was approved. "The proposition to maintain such a laboratory at the university has come about because of recent valuable work done in the present imperfect laboratory at the university, by Professor Vaughan, who lectures in sanitary science, in the school of political economy, at the university, and whose original investigations into the nature of the cause of numerous cases of poisoning in this state have resulted in learning, not only of the nature of that cause, but probably also of the cause of one of the most important diseases of mankind. Professor Vaughan's important researches are already known and acknowledged throughout the civilized world. It is a mistake, therefore, to suppose that it is an entirely new scheme to establish a laboratory of hygiene at the Michigan university. It is not an untried experiment. It is a proposition to give proper room, opportunity and support to a laboratory which has already made contributions of incalculable value for the promotion of human welfare; and a proposition to provide for better instruction in a subject now imperfectly provided for, but which is the most important of all subjects which receive attention at the state university."[20]

Approval for the establishment of a hygiene laboratory, presumably on the campus of the University of Michigan, was one thing. Funding for building such a laboratory was something else. The Board of Health then unanimously passed and placed a request before the Michigan legislature:

> To the Honorable the Senate and the House of Representatives
> Your memorialists, the members of the State Board of Health, respectively represent that:
> *Whereas*, The highest education and that of the most use, is that which bests fits mankind for right living, that which tends directly to the preservation of life, and to the perfection of physical and mental health and strength; and,
> *Whereas*, The teaching of knowledge "of most worth" at the University of Michigan is not yet well provided for; therefore,
> *Resolved*, That we earnestly memorialize your honored bodies to take such action as shall lead to the maintenance of a well-equipped laboratory of hygiene at the University of Michigan, and of such instruction in sanitary science at that Institution, as shall place that subject on a plane not inferior to that of any other subject taught at the university.[21]

Placing the laboratory on the University of Michigan campus would require approval by the Regents. Vaughan's lobbying directed at that body emphasized the scientific advantages to the university. "This laboratory should naturally belong to the University and have all the advantages of the association with the other departments.... In the association of these departments there will be felt an influence in the direction of scientific thought and investigation which will redound to the interest of the University and the state at large."[22]

Both Vaughan's request to the university Regents, and that by the State Board of Health before the legislature, were approved. While the initial request by the Regents before the legislature was for an appropriation of $75,000, to be used for several programs in science, including physics and hygiene, the actual amount approved by the legislature was for $35,000, to be used "for the construction of a building to be used for scientific laboratories and for the equipment of the same for the year eighteen hundred and eighty-seven."[23]

The appropriated sum was clearly not sufficient for construction of an entirely new building, and a compromise within the university would be necessary. Vaughan, along with Professor Prescott and Dr. John Langley, also a professor of chemistry, presented to the Board of Regents two requests: that a department of hygiene be established, that the new department would include physiological chemistry under a single chairman, with the title of professor of hygiene and physiological chemistry, and that an instructor in hygiene and physiological chemistry be appointed. The Regents accepted the request, and Vaughan was appointed as head of the department.[24] His colleague, Novy, by then having graduated with his doctorate, received the appointment as instructor. (See below.)

The question of where to house the laboratory was also settled with a compromise. Regent James Shearer, chairman of the Committee on Buildings and Grounds, pointed out that the $35,000 appropriation from the legislature was not adequate to construct a building for the new department. Instead, one-fifth–$7000—was to be used for purchase of equipment. With the remaining $28,000, Shearer's committee recommended "that a brick building be erected, three stories in height, and on a plan suitable to accommodate at least two of the laboratories, those of hygiene and physics, and that this proposed building be respectable and appropriate in design, and not to exceed in cost the sum of "28,000 [a sum increased to $30,000 by the Regents]."[25] The final resolution passed by the board stated "That the Committee on Buildings and Grounds be and are hereby authorized to procure and decide on designs and specifications for the two buildings intended for physics and hygiene in the one case and for anatomy in the other."[26] Construction was completed by the time Vaughan (and Novy) returned from Europe (see below), and ready for occupancy by January 1889. The building remained in use until it was demolished in 1966. The two appointments, along with their recent work on the subject of ptomaines, arguably represented the official beginning of the long collaboration between Vaughan and Novy.

Frederick George Novy (1864–1957)

Unlike Victor Vaughan, whose family had lived in the United States for generations, Novy was a first-generation American. He was born December 9, 1864, at 450 DeCovin Street in Chicago's West Side, notably only because, among the neighbors, was the family of Patrick and Catherine O'Leary, whose cow, according to legend, knocked over the lantern which started the Great Chicago fire in 1871.[27] His parents had emigrated from Bohemia in central Europe earlier that year, a time of significant political turmoil in the region. Bohemia, later to become a region in Czechoslovakia following World War I, was then part of the Austro-Hungarian Empire. During the 1860s, Bohemian nationalists attempted to establish a level of autonomy within the region, one of the most prosperous within the empire. Though a compromise of sorts was reached in 1867, with Bohemia, along with Moravia and Silesia becoming crown lands, the issue of nationalism would continue for another generation.

Novy's father, Joseph, born about 1825, was by profession a master tailor, a trade he continued in Chicago. He had served as a sergeant in the Austrian army, and possibly among those favoring Bohemian independence, found it preferable to emigrate to a safer country. Novy's mother, Francis, had been a milliner of some means in their homeland, and would continue such work in Chicago. Frederick was their third son, following Theodore and Bohumil, born while the family lived in Europe.

Education

Frederick's first formal education was a year spent at the "Mission School," a small one-story building in a largely immigrant area known as "The Fields." Now known as the "Near West Side," the area had originally been settled by Irish immigrants during the 1830s. During the period in the 1860s and 1870s in which the Novy family arrived, the area included large numbers of emigrants from Bohemia and the German States.[28]

Novy's interest in academics developed early. When he was seven, Novy transferred to the nearby Union School. As a result of one of the teachers discussing the works of Washington Irving—in particular, the story of Rip Van Winkle—he spent long periods at the public library reading the works of that author. Novy's secondary education continued at West Division High School, developing interests in history, particularly classes in classical Greek and Roman history taught by a veteran of the Civil War, Dr. Sam Willard. It was as a student in West Division High that Novy was exposed to classes in the sciences, including participating in a physics course taught by a recent (1869) graduate of the University of Michigan, George Clayberg.[29] But it was the field of chemistry to which Novy was particularly attracted.

Novy's chemistry instructor was a Swiss Frenchman, Marc de la Fontaine, an instructor who did more than "just" teach, but one who carried

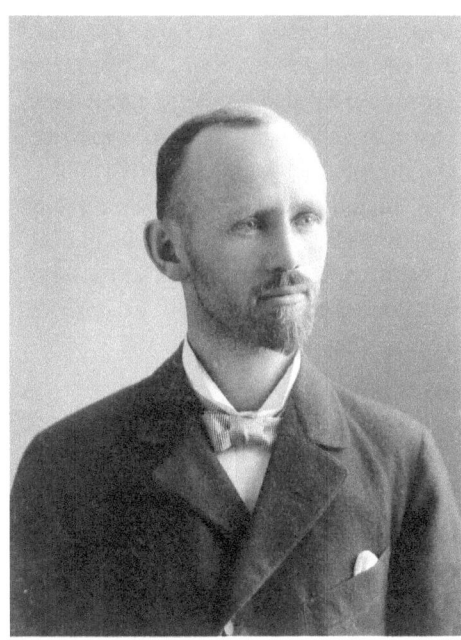

Frederick George Novy (1864–1957). Student and then a professional colleague of Victor Vaughan, with whom he collaborated on numerous medical topics, Novy served the university as a member of the faculty from the late 1880s until his retirement in 1935. He was the first chair of the newly established Department of Bacteriology at the university (1904), later serving as dean of the medical school (1933–1935) (Frederick G. Novy file, Bentley Historical Library, University of Michigan).

out original experimentation.[30] Novy was inspired by de la Fontaine to develop and carry out chemistry experiments on his own, building a small laboratory under the wooden back porch of his home. Among his amateur experiments was one which created an explosive gas, phosgene. Fortunately, no one was injured when the gas exploded, nearly setting the house on fire. But from that time on, Novy's experiments were confined to a separate woodshed.

Novy's interest in the sciences, and particularly in chemistry, was reinforced when de la Fontaine invited him to his home where he had a collection of laboratory instruments, including a microscope. With his eyes potentially opened to additional areas of science, Novy decided he wanted to purchase a microscope for himself. In order to earn the money, he accepted a job with the Chicago Public Library, working in the stacks during the evening and Saturdays; it required two years, but he earned enough to purchase an R & J Beck microscope for sixty dollars.[31] With his newly purchased microscope, Novy began an investigation of organisms found in the ponds and swamps around Chicago. He also received an invitation to attend meetings of the Chicago Microscopical Club, which met on Wabash Avenue downtown, at a site later occupied by the Marshall Field Store.[32] Not satisfied with merely observing microscopic organisms, Novy also studied in the literature the characteristics of his findings. Among his discoveries was a *Volvox*, found in a South Chicago pond, an organism formerly thought to be found only in Europe. Among the presentations by other members, was that of an organism thought to be a cause of hog cholera. Ironically, this would be a subject later studied by Novy for his doctoral presentation.[33]

Novy also used a portion of his earnings for the purchase of books, helped out with discounts when purchased through the library. While most of his purchases were related to microscopy, he also wrote to Dr. Albert Prescott, the organic chemist at the University of Michigan, and by then an acquaintance of Victor Vaughan, for a recommended list of chemistry books. Prescott responded with a list of books, including the three volume set *A Treatise on Chemistry* by Henry Roscoe and Carl Schorlemmer, several of which Novy subsequently purchased. Despite resistance from his father, who preferred Frederick follow him in the tailoring business, as did Frederick's older brothers, Novy decided on a career in chemistry.

The University of Michigan

De la Fontaine had highly recommended Professor Prescott as a possible mentor to Novy. Consequently it was the University of Michigan in which Novy decided to enroll for his college education. In 1882, he moved to Ann Arbor, accompanied by his parents in support of his education. Novy's study of chemistry began in earnest in his sophomore year, and by the time he graduated in 1886 with a bachelor's degree in that subject, he had taken every chemistry course officially offered at the university, including a course in physiological chemistry taught by Prescott himself, and some that were established specifically for his interests. Among these was a course in gas analysis, in which Novy worked with John Langley, professor of chemistry and metallurgy, in the study of gasses found in a Bunsen burner flame. While carrying out an independent study with Langley, Novy also designed his own apparatus, which he used as part of his analysis of the gasses.[34] Novy's abilities and potential were highlighted in a letter of recommendation later provided by Prescott: "I regard Mr. F.G. Novy as a student of unusual ability and a young man who gives excellent promise of success both as a teacher and as a worker in science."[35] Novy also had the opportunity to experience teaching directly, when, with the absence of two chemistry instructors during his junior and senior years, Novy was placed in charge of their respective courses.

Long an advocate for public health reform, Albert Prescott (1832–1905) played a significant role in Novy's future career. Born in Hastings, New York, his lineage included a grandfather, Colonel William Prescott, a commander at the battle of Bunker Hill in Boston. After earning his medical degree, Prescott came to Ann Arbor in 1860, joining the Department of Medicine and Surgery. Enlisting in the army during the Civil War, Prescott was subsequently appointed to the position of chief surgeon at Jeffersonville General

Hospital in Indiana, the third largest military hospital in the war. In 1865, Prescott returned to Ann Arbor, where he was appointed assistant professor of chemistry. When a School of Pharmacy was established at the university in 1868, Prescott was among its administrators. In 1876, he was appointed dean of the school. A further honor was conferred in 1884, with Prescott's appointed as director of the chemical laboratory, the position he held at the time of his association with Novy.[36]

Novy was one of three recipients in 1886 of the newly created Bachelor of Science degree in chemistry.[37] Following graduation, Novy returned to Chicago where he hoped to find a job as an analytical chemist, either teaching in a high school, or in an industrial position. He had little success. Novy found a total of three analytical chemists in the city, none of whom could make a living in that field. Partly in desperation, he contacted Philip D. Armour, president of the meatpacking company Armour & Company, offering to analyze waste products producing through the slaughter and processing of hogs. Armour was less than enthusiastic—asking at one point in the interview, "What's a chemist?"—but agreed to hire Novy on the condition that his salary would match any earnings the company accrued from his work. As it turned out, the offer was not a decision which Novy had to make. A proposal was made by Dr. Prescott at the university, offering Novy a position as assistant to Prescott in organic chemistry, replacing Theodore Wrampelmeier. The position came with a salary of two hundred dollars a year. Novy accepted the offer, and for the next two years taught courses in toxicology and organic chemistry, at the same time working on a Master of Science degree. In 1887, Novy received his degree, with his thesis titled "Cocaine and Its Derivatives," work which included the first synthetic alkaline derivatives produced on the Ann Arbor campus. His professional focus, to this point, was purely in the area of chemistry.

Novy's work with cocaine caught the attention of chemists associated with the Detroit pharmaceutical firm Parke, Davis & Company.[38] Established in 1866 by the Michigan businessman Hervey Parke, and chemist Samuel Duffield, and joined a year later by salesman George Davis, the company initially focused on marketing medicinal herbs. By the early 1880s, however, increasing demand for cocaine and its derivatives, allegedly for treatment of everything from pain to hysteria, caused the company to move towards manufacturing that drug from coca leaves. Novy's studies appeared to contribute to those goals, and the company subsequently published his work in 1887, the publication providing a detailed background of the discovery and use of cocaine, and the methodology involved in the manufacture of its derivatives; the publication would proceed through several editions. An additional half dozen studies of cocaine were also published that year, in a variety of pharmaceutical journals under Novy's name.

With an advanced degree in hand, Novy was offered a position at the University of South Dakota, as assistant professor of physics and pharmacy. Hesitant at accepting an offer in a field distinct from that for which he was trained, the decision became moot when Victor Vaughan, by then professor of hygiene and physiological chemistry, persuaded Novy to remain at Michigan as an instructor in hygiene. Novy would remain with the school for another six decades.

Along with the teaching position, Novy continued to pursue studies towards a doctorate in science (Sc.D.) degree, which he received in 1890; His thesis was titled "The Toxic Products of the Bacillus of Hog Cholera."

Focus on Bacteriology

It was during these first years working directly with Vaughan, 1887–1888, that Novy's interests gradually evolved into merging his chemistry background with the growing field of bacteriology. As described above, Vaughan himself had developed an interest in that field, and their collaboration on the tyrotoxicon study had already resulted in the book published in 1888, *Ptomaines and Leucomaines*. Novy's duties as an assistant to Vaughan included the chemical and bacteriological analysis of water. He could readily apply his knowledge of chemistry in examining the chemical factors which might be present, but he had only a minimal background in the new field of bacteriology. Further compounding the problem, nobody else at the university had the necessary knowledge of the field from which Novy might draw. Nor were there any sizable collection of handbooks on the subject. Novy was at least able to locate one book which proved significantly helpful: *Die Methoden der Bakterien-Forschung* ("The Methods of Bacterial Research"), written by Dr. Ferdinand Hueppe, a colleague of Robert Koch in Berlin, and only recently published in Wiesbaden. (A translation of Hueppe's textbook would later form a staple in American bacteriology courses.) Using the handbook as a guide, Novy prepared his first gelatin plates. By this time, Novy was also aware of the significant laboratory research carried out in Europe on the subject of bacteria and their role in infectious disease. Clearly this would have an impact for medical students interested in the etiological basis of disease.

Hueppe planned to offer a course in bacteriology during the summer of 1888 in Wiesbaden, and Novy proposed to Vaughan that they use their vacation time to participate in that course. Vaughan agreed that first-hand exposure to the methodology would provide the necessary expertise for their future work, but suggested that rather than going to Wiesbaden, they attempt to enroll in the course offered by Koch himself.

Vaughan and Koch in Berlin

Vaughan was initially informed that if they wished to participate in Koch's course, in light of the large number of worldwide applicants for admittance into the course, they would first have to obtain supporting letters from the President of the United States, or from the Secretary of State. Vaughan decided to ignore the advice, hoping the two of them would have no problem in enrolling once they appeared in Berlin. Vaughan was proven correct, as both he and Novy were able to immediately participate in the course without any problems.

Novy and Vaughan took full advantage of the opportunity to learn the principles and methodology of bacteriology, expertise which they would subsequently apply in their own laboratories back in Michigan. Novy, in particular, was now moving from a scientific filed largely consisting of chemistry, to one which applied chemical principles in the study of bacteria. Once he returned to Ann Arbor, he published an account of the daily routine taking place in the Berlin laboratory, much of which is described in Chapter 5.[39] Koch himself, while not personally working directly with the students in the class on a daily basis, did provide several lectures. Classes were small, which allowed for greater interaction with the instructors. Most of Novy's training involved working with Koch's assistant, Dr. Carl Fraenkel, the impact evident in Novy's future research. Novy had nothing but praise for Koch's Institute itself, expressing hope that in the future, equivalent research and educational facilities could be transplanted to Ann Arbor. "The Hygienic Institute of Berlin, known better to the world under the title of Koch's Laboratory, has attracted, by the wonderful series of brilliant discoveries made by Koch and his pupils, the close attention of medical and scientific men. It is one of those typical institutions of our day which are called into existence by, and owe their prominence to, the master-minds of their creators. The names of Pasteur and Koch are inseparably connected with the evolution and progress of the germ theory of disease which, ridiculed perhaps at first, has nevertheless, step by step, earned a reluctant recognition, till today it may be said to be an established fact. The classical researches of Koch, and the simplicity and extraordinary precision of his methods, are known and valued throughout the world. It is no wonder then, that students should flock, even from very distant lands, for the express purpose of receiving instruction at the hands of the master.... As already stated, the facilities for study at this Institute are unsurpassed, and up to within a few years, it was the only one of its kind where such instruction was imparted. Of late the importance of this department of study has been so well recognized that even most of the conservative universities in Europe have introduced it into their curricula. In our own country practical instruction in this important field of work is given at only a few educational institutions. It is expected that suitable courses in the study of bacteriology will be given before long in the new Hygienic Laboratory of the University of Michigan."[40]

Vaughan's impression of Koch on a personal basis was, to put it nicely, less laudatory, even antagonistic. The underlying basis for the latter's attitude towards Vaughan and, by extension, the entire scientific program at the University of Michigan, was clear. "While I [Vaughan] was at work in the laboratory, Professor Koch summoned me to a conference in his private room. I felt highly honored to be thus distinguished, but the burden of his talk was the condemnation of the University of Michigan for retaining as its professor of pathology a man who did not accept the well established fact that bacteria cause disease, referring to Professor Gibbes, whose name Koch pronounced with bitterness, biting it into two syllables. I tried to explain that I was an antagonist of Professor Gibbes' teaching and that my purpose in seeking instruction in Koch's laboratory was to fit me better to combat my colleagues' erroneous teachings, but I did not succeed in mollifying his anger. Robert Koch was a great man, but in many respects a typical German, ready to stamp upon those who did not acknowledge his authority. While I admired his work I could not be altogether pleased with his personality."[41]

Some of Gibbes' objections to Koch's ideas, particularly as they applied to the etiological agent of cholera, have been outlined in Chapter 8. Certainly he was not the only dissenting voice—witness the arguments expressed by Koch's countryman, Max von Pettenkofer. But Gibbes was more strident in his objections to many of the scientific advances taking place in the field; his doubts included Joseph Lister's antiseptic practices, vaccines as protective against infectious disease, and, of course, bacteria as etiological agents of specific diseases. Despite his brilliance in areas of histology and pathology, including his authorship of a recommended textbook on that subject, Gibbes' ideas continued to stir controversy in the medical school until his resignation in 1895.

In the tradition of the time, following the completion of the course, Professor Fraenkel and his assistants for the course were treated by the students to what was called a *kneipe*, the term referring to a pub, but to Vaughan represented a "drinking bout." Vaughan managed to remain reasonably sober—there is no record of the situation with Novy—and was among those who brought an inebriated Fraenkel home, and put him to bed.

Novy and Vaughan went their separate ways after leaving Berlin. Novy traveled to Paris, hoping to meet with Pasteur, but was unsuccessful. Vaughan spent the remainder of the summer traveling throughout Europe, visiting a number of cities in Germany and Austria, and also spending some time in Switzerland. He returned to Ann Arbor in the fall, in time for the completion of the building for the new Hygienic Laboratory.

Aftermath

Establishment of the Hygienic Laboratory, the first of its kind in the United States, represented the growing recognition of bacteriology nation-

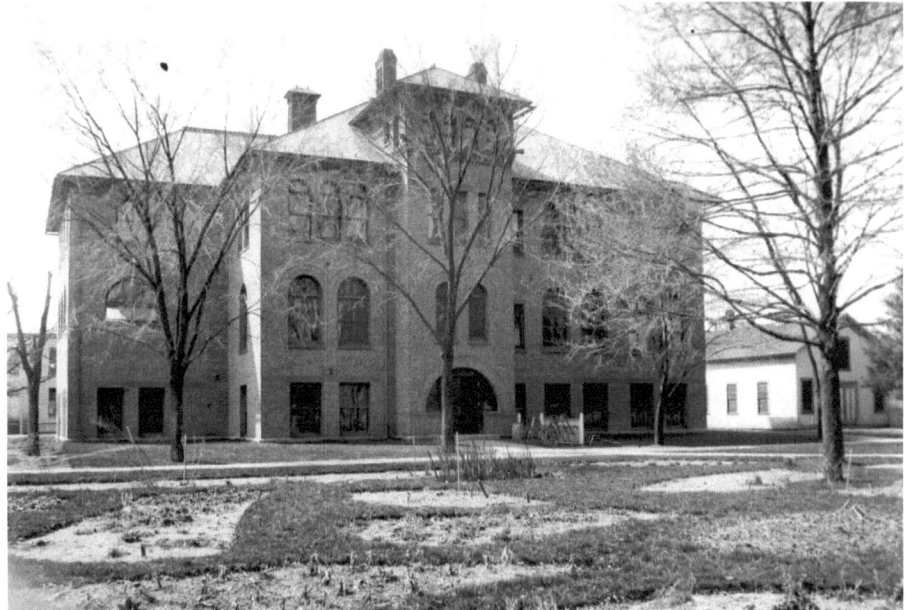

Hygienic Laboratory, University of Michigan. Constructed during the late 1880s, during the period in which Vaughan and Novy participated in Koch's bacteriology course, the facility served as both the site of medical investigations carried out on behalf of the state and teaching laboratories for medical students. A portion of the building also served as a physics laboratory. In 1903, a branch of the Pasteur Institute was established in the building for investigation of rabies outbreaks. The building was demolished in 1966 (Bentley Historical Library, University of Michigan).

wide as a discipline. It was quickly followed by others. The United States Marine Hospital had been established in New York the year before, moving to Washington, D.C., in 1891 where a hygienic program was developed. During the 20th century, the institution evolved into what is now the National Institutes of Health.

In 1900, a decade after the Michigan Hygienic Laboratory was established on the Ann Arbor campus, Novy summarized its impact on public health in the state. If one believes imitation to be the better part of flattery, Novy pointed out that in the wake of the establishment of the laboratory, other states followed, though "none have laid a broader and more thorough foundation for work in hygiene."[42] Twenty years prior, only the University of Munich in Germany—a laboratory established under the direction of the "father of modern hygiene," Max von Pettenkofer—possessed such a laboratory. Analysis of food or water was based purely on chemistry, including "metallic or vegetable poisons," though it must be conceded that, at the time, germ theory was only just being developed. "Epidemic diseases ... received only such consideration as could be obtained from a purely epidemiological standpoint."[43]

Novy summarized the importance of the Hygienic Laboratory in justifying its creation on the Ann Arbor campus. "The scope and usefulness of a hygienic laboratory is three-fold. It was called into existence by the desire or demand for a knowledge of the hidden facts which bore upon the causation of disease. The first object, therefore, of such an institute is to carry on original investigations whereby the bounds of knowledge will be materially widened. The practical application of known facts in elucidating health problems and in preventing disease constitutes another aim of a hygienic laboratory. The sanitary analysis of water, milk, butter and foods in general; the identification of disease-producing organisms in suspected tuberculosis, diphtheria, typhoid fever and in other affections render such a laboratory useful to the community. The third, and by no means the least important object of a hygienic laboratory, is that of instruction."[44] While several of the subsequent uses for the hygienic laboratory fell within the category of chemical analysis—most notably adulteration of milk by dairy operators[45]—the ability to grow, analyze and identify disease-causing organisms required the type of expertise acquired in Berlin.

The following January 1891, Vaughan offered a three-month elective course, based in part on the knowledge developed while enrolled in Koch's course. Vaughan's course was initially designated Sanitary Science, a continuation of that which had been taught since 1884, then simply named Hygiene, but focusing on bacteriology. Few students enrolled that first year, and even

10. Victor Vaughan and Frederick Novy

these were largely from the liberal arts program. There were two notable exceptions: Aldred Scott Warthin (1866–1931), later to become professor of pathology at the University of Michigan, and known as the "father of cancer genetics," and Dr. Henry Sewall (1855–1936), a professor of pathology.[46] Sewall at the time was suffering from tuberculosis, a disease which would shortly force his resignation, and wished to isolate and study the organism responsible for his disease. The course proved a success, and when Vaughan was appointed Dean of the Medical School in 1891, among the changes which he instituted was to change the bacteriology course from an elective to a course which was now required.

Vaughan's tenure as dean lasted until his retirement in 1921. During these decades, he oversaw the modernization of medical education, not only at Michigan, but in medical schools nationwide. Vaughan served his country in two wars, investigating outbreaks of typhoid fever among the troops during the Spanish-American War (1898), and the influenza pandemic during the First World War. A summary of his many accomplishments prior to his death in 1929 can be found elsewhere.[47]

In 1891, Novy received his medical degree from Michigan, his thesis titled "The Toxic Products of the Bacillus of Hog-Cholera," shortly afterwards being appointed assistant professor of hygiene. Still closely associated with Vaughan, with the latter's appointment as dean, Novy took increasing responsibility for the bacteriology program in the medical school. Arguably, no two individuals were as responsible for the development of the medical school at Michigan between 1891 and 1914, the beginning of the First World War, as were Vaughan and Novy. During these decades, the University of Michigan Medical School rose to elite status in the country, a school modeled in great part on the medical programs in Berlin and elsewhere.

In the years immediately following his attainment of two professional degrees, Novy devoted his time to both service in the area of public health, much of which involved collaboration with Vaughan, and in development of teaching newly instituted coursework in bacteriology for the medical program. It was in this realm that his time spent in Koch's laboratory was most beneficial. Even as late as the 1890s, few textbooks were available to students of bacteriology, and even these were primarily translations of those published in German. Novy had already written one text in the area of physiological chemistry, *Directions for Laboratory Work in Urine Analysis* (1892), which would eventually be printed in several editions, and two years later he produced *Directions for Laboratory Work in Bacteriology* (1894), which would also run through several editions. In his *Preface*, Novy outlined the course in bacteriology, while acknowledging his predecessors: "The subject-matter has been arranged entirely with reference to progressive work in the laboratory and, more especially, corresponds with the work as carried on in the Hygienic Laboratory of the University of Michigan. The course covers a period of twelve weeks of daily afternoon work. Illustrations of the various bacteria and of their cultural characteristics have been expressly omitted, as the student is expected to sketch from observation the form of each organism and its peculiarities of growth in the colony, and in tube culture.... The works that have been drawn upon freely in the preparation of these pages are Fraenkel's *Grundriss der Bakterienkunde,* Eisenberg's *Bakteriologische Diagnostik,* and Flügge's *Die Mikroorganismen.* The larger works of Baumgarten and of Sternberg were likewise frequently consulted, and in many instances recourse was had to the original sources."[48]

Each of these books would be well received:

Aug. 1, 1898; William Welch

I thank you very much for the copy of your "Laboratory Work in Physiological Chemistry." It seems to me a very useful, practical guide for students, and I am sure your students must receive an exceptionally good training in this important subject.

Very sincerely yours,
William H. Welch

May 1, 1899; Welch

I thank you very much for the copy of your "Laboratory Work in Bacteriology" (2nd edition). It seems to me a very helpful work and to cover the essentials of a laboratory guide. I shall take pleasure in calling the attention of my students to the book.

With best regards, I am,

Sincerely yours,
William H. Welch

May 6th, 1899; Edwin O. Jordan, Univ.of Chicago
My dear Prof. Novy:

Please accept my cordial thanks for the copy of your Laboratory Work in Bacteriology which you have so kindly sent me and allow me to offer my congratulations upon the completion of such an admirable work. I am sure that all practical workers will find, as I find myself, many suggestions of great value, not the least important of which are the hints and descriptions based upon your own laboratory experience...

I remain, Very sincerely yours,
Edwin O. Jordan[49]

Novy returned several times to Europe, including time spent studying at the University of Prague in 1894. That same year, Novy and Vaughan attended the International Congress of Hygiene and Demography in Budapest, where they had firsthand opportunity to hear Alexandre Yersin describe his isolation of the bacillus of bubonic plague, and Emile Roux and Emil von Behring describe their development of antitoxin for combatting diphtheria. He returned to the Pasteur Institute in 1897 for the study of the rabies vaccine. Pasteur had died several years earlier, but Novy did have the opportunity to develop a lifelong friendship with Pasteur's associate, Roux.[50]

By the end of the decade of the 1890s, Novy was a nationally recognized authority in bacteriology. In 1901, he was appointed to the United States Plague Commission in California, their task being to ascertain the presence of an outbreak of plague among the Chinese community in San Francisco. Their report stressed the importance of bacteriological examination of buboes (lymph nodes), observing the presence of the plague bacillus necessary for firm diagnosis of the disease. In 1902, Novy was promoted to professor of bacteriology, becoming chairman of that department. His research evolved into the study of trypanosomes, protozoans involved in several diseases, becoming the first to develop artificial media for their study in the laboratory. During the next decades, Novy carried out what is considered by many to be groundbreaking work in the study of anaphylaxis (with Paul de Kruif, and two of Novy's sons, Robert and Frank), as well as studies in microbial metabolism of bacteria, particularly that of the tubercle bacillus.[51] Among the extraneous events in his professional life during this period, Novy had been considered as the model for Max Gottlieb, a character in the 1925 medical novel *Arrowsmith*, written by Sinclair Lewis. In 1922, Lewis had been introduced to de Kruif, likely by Dr. Morris Fishbein, editor of the *Journal of the American Medical Association*. De Kruif, at the time,

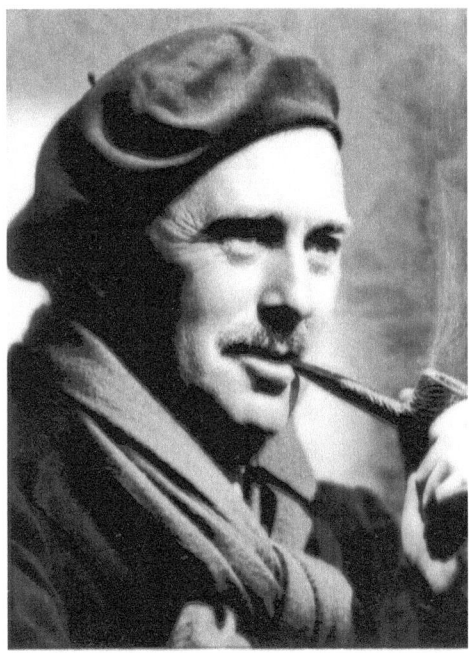

Paul Henry de Kruif (1890–1971). A doctoral student and colleague of Frederick Novy at the University of Michigan, De Kruif published works with Novy including studies of anaphylaxis as well as the toxicity of serum. Following his graduation and service in World War 1, de Kruif became a full-time writer. His most famous work was *Microbe Hunters* (1926), a staple for those interested in a career in microbiology. De Kruif collaborated with writer Sinclair Lewis in the latter's novel *Arrowsmith* (1925), basing several characters on professional colleagues (Paul de Kruif file, Bentley Historical Library, University of Michigan).

was just developing into the prominent author he later would become. Lewis and de Kruif decided to collaborate on the medical novel, which they wrote while on a ship traveling to the West Indies. While *Arrowsmith* was fictional, several of the events described in the book, as well as characters such as Gottlieb, had some historical basis.[52]

Novy retired in 1935, by then dean of the medical school, and the recipient of numerous honors. Despite his advancing age, Novy continued to contribute. With de Kruif as one of his co-authors, Novy's last scientific paper was printed in 1953. Novy was eighty nine years old by then. The article consisted of the description of a re-discovered rat virus, and was published four years before his death in 1957.[53]

11

Lydia Rabinowitsch-Kempner

In the final decades of the 19th century, many American physicians traveled from the United States to study with Koch in Germany. Rabinowitsch's career went in the opposite direction—it began with Koch, then shifted to the United States where she established research and pedagogical programs in bacteriology.

Dr. Rabinowitsch's career in the United States was ground-breaking in several aspects. First, of course, was that she was a woman in a field, medical research, dominated almost exclusively by men. When she was appointed director of the newly established Bacteriological Laboratory at the Woman's Medical College of Pennsylvania in 1895, she became the first woman in the United States to hold such a position. Also to her disadvantage was that unlike most scientists studying in that field, Rabinowitsch was not a physician; her Ph.D. degree was in a peripheral area of medical science.

Lydia Rabinowitsch was born on August 22, 1871, to Leo Rabinowitsch, a prosperous merchant and owner of a brewery, and Minna Werblunsky. Lydia was the youngest of nine children. Kovno, her birthplace, is now a city in Lithuania, but at the time was part of the Russian Empire following the absorption of the region in 1795. When she was born, the Jewish population of Kovno was approximately 36,000 persons, representing roughly half of the city's total population.

Unlike the situation in the United States in the latter part of the century, during the 1870s, within the Russian Empire, education of women in the medical field—indeed in the sciences in general—was much more commonplace; many of these students were Jewish, and at least within the Jewish middle-class, were encouraged to take advantage of the opportunities for higher education.[1]

The advent of Alexander II as Tsar in 1855 led to the institution of a number of significant reforms in the empire, not least of which was the emancipation of the serfs. In the fields of education, special programs were established specifically for the education of women, including state schools and *gymnasia* that taught the medical sciences. While the Jewish population was still restricted to living in the Pale of Settlement—the western portion of the Russian Empire—children of the middle-class were usually able to obtain permission to attend universities elsewhere.

This was certainly the situation for the Rabinowitsch family. Her father, Leo, died in an accident while Lydia was still a child, but his successful business left the family in an excellent financial state. Unfortunately, the greater acceptance, at least relatively speaking, of the Jewish population by the authorities would only be temporary. The assassination of Alexander II in 1881 by a member of the left-wing revolutionary group *Narodnya Volya* ("People's Will") was followed by a series of pogroms, and also resulted in many of the more liberal policies relevant to the Jewish population being revoked.

But despite the increase in terror directed at the Jewish population, utilizing the resources provided by her late husband, Minna was able to send five of her children to universities: three sons graduated from the German university in Konigsberg in East Prussia, becoming a physician, dentist and merchant, respectively; Lydia's older sister entered the field of law, while Lydia herself would enter the medical field.[2]

Lydia's (and her sisters') education began with their attending the local public school, followed by enrollment in the girls' *gymnasium*. While the school itself was non-Jewish, of the 310 students enrolled, 115 were Jewish.[3] Though the primary purpose of the girls' *gymnasia* was for the training of teachers, students nevertheless received rigorous training in the sciences and classics, as well as the opportunity to elect courses in Greek, Latin or German. This was the situation which proved advantageous to Lydia. In addition to becoming fluent in German, which included the study of German classics, she became particularly interested in the field of botany.

As a Jewish woman, Rabinowitsch found herself in the 1880s unable to enroll in Russian universities. Indeed, women in general had been unable to enroll in Central European institutions of higher education without special permission until nearly the time of her birth. The first institution to alter this policy was the University of Zurich in Switzerland, to be followed soon after by universities in Bern and Geneva. The Swiss policy was almost unique for this part of Europe. By the end of the 19th century, some five thousand women from Tsarist Russia were studying at Swiss universities, representing the majority of the students. Most studied medicine, and most were Jewish.[4]

So in 1889, at the age of 18, Rabinowitsch enrolled in the University of Bern, where she would begin her studies with an emphasis on botany.

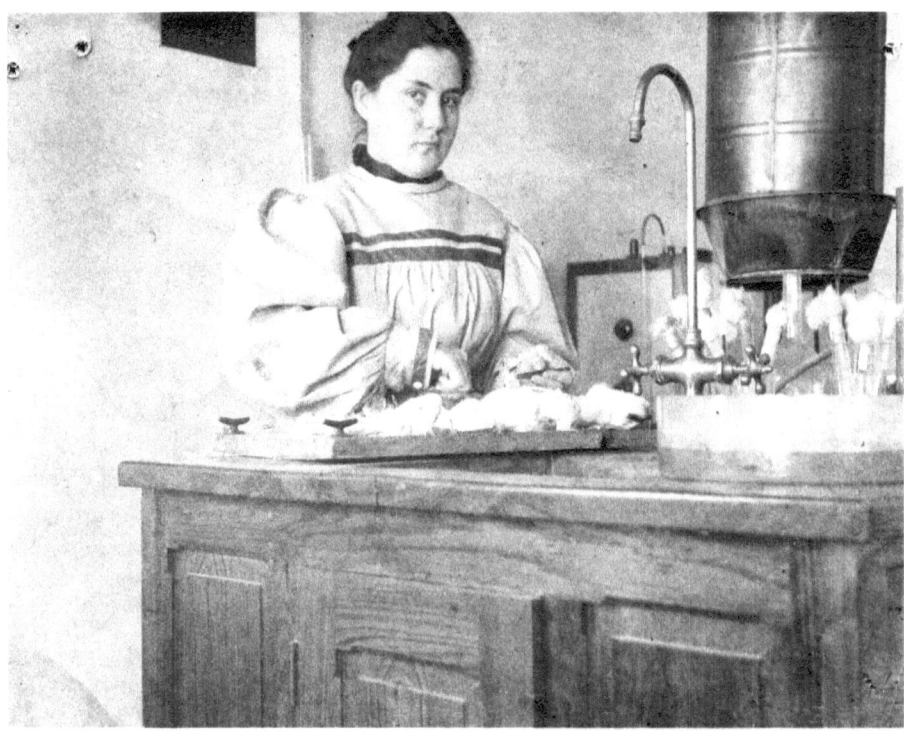

Lydia Rabinowitsch-Kempner (1871–1935). A German-born physician and bacteriologist, Rabinowitsch received much of her early training with Robert Koch. As a member of the faculty at the Woman's Medical College of Pennsylvania, now part of Drexel University College of Medicine, Rabinowitsch established the first bacteriology laboratory at that institution (Legacy Center Archives, Drexel University College of Medicine, Philadelphia).

Whether her "education" included an evolution in her political views during this period is unknown. But it would have been unusual if her friends—Russian Jews or otherwise—did not include those with left-wing tendencies.

One member of the faculty Rabinowitsch encountered in Bern was Dr. Eduard Fischer, one of the most important figures in the field of mycology (study of molds). Fischer was the son of Dr. Friedrich Ludwig Fischer, the late director of the St. Petersburg botanical garden from 1823 to 1850. Eduard Fischer himself later became director of the botanical garden in Bern.

In 1891, Rabinowitsch moved to Zurich, where at the university in that city she continued her studies in botany and mycology. Among the faculty with whom she interacted was Dr. Arnold Lang, professor of zoology and comparative anatomy, who expanded her training beyond that of the study of molds. While the extent of Rabinowitsch's exposure to the political views of her classmates in Bern is uncertain, while in Zurich she made the acquaintance of numerous women whose liberal views would influence her later beliefs. Among these women were Anita Augsburg, future lawyer and a leader in both the pacifist and feminist movements in Germany, and the revolutionary Rosa Luxemburg.[5]

Rabinowitsch returned to the University of Bern in 1893, earning her doctorate, *summa cum laude*, the following year for her thesis in mycology: "Beitrage zur Entwicklungsgeschichte der Fruchtkorper einiger Gastromyceten" (Contributions to the Development of Fruiting Bodies of Gastromycetes), once again under the guidance of Eduard Fischer.[6] Following her graduation, Rabinowitsch joined the laboratory of Robert Koch as an unpaid trainee at the newly established Royal Prussian Institute for Infectious Diseases in Berlin, where she began her research in a field more directly involved in medicine. As described in an earlier chapter, Koch and his colleagues by this time had developed many of the early techniques for growing and studying micro-organisms in the laboratory; Koch himself was already credited with the identification of the etiological agents of cholera and tuberculosis.

As a member of his laboratory (and the only woman at the institute) Rabinowitsch's work initially focused on the isolation and identification of thermophilic bacteria from sites around Berlin—organisms which grow best at temperatures above 54°C. She then applied her previous expertise in the study of yeast in observing the pathogenic properties of these organisms. This work resulted in two publications during her year working in Koch's laboratory: one dealing with her studies of thermophilic bacteria, the other a summary of her investigations of pathogenic yeast.[7] In September 1895 Rabinowitsch accepted an offer for work as demonstrator in a newly established bacteriology department at the Woman's Medical College of Pennsylvania in Philadelphia. As discussed in greater detail below, both the offer and level of support were associated with no shortage of controversies.

Establishment of the Woman's Medical College of Pennsylvania

> "That the exercise of the healing art, should be monopolized solely by the male practitioner ... can neither be sanctioned by humanity, justified by reason, [nor] approved by ordinary intelligence; prejudice, bigotry, and selfishness may dispute woman's claim to the high calling, but an enlightened liberty, and intelligent sense of justice, never. That woman, from the acuteness of her perception, correctness of her observation, her cautiousness, gentleness, kindness, endurance in emergen-

cies, conscientiousness and faithfulness to duty, is not equally, nay, by nature abundantly better qualified for most of the offices of the sick room, than man, very few will venture to contradict."[8]

The Woman's Medical College of Pennsylvania was officially founded March 11, 1850, when the Pennsylvania Assembly incorporated the college: "Be it enacted by the Senate and House of Representatives of the Commonwealth of Pennsylvania in General Assembly met., and it is hereby enacted by the authority of the same; That William J. Mullen, Frederick A. Fickard. M. D., Henry Gibbons, M.D., Jos. S. Longshore, M.D., Ferdinand Dreer, William J. Birkey, M.D., R. P. Kane, John Longstreth, and their associates, be incorporated under the name, style and title of 'The Female Medical College of Pennsylvania,' for the purpose of instructing females in the science and art of medicine; the said college to have all the powers and be subject to the restrictions contained in the act, entitled "An Act to incorporate the Franklin Medical College," approved the twenty-eighth day of January, one thousand eight hundred and forty-six."[9] The aforementioned Franklin Medical College had been chartered that day in 1846, only to cease to exist three years later.

The Female Medical College of Pennsylvania, forerunner of Woman's Medical College, was considered to be the first such institution in the world established specifically to educate women in the medical profession; as the name implied, women were the only prospective students admitted for training. The original idea for the college is generally attributed to Dr. Bartholomew Fussell (1794–1871). In a meeting with five other physicians at his home, The Pines, in Kennett Square, Pennsylvania in 1846, Fussell proposed the establishment of such a facility. Fussell, a member of the Friends (Quakers), was an ardent abolitionist; indeed, Kennett Square was an important stop on the Underground Railroad. For some time previously, Fussell had been providing medical training to women, and it was only logical, given his liberal leanings, that he would support the establishment of a more formal means for training female physicians. Fussell believed his sister Esther would have had the makings of a fine physician had she been given that opportunity. Esther, who married John Lewis in 1818, had four children (a fifth died in infancy), one of whom, Graceanna Lewis, was present at that meeting, later providing a description of the ongoing discussions.[10] Attesting to his support for the education of young women, Fussell also ran a boarding school for girls in York, Pennsylvania during the 1840s where Graceanna taught astronomy and botany.[11]

Dr. Joseph Skelton Longshore (1819–1879), along with William James Mullen (1805–1882), jeweler, philanthropist and practitioner of dentistry, are considered the key figures in the establishment of the medical college. Longshore had obtained his degree from the University of Pennsylvania at the age of 24, and in keeping with the Quaker tradition (including that in support of the abolitionist movement), was a strong believer in the education of women. Longshore's publication of *The Principles and Practice of Nursing* (1842) was his initial attempt to rectify the lack of medical training available to women at the time. In 1849, he helped draft the proposal for the Pennsylvania assembly which led to the establishment of the medical college. The original location was at 229 Arch Street, now 627 Arch Street following the renumbering which took place in 1858, which is just north of 6th and Market Streets, and the Liberty Bell—perhaps fitting—in modern downtown Philadelphia.

The first class when the college opened in October of 1850 consisted of forty students and five faculty members; Longshore taught the lecture in obstetrics. Both Longshore's sister Anna, and his brother Thomas' wife Hannah Myers Longshore, would become members of the first graduating class of that medical college in 1851.[12] At that commencement, held December 30, 1851, Longshore presented the address to the eight graduating students, noting the occasion with the statement, "this day forms an eventful epoch in the history of your lives, in the history of woman, in the history of the race."[13] The dean, anatomy professor Dr. Nathaniel Moseley, presented the eight women with their doctor of medicine degree.

While not a physician, Mullen's philanthropy was a key motivation for establishment of the college. As director of the Philadelphia Society for the Employment and Instruction of the Poor and its House of Industry, he provided food, a place of refuge, and job training for the poor of South Philadelphia. Much of his work was in the area of prison reform, where he was instrumental in promoting proper treatment of the incarcerated.[14]

Among the women initially enrolled in the college was Ann Preston (1813–1872). Preston had previously carried out an apprenticeship under the guidance of Moseley. But after being rejected in her applications to other schools because she was a woman, she enrolled in the Female Medical College, graduating at age 38 in 1851. In 1853 she became professor of physiology and Hygiene at the college, and in 1866 she was appointed as the first female dean.[15]

Joseph Longshore's sister-in-law, Hannah Myers Longshore (1813–1902), likewise was a member of the first class. Following her graduation, Dr. Longshore was appointed "demonstrator in anatomy," the first woman to become a member of the faculty at the college. Despite her expertise in that subject, she did not receive appointment to a professorship, likely because that position in anatomy was already filled by Moseley himself.[16]

The name of the college remained unchanged until 1867. Following the recognition of the ten graduates of the class of 1867 and the valedictory address, an announcement was presented, stating that "the Woman's Medical College of Pennsylvania is but an amended title for the Institution already well known as the Female Medical College of Pennsylvania.... In making this announcement, the Corporators and Faculty take pleasure in assuring the friends of the College of its increasing prosperity. A larger numbers of students attended its last sessions of lectures than had attended in any previous year, and a greater proportion were women of good preliminary education, and possessed of the determination and the means to make their studies thorough...

"The change in the title of the College, is accompanied with no change in its chartered rights or privileges. It is designed to be a simple recognition of the growing purity of our English tongue, which demands that terms shall be distinctive in their signification; and of the increasing regard for the dignity of woman—the co-worker with man, and his companion in the noblest thoughts and pursuits."[17]

The reason for the change in the name is uncertain, but likely originated with the perceived pejorative nature of the term "female." Peitzman, in his extensive history of the medical college, has suggested the change originated with the contemporary campaign of author Sarah Josepha Hale and her "zeal for the eradication of the term 'female' when applied to women."[18] Hale initially directed her campaign against Matthew Vassar, a friend of Hale's, who in 1861 founded what was then known as Vassar Female College. As cited by Peitzman, among the comments Hale directed at Vassar was "Female! What female do you mean? Not a female Donkey? Must not your reply be, 'I mean a female woman?' Then ... why degrade the feminine sex to the level of animals?... I write thus earnestly because I wish to have Vassar College take the lead in this great improvement in our language."[19] Mrs. Hale's campaign was successful; the term "female" was deleted from the name. Whether Hale's campaign was the key factor in the name change from Female to Woman's Medical College—which Peitzman thinks likely since Hale lived much of her life in Philadelphia—or a response to a general "feminist" movement is unknown.

The institution was stilled called the Woman's Medical College when Rabinowitsch joined the faculty nearly three decades later, and would be unchanged until it was renamed the Medical College of Pennsylvania in 1970, when admission was opened to men. In 2003 the institution, which had since merged with Hahnemann Medical School, became part of the Drexel University College of Medicine.

Member of the Faculty

> "A brilliant Russian who, with her slight accent and blue-checked bib aprons was the delight of all her students."[20]

The specific reasons as to why Rabinowitsch left Koch's laboratory in 1895, traveling across the ocean and accepting a job in a new facility, are unknown. However, in her study of European women in science in this period, Creese speculated as to several possibilities.[21] Rabinowitsch's association with Koch at that time was largely that of an unpaid post-doctoral position. She may very well have been searching for a more permanent, or at least a paid, position elsewhere, and such positions in Europe were few. Rabinowitsch may also have wished to establish her own credentials as an independent researcher. The possibility of setting up a new research program, while at the same time having the opportunity to teach (particularly women?), may also have had a strong appeal. Whatever the case, when the position became available, Rabinowitsch applied.

The establishment of a bacteriology department, even in the years prior to Rabinowitsch's application for the position of director, generated a significant amount of controversy within the college. The context of the time is important in understanding some of the reasons. The germ theory of disease, the idea that unseen micro-organisms might be involved in disease, had only recently been acknowledged; Koch of course was at the forefront of this theory. Physicians had not yet universally accepted this idea; the concept of miasmas, something in the air, as the basis for disease pathology was still prevalent. And even if medical schools had good intentions in introducing bacteriology into the curriculum, microscopes and other basic forms of equipment were expensive.

Thus the training of physicians in the nascent field of bacteriology in medical schools, particularly in the United States, was still new when Rabinowitsch came to the Woman's Medical College. While the WMC was not unique in adding the curriculum, it was still the rare exception. The University of Pennsylvania, also located in Philadelphia, had been among the first to provide such instruction for prospective students and visitors. In February of 1892 the Laboratory of Hygiene in their medical school announced a sequence of courses in elementary bacteriology: "Through the liberality of a number of citizens of Philadelphia, the University of Pennsylvania has been enabled to establish a Laboratory of Hygiene." That first year (1892) the curriculum consisted of two courses: "A Course in Practical Hygiene, and An Elementary course in Bacteriology." The four instructors came from the Johns

Hopkins Hospital. Among the first eleven matriculates in the program was Dr. Adelaide Ward Peckham, who some years later would become a major figure at the WMC. The 1895–1896 class consisted of thirteen students. Among the visiting students taking part in this program was Lydia Rabinowitsch.[22] Other schools had already incorporated similar bacteriological laboratories in association with hospital affiliates. In 1889, Dr. Edward Shakespeare (1846–1900) was hired as a bacteriologist at Philadelphia General Hospital. Shakespeare, a pioneer in ophthalmic surgery, was also well known for his investigations of cholera outbreaks around the world.[23] Likewise, in 1892, Dr. Henry Middleton Fisher, pathologist, "Curator of the Pathological Museum, and Microscopist" at the Pennsylvania Hospital in Philadelphia was granted a laboratory for bacteriology for "absolutely trustworthy diagnosis of some of the infectious diseases."[24]

In spite of those schools' successes in doing so, there were these challenges, and therefore arguments opposing the institution of a new program at WMC weren't unique to that school. The cost of the department would remain a real concern. Sources of revenue were always a challenge, and if funds were provided for this new department, would the funding in other programs at the college have to be reduced as a result? There was also the problem associated with what might be called inertia—the desire to maintain things as they already were. Bacteriology would represent a new area. The college had functioned perfectly well without instruction in this field, and in the minds of some faculty, could continue to function just as well in its absence. Another example of the controversies generated and pointed out by Walsh was that of the role of bacteriology *vis-à-vis* clinical instruction.[25] Dr. Frederick Porteous Henry, a professor of pathology and consulting physician at Woman's Medical Hospital, incorporated in 1861 and affiliated with WMC, visualized the integration of bacteriology with clinical instruction. Others saw this only as an interference with their own methods of diagnosis which were often based largely on observations.

The first discussions pertaining to whether the WMC should establish a bacteriology laboratory, and along with it, the hiring of a demonstrator, began late in 1890. Dr. Helen L. Betts (1845–1910) was sent to Berlin by a committee of the faculty to observe the bacteriological techniques in the laboratory of Robert Koch. Koch, in addition to isolating the etiological agent of tuberculosis, had recently reported the development of a (later discredited) vaccine against that disease using an extract called tuberculin. Betts, an 1872 graduate of the WMC now practicing in Boston, was considered an expert in pulmonary diseases of children as well as women's health. As the first woman sent on such a mission, Betts' experience in dealing with pulmonary diseases, and of course as a graduate of the college, made her an ideal choice for the endeavor. With its description emphasizing the importance of the advanced techniques developed by Koch and his associates, Betts' 1891 report played a significant role in the decision to establish such a laboratory.[26]

By December 1893 the decision had been finalized to establish a new department in bacteriology. The new laboratory for the program would be housed in a nearby row house owned by the college at 2106 Henrietta Street, not far from the orphan's school of Girard College. Several months later the faculty agreed on the hiring of a demonstrator to oversee the laboratory and instruct students in that discipline, a position which included a salary for the seven-month academic year. The candidate should be "a suitable person as Demonstrator in these branches who shall be able to give the necessary time to work through the entire seven months of the session, such work to be carried on in the present Pathological laboratory until the college shall have the funds for the erection and equipment of a building especially devoted to the practical departments of our school. The salary for this demonstrator will be $500.00 for the College year [18]95–96."[27]

By October 1895, three candidates were considered for the position. In the order in which the applications were received: Dr. Arthur Albert Stevens (1865–1944), Dr. Michael Valentine Ball (1868–1945), and Rabinowitsch, the only one among the three who was not a physician. Stevens was a local practitioner and auxiliary instructor, well known to the faculty at WMC. Ball, who had graduated from Jefferson Medical School in Philadelphia at the age of eighteen, had carried out postgraduate work in the laboratories of Koch, Emil von Behring, and the German physician and biologist Rudolf Virchow, who is considered the "Father of Pathology." On the surface it appears that simply on the basis of experience, preference would have been given to Dr. Ball. He had previously been an instructor in histology and microscopy at Niagara University in Buffalo, the city in which he had had his early schooling. Prior to applying for the position at WMC, Ball had lectured on bacteriology at the Academy of Natural Sciences (now part of Drexel University) and at the Franklin Institute in Philadelphia. He had also authored a textbook on the subject (*Essentials of Bacteriology*).

Despite the imposing credentials of the other two applicants, it was clear in retrospect that Rabinowitsch had the "inside track" for the position, one for which she had apparently not formally applied: "The Committee on Auxiliary Instruction would respectfully report.... Dr. Rabinowitsch has the degree of Doctor of Philosophy from the University of Berne, but not that of M.D. She has studied with Koch, [Ludwig] Brieger, [Paul] Ehrlich and others and is at present at work in the Laboratory of Hygiene of the University of Pennsylvania. She has published several articles on bacteriological subjects which I lay before the Faculty. One is her Inaugural Dissertation for the Doctorate [the aforementioned study of development of the molds of basidiomycetes], and the other two upon 'Thermophilen Bacteria ['Heat-loving Bacteria'] and 'Pathogene Hefearten' ['Pathogenic Yeast']. She is at present engaged in a research upon the pathogenic varieties of yeast, especially with reference to the etiology of tumors; a work which she has undertaken at the suggestion of Professor Koch."[28]

The decision to hire Rabinowitsch was further influenced by the alumni of the college who also favored her over the other candidates. Rabinowitsch joined the department that December. As expected, funding for purchases of equipment and supplies was the immediate problem. Much of her needed supplies—glassware and microscopes—had to be imported from Germany, though some materials were obtained "in house." The college appropriated $175.89 worth of supplies from other areas of the institution, which included eight microscopes from the department of embryology.[29] Cultures of microorganisms for use in the teaching laboratory were included among the supplies. Rabinowitsch spent the first months of 1896 preparing her laboratory for teaching. The question of when, in the course of their studies, medical students should enroll in the new bacteriology course had also been debated. As Walsh has pointed out, among the sources of contention was the role of clinical work carried out during the fourth year of study versus that of "practical medicine"—the underlying purpose of the bacteriology course. The dean, Clara Marshall, decided to include Rabinowitsch's course during the third year in hopes of avoiding any sort of conflict.[30]

In March 1896 the new course was taught for the first time, with Rabinowitsch as the instructor for the third year students; the fee was $10, with an additional deposit to allow for breakage. Rabinowitsch was an immediate success with the students as well as with Dean Marshall and other faculty. In the words of Marshall, also quoted above, Rabinowitsch was "a brilliant Russian who, with her slight accent and blue-checked bib aprons was the delight of all her students."[31] As a student in her class described her: "one of the sweetest, prettiest and smartest of women."[32]

This is not to say that all went smoothly during this time. It was routine to melt tubes or flasks of agar, the solidifying substance used to culture bacteria, over an open flame. "Agar that was heated too long had boiled over, resulting in a lot of broken glassware."[33] Another student recalled a potentially hazardous accident when "someone dropped a culture of typhoid bacilli on the floor. It was much more impressive than the lectures."[34]

Establishing the teaching laboratory was not the only challenge encountered by Rabinowitsch. Disappointed by neither having the time nor proper facilities to develop the research program she hoped to include, Rabinowitsch obtained leave to return to Koch's laboratory that August and September.[35] Koch had continued his research during the interim on the disease tuberculosis, attempting to answer the question of whether contamination of milk by a microbe similar to that which caused tuberculosis also posed a health hazard. Koch's initial thought was that the agent posed no significant threat to humans, but when he was unable to show whether or not the milk-borne agent was associated with human disease, controversy resulted.

The result was the so-called "Milk War," the competition between milk cooperatives for the lucrative profits from the sale of milk to the German public.[36] Hygienic principles often came secondary to companies' desire to sell their milk, and infections from milk or milk products were common. Rabinowitsch entered the fray, subsequently demonstrating and publishing that contamination of milk products did indeed pose a threat to public health.

When Rabinowitsch returned to the WMC, she expanded her lectures to include second and third year students. That her interests went beyond that of simply teaching and carrying out research in bacteriology, limited at present to her work in Germany with Koch, is attested to by a lecture she presented in the spring of 1897 at the Berlin International Congress on Women's Work before some 1700 participants. The title of her presentation was "American Women and Their Achievements," in which she noted "the freedom of young women, of family life, the women's rights movement, higher education, social life, women's clubs, the voluntary welfare system, etc." She also noted that "in 1892 there were 4555 women physicians and surgeons in the United States."[37]

The success and popularity of the bacteriology course developed by Dr. Rabinowitsch meant that within a year, the program had outgrown its facilities. In response, the faculty agreed to increase the size of the laboratories by erecting a new three story building, one which would include a "gymnasium, a laboratory of Hygiene and a lecture room."[38] The new facility would be the Hiram Corson Memorial Laboratory of Hygiene, named for Dr. Hiram Corson (1804–1896) who, at the time of his death, was the oldest practicing physician in the United States. Corson, like Longshore and others involved in the establishment of the college, had been a longtime advocate for the training of women as physicians, as well as an ardent abolitionist before the war. The new facility was ready for occupancy in 1898. By that time, Lydia Rabinowitsch was no longer associated with the Woman's Medical College.

The loss of Dr. Rabinowitsch to the college was the result of what almost could be called a comedy of errors, had it not been so important an issue. Part of the problem was that the desire to carry out independent research on her part was never truly acknowledged on the part of her peers on the faculty. There also remained the question of the nature of her appointment. The faculty had no difficulty with her serving as demonstrator; the promotion to a professorship, in the absence of a medical degree, was another issue entirely. "They were leery of the 'necessity of a professorship of a subdivision of a great department of medicine' and the 'advisability of a teacher without the training and the degree of Doctor of Medicine, becoming a Faculty member with the right to reject by examination candidates for promotion or graduation.'"[39] Faculty in the Department of Pathology likewise objected, viewing the subject of bacteriology as more appropriately a subdivision of pathology. In time honored fashion, an *ad hoc* subcommittee of faculty was set up to address the issue. The committee consisted of three physicians: Dr. Arthur Stevens, the same person who had previously applied for the position now held by Rabinowitsch, Dr. John B. Roberts, professor of principles and practice of surgery, and Dr. Anna Elizabeth Broomall, an 1871 graduate of the WMC and professor of obstetrics. The outcome was an unwillingness to provide "undue prominence to bacteriology by creating a professorship of that subdivision of pathology, since now [bacteriology] is the only department with good laboratory accommodations ... [it is wrong] to further emphasize bacteriology by raising it to the dignity of a Professorial chair ... unwarrantably to the relative importance of that department."[40]

Within two months, however, the faculty reversed their decision, not once but twice. In the April 16 meeting, Rabinowitsch received her first promotion, which included a significant increase in salary: "in view of the importance of the instruction involved, and of our present ability to secure an especially competent person to fill the position, it is for the best interests of the college to recommend to the Corporators that Dr. Lydia Rabinowitsch be appointed Associate Professor of Pathology in charge of the bacteriological department as Director of Bacteriology, with a seat in the Faculty, at the same salary paid the other professors, $1150 for the [academic] year 1898 and 9."[41] Her second promotion came two months later when her title became professor of bacteriology. Rabinowitsch accepted the offer, prepared to return to the college during the fall of 1898.

Why the sudden change in the decisions made by the faculty? We can probably ignore any altruistic explanation for their decision. More likely it had to do with her growing international visibility. During the second week of April, Rabinowitsch attended the Ninth International Congress of Hygiene and Demography in Madrid, Spain. Included among the attendees were a large number of German physicians and scientists, in addition to those from France, England and the host country. By providing Dr. Rabinowitsch with a more impressive title, the college could significantly increase its visibility and prestige.

With the close of the international meeting, Rabinowitsch returned to WMC for the completion of the session, after which she once again traveled back to Koch's laboratory to continue her work on tuberculosis. In particular, she focused on the question of whether the agent of bovine tuberculosis could infect humans. This time it was more than simply the opportunity to carry out research which drew her back to Germany. While attending the Madrid conference she married Walter Kempner (1864–1920) at the German consulate in that country. Their marriage and collaboration in the field of science would continue until his death—ironically from tuberculosis—in 1920. Walter and Lydia would have three children. Their son Robert (1899–1993), named for Lydia's mentor Robert Koch, would become a prominent American jurist who served as assistant U.S. chief counsel during the military trials at Nuremberg after World War II. Their two other children were Nadeshda, who in 1932 also succumbed to tuberculosis, and another son, Walter (1903–1997), who would as a scientist study metabolic diseases at Duke University.

While working in Koch's laboratory that summer Rabinowitsch agreed (in principle) to accept the WMC offer of a professorship, but requested she be granted leave until January 1899. The faculty refused. After a second request Rabinowitsch was informed that if she did not return by mid–October her appointment would be canceled. She didn't, and it was, severing her ties with the college. Rabinowitsch's vacated position as director of the bacteriology laboratory was filled by Dr. Adelaide Ward Peckham. Peckham (1848–1944) would prove to be a wise choice. In her own professional career, Peckham would become well known for her work with colon bacilli, more specifically for her studies of the effect of the intestinal environment on the etiological agent of typhoid fever.[42]

Rabinowitsch-Kempner ultimately had a long and successful scientific career despite having to deal with the increasing level of anti–Semitism in Germany. Her scientific pursuits would take her far afield. In 1902 she and her husband traveled to Odessa to investigate an outbreak of plague which had begun the previous December. Later, she accompanied Koch to East Africa to study an outbreak of sleeping sickness. Eventually, however, the primary focus of her research would become the study of the etiological agent of tuberculosis: a species of mycobacteria. In at least one area, the student taught the teacher. Koch's belief was that human and bovine tuberculosis were caused by different species. Rabinowitsch-Kempner's "unitary theory" proposed that the diseases were caused by variations of the same species. Rabinowitsch was able to isolate several bovine-type mycobacteria from patients with tuberculosis, evidence in favor of her theory. As a result physicians and other healthcare workers became more aware of the danger of ingesting the micro-organisms for a disease previously thought to be entirely airborne.[43] In 1903, Dr. Rabinowitsch-Kempner became an associate at the Pathology Institute of Charité Hospital in Berlin.

Rabinowitsch-Kempner was further honored in 1912 by Kaiser Wilhelm II himself, who awarded her with the title of Professor. With Koch's death two years previously she had lost an advocate whose prestige might have helped her overcome the anti–Semitic attacks which prevented her from attaining a position at the University of Berlin. She was forced to rely on grants to continue her research. In 1918 she became director of the bacteriology laboratory at the Berlin-Moabit Hospital Biological Institute, a position she held until the Nazi takeover in 1933. With increasing attacks on the Jews making their lives more hazardous, both sons escaped to the United States. Rabinowitsch-Kempner died in August 1935.

Lydia Rabinowitsch served as demonstrator in bacteriology at the Woman's Medical College only slightly more than two years, with some of that time being spent in Europe. Nevertheless, she still had a significant impact on the school. As the first Director of the Bacteriology Laboratory, she helped establish a teaching laboratory in a discipline which was only going to grow in the ensuing years. As an instructor, she helped develop a new generation of women physicians, imparting her knowledge of bacteria and their role as etiological agents of disease. The question remains, however, as to why she accepted this position in the first place. As suggested earlier and alluded to by Creese, she may have been motivated by the promise of a salary. Rabinowitsch's marriage to Walter Kempner, an independently wealthy member of a family of bankers as well as a physician and researcher, afforded her financial stability which allowed her to pursue her true interests in research.[44]

12

American Bacteriology After Koch

During the late 1870s, about the time Koch was carrying out his studies on the anthrax bacillus in Germany, few investigations, and even fewer courses in the medical curricula at American universities, dealt with the (then) new germ theory of disease. Welch, for one, felt the only means to address this problem was to study directly with the European pioneers in the field. "I am glad that I did not attempt to dabble at the subject in New York, for I might have made as melancholy a failure of my cultivations and experiments as [Henry] Formad. The methods can be learned only by personal observations in a laboratory."[1] The exceptions stand out simply because they were uncommon. This is not to say all American bacteriology was nondescript. Some examples are described in Chapter 3. Thomas Burrill, plant pathologist at the University of Illinois, identified in 1877 the etiological agent of the plant disease pear blight as a bacterium, naming the agent *Micrococcus amylovorus*. His knowledge of bacteriology played a significant part in the botany course which he taught, in addition to publishing, several years later, one of the first manuscripts in the United States which described the state of bacteriology.

Another notable exception was George Sternberg, some of whose work was previously outlined in Chapter 3. In addition to publishing the first significant works in America dealing with bacteriology, a translation of the Antoine Magnin work *Les bactéries* (*The Bacteria*), he is credited with identifying, in 1881, the pneumococcus as the etiological agent of bacterial pneumonia, the first (and to then only) organism associated with a human disease to be isolated by an American bacteriologist. *The Bacteria*, expanded as *The Manual of Bacteriology*, updated with numerous editions, would be a standard text used in bacteriology courses for decades.

Then there were those who did not have the immediate opportunity to participate in Koch's courses, but nevertheless were indirectly influenced by his work. Dr. Theobald Smith, a bacteriologist and first inspector of the Bureau of Animal Industry which was established in 1884, has been considered by some as the first American research scientist. Smith's superior at the BAI, Dr. Daniel Salmon, was the Chief of the Bureau, and often the recipient of honors for work carried out by those working under him. Smith enrolled in the Albany Medical College in 1881, receiving his medical degree two years later. During these years, Smith had the opportunity to participate in laboratory work, spending a spring at the Johns Hopkins University. Shortly afterwards Smith was hired as a laboratory assistant with the Veterinary Division at the United States Department of Agriculture in Washington, D.C. Though his training was primarily that for the study of human disease, he became more interested in the veterinary application of his training. When the BAI was created in May of the following year, with Salmon as its Chief, Smith was hired as Inspector. The function of the Bureau was to investigate the bacteriological basis of animal diseases and to ensure meat was safe for the general public. In his career, lasting from 1886 to 1932, some 75 of his more than 300 publications addressed subjects in bacteriology.[2]

Smith had received little training in bacteriology as a medical student, and when he went to Washington as a member of the BAI, he knew little of the methodology of the subject. He did not have the means or opportunity to travel to Europe at the time, but this did not hinder his growing interest in learning bacteriology. As it turned out, Smith

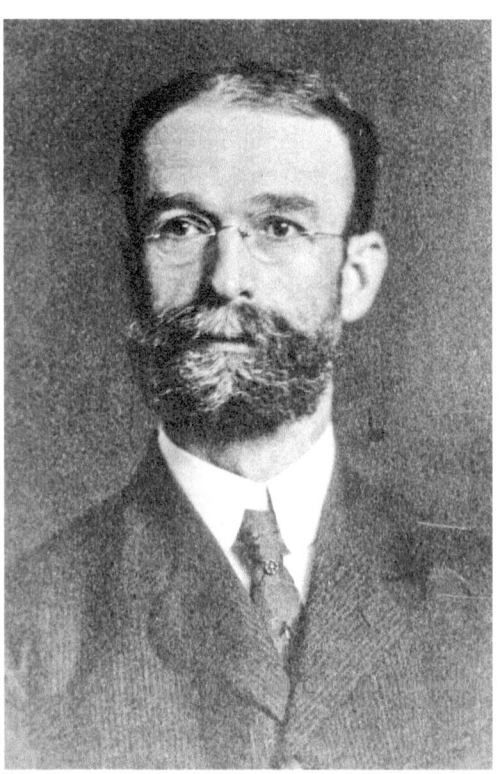

Theobald Smith (1859–1934). A bacteriologist and first inspector of the Bureau of Animal Industry, Smith has been considered by some as the first American research scientist in the field of bacteriology. In 1893, he identified the protozoan which was the etiological agent of what was called Texas Fever. He later identified the bacterium subsequently named *Salmonella*, after Daniel Salmon, his superior at the Bureau of Animal Industry (National Library of Medicine).

was conversant in speaking and reading both French and German. To address his deficit in the field of bacteriology, Smith translated some of the significant works of Pasteur's and Koch's, particularly those from the latter which dealt with tuberculosis. With practice in the laboratory, Smith was able to apply Koch's methods in his own work, as a side effect introducing those procedures to American laboratories. "In the examination of sputum for the *Bacillus Tuberculosis*, it is essential that the sputum be from the proper source, that the method of staining be properly applied, and that the microscope employed be of sufficient power to bring the bacillus distinctly into view. Among the many methods and modifications of methods that have been suggested, or are in actual use, I select the one now employed by the discoverer of the bacillus himself [i.e., Koch]."[3] Smith continued with a detailed description of the method utilized by Koch for the identification of the etiological agent. The use of hot fuchsin as the stain, followed by decolorization using an acid-alcohol mix, is identical in principle to the modern acid-fast staining procedure. In 1896, during a trip to Europe, Smith had the opportunity to meet with Koch in person. Smith had already demonstrated by this time, the distinctive relationship between the agents of bovine tuberculosis, and that of humans, a distinction disputed by Koch. "We may now maintain without fear of contradiction that the bovine bacillus presents certain traits which serve to distinguish it from the great majority of bacilli isolated from the human subject. These traits or characters are not the exclusive property of the bovine bacillus as contrasted with those from human sources. I am merely emphasizing the constancy of such characters and not their peculiarity."[4] Smith turned out to be correct, though it would be some time before this was acknowledged by Koch.

Smith's most notable work during these years, which he published in 1893, was the demonstration that the etiological agent of Texas Cattle Fever was a protozoan, *Pyrosoma bigeminum*, and transmission was carried out by a tick, *Boophilus bovis*, the first animal disease shown to be arthropod-borne.[5] While it was therefore true that Smith's initial training was not directly at the hands of either Koch or his associates, he still was part of the 1880s cohort whose developing expertise was the direct result of Koch's research and influence.

But it was arguably the group of American physicians who traveled to Berlin for direct laboratory training who, if one looks at actual numbers, ultimately had the greatest long-term ("scientific genealogy," if you will) influence in creating future generations of American researchers. William Welch, Theophil Prudden, and Harold Ernst, as related in previous chapters, all spent some time during the mid–1880s learning directly from Koch. After completing his training in Berlin, Welch returned to Baltimore, bringing with him cultures of bacteria—which did not include the cholera bacillus—and the knowledge and expertise necessary for developing a course in bacteriology for the new medical school. George Sternberg was among the first to study with Welch at Johns Hopkins. Among Sternberg's contemporaries who either learned bacteriology under Welch's tutelage, or received more advanced training in the subject, was Dr. Walter Reed (1851–1902), army physician and member of both the 1898 Typhoid Commission investigating the epidemics of that disease in army camps during the Spanish-American War, and head of the Yellow Fever in Cuba, which confirmed the role of the mosquito in transmitting that disease.

Dr. Simon Flexner (1863–1946), the first and long-time (1901–1935) director of the Rockefeller Institute for Medical Research, and Welch's biographer, carried out postdoctoral work in pathology and bacteriology—the latter rather reluctantly on Welch's part to be more accurate—under Welch's tutelage in 1890. Flexner later pointed out, that while Welch followed the European model in the sense of stressing the importance of research in applying scientific knowledge, he also imparted his own adaptations in merging that model with American ingenuity. "He [Welch] had come to the Hopkins eager to establish the German system of laboratory education there, but the result was very different. In Germany, a laboratory entered on the investigation of a large subject which provided a variety of separate problems that were parceled out among the advanced students, the professor keeping the many threads in his own hands. The nature and comprehensiveness of the general subject reflected the inventiveness, fertility and technical skill of the professor, which also determined the results achieved.

"This was not Welch's way. He never devoted his laboratory to the investigation of any single subject, nor did he show any special fertility in the choice of problems for himself or others; his own choices ... were determined by fortuitous circumstances, not any plan. And he never set a student to work on a concrete problem, seeming rather to avoid any such commitment; he held that men did not work well on assigned tasks."[6]

Alexander C. Abbott had the opportunity to train under two American pioneers, Sternberg and Welch. Though initially trained in bacteriology with Sternberg, he joined Welch as an assistant when the latter became director of the Pathological Institute, where the two confirmed Friedrich Loeffler's identification of the diphtheria bacillus. Welch's isolation of the gas gangrene bacillus, *Clostridium welchii*, with his student and colleague George Nuttall, has previously been described (Chapter 7). Nuttall had a long distinguished career in which his research focused on studies of tick-borne diseases. Among others during these years was Harry Lumen Russell, who received his Ph.D. at Hopkins in 1892 while studying under Welch after studying with both Koch and Pasteur several years earlier. Russell became a significant figure at the University of Wisconsin in the field of agricultural bacteriology (Chapter 3).

Welch's teaching and influence was, of course, not confined solely to the field of bacteriology, but included pathology as well. At least two Nobel laureates spent time with Welch: Drs. George Whipple and Peyton Rous. Whipple (1878–1976) was awarded the Nobel Prize in Physiology or Medicine for his application of liver extracts in the treatment of certain forms of anemia, and Rous (1879–1970) was awarded the 1966 Nobel Prize in Physiology or Medicine, for his work in the transmission of certain types of tumors using cell-free extracts (viruses). Interestingly enough, Rous' son-in-law, Sir Alan Lloyd Hodgkin, was also a Nobel laureate, being awarded the 1963 Nobel Prize in Physiology or Medicine for his role in studies of nerve transmission.

Theophil Prudden, following the completion of his participation in Koch's laboratory course, returned to New York and developed his own programs in the field of bacteriology, some of which involved collaboration with Biggs in the city's health department. An account of Prudden's career is found in Chapter 6. Prudden's 1885 report to the Connecticut Board of Health of his experience in Koch's laboratory was a major factor in bringing him to the forefront in the field of public health. The report produced in the early 1890s by Prudden, Biggs and Loomis, which outlined the nature and spread of tuberculosis in New York City, and recommendations for its control, became a classic in that field. Both Prudden and Biggs, in turn, were major influences in the career of William Hallock Park (1863–1939), the New York City bacteriologist who became the long-time director of the city's Board of Health Division of Pathology, Bacteriology and Disinfection, serving from 1893 to 1936. Park had already received training in bacteriology under Prudden in 1890, investigating the bacteriological diagnosis of diphtheria prior to his appointment. Biggs had recently been appointed to the position of Chief of that division of the Board of Health, and in turn, in May 1893, appointed Park for the purpose of developing a laboratory. Focusing on diphtheria, before the end of that year Park would produce a definitive report on the diagnosis and spread of that disease, demonstrating "(1) the validity of the culture test as the only reliable criteria for the diagnosis of diphtheria; (2) the persistence of virulent diphtheria bacilli in the throats of convalescents; and (3) the importance of the well carrier in the transmission of the disease."[7] Application of the report included the use of diphtheria antitoxin by Park and Biggs, under the auspices of the Board of Health, in treatment of the disease. It was said in his lifetime, "Park contributed more than any other living man to the development of bacteriological diagnosis and serum treatment which has made possible the conquest of diphtheria."[8] Park would subsequently establish the nation's first municipal bacteriological department used specifically for diagnosis of disease, not only addressing diphtheria, but in the prevention and treatment of other infectious diseases.

The careers of both Vaughan and Novy, and their professional contributions have been recounted in Chapter 10. Once appointed Dean of the University of Michigan Medical School, Vaughan spent much of his time immersed in administrative work, modernizing the curriculum of the program, and hiring those instructors who could teach, carry out research, and become involved in clinical practice. Both he and Novy, in the years after the latter received both his doctorate and a medical degree, dedicated much of their research on toxic products produced during bacterial growth or infection. Novy also focused on the application of his studies in improving public health, educating the general public (and medical students as well) on germ theory of disease, food poisoning and disinfection.

With the improvement in medical education in the United States, including the incorporation of bacteriology often taught by the 1880s "alumni" of Koch's courses into those programs, one might have expected a rapid decrease in the number of American students traveling to Europe; such was not the immediate result. Several events associated with Koch served for a time to maintain the interest of prospective American physicians. In 1890, Koch announced a "cure" for tuberculosis, an extract prepared from the bacilli called tuberculin. Though based on a similar premise used for some other vaccines, tuberculin subsequently proved to be largely useless. Colleagues of Koch, in particular Emil von Behring and Paul Ehrlich, were more successful in developing a diphtheria vaccine and antitoxin treatment of the illness. It was an application of this development which Biggs and Park applied in New York. At the same time, the building and opening of Koch's Institute for Infectious Disease as part of the University of Berlin continued to stimulate the interests of American students, as well as those from other countries. In Koch's 1891 course taught at the new Institute, of the thirty-three students enrolled, fourteen were German, while among the nineteen foreign students were ten Americans. Between 1891 and the beginning of the war in 1914, twenty American students participated in the course.[9]

One example was Dr. Rufus Cole (1872–1966), who bridged a number of those individuals taught by, or were influenced by, Koch. Born in Rowsburg, Ohio, Cole received his undergraduate degree from the University of Michigan in 1896. Though his initial inclination was to enter the medical school of that University, he decided instead to enter the Johns Hopkins

School of Medicine, graduating in 1899. During the period of 1903–1904, Cole traveled to Berlin where he spent the year at Koch's Institute, working with August Paul von Wassermann in a study of the typhoid bacilli. Wassermann himself would later develop a test for the presence of syphilis. In 1908, Cole was appointed Director of the Hospital of the Rockefeller Institute, while both maintaining and directing research into pulmonary diseases such as pneumococcal pneumonia and tuberculosis. Among the co-workers he appointed at the hospital was Dr. Oswald Avery, who during the 1940s would identify DNA, rather than protein, as the hereditary material in cells.[10]

Koch's laboratory was certainly not the only attraction in Germany for American students interested in bacteriology; several others have been described in earlier chapters. The German climate for research, aided in no small measure by government support, and not limited to bacteriology among the sciences, provided fertile grounds for several generations of scientists. Some were colleagues or associates of Koch's; many were not.

While we think of American or British physicians as those who most disputed Koch's ideas as pertaining to germ theory—Henry Formad and Heneage Gibbes come immediately to mind—acceptance was not universal even among German scientists. Some were hosts to American students as well. Max von Pettenkofer from the University of Munich, arguably among the most important figures in areas of hygiene and public health, disagreed so strongly with Koch as to the bacterial agent of cholera, that in 1892, long after most physicians had accepted Koch's identification, he swallowed a beaker full of bacillus to support his contention. He had at least one American student: Alexander Abbott. Pettenkofer's Institute of Hygiene, which had been established in 1879, served as a model for similar institutions established in the United States in later decades.

But 1900 also served as a breaking point for American interests in European bacteriology. By that year, a second generation of American students was being taught by American professors, trained and experienced in European methods. Medical curricula, which included courses in bacteriology, were becoming more rigorous. In upcoming years, the Flexner Report, a description of American medical education produced by Abraham Flexner, brother to Simon Flexner, included specific recommendations necessary for proper training of physicians. Published in 1910, the impact included the closing of most so-called medical schools in the country. While the upcoming world war would finally put an end to American travel to Germany for scientific training, the conflict merely hurried a process which had already become inevitable.

Chapter Notes

Preface

1. A more personal description of events surrounding Vaughan's visit can be found in his autobiography, *A Doctor's Memories* (Indianapolis: Bobbs-Merrill, 1926).
2. This is not meant to discount the contributions of scientific researchers in France or elsewhere, obvious examples being Louis Pasteur or the Curies in their respective fields. This author merely wishes to make the point that a disproportionate level of scientific contributions originated in Germany during these years.

Introduction

1. R.M. Jones, "American Doctors and the Parisian Medical World, 1830–1840," *Bulletin of the History of Medicine* 47, no. 1 (1973): 40–65; cited by David McCullough, *The Greater Journey: Americans in Paris* (New York: Simon & Schuster, 2011), p. 106.
2. The modern concept of a virus, a microscopic infectious entity unable to be observed with the instrumentation of that period, would not appear until the following century. To a bacteriologist of the 1870s or 1880s, the term virus was either used generically to denote an infectious agent, or meant a poison, the original definition of the term.
3. James R. Manley, *Letters Addressed to the Board of Health and to Richard Riker, Recorder of the City of New-York* (New York: Peter van Pelt, 1832), p. 15. Also cited by Sonia Shah, *Pandemic* (New York: Farrar, Straus and Giroux, 2016), pp. 104–105.
4. Richard Adler, *Cholera in Detroit: A History* (Jefferson, NC: McFarland, 2013), p. 67.
5. Thomas Neville Bonner, *Becoming a Physician: Medical Education in Great Britain, France, Germany and the United States, 1750–1945* (New York: Oxford University Press, 1995), p. 176.
6. *Ibid.*, p. 178.
7. William M. Hubbard and Nicholas H. Steneck, *The Origins of Michigan's Leadership in the Health Sciences* (Ann Arbor, MI: Historical Center for the Health Sciences, 1995), p. 38.
8. http://elane.stanford.edu/wilson/html/chap22/chap22-sect3.html.
9. Simon Flexner and James Thomas Flexner, *William Henry Welch and the Heroic Age of American Medicine* (Baltimore: Johns Hopkins University Press, 1941), p. 113.
10. Bonner, *Becoming a Physician*, pp. 159–160.
11. *Ibid.*, p. 160.
12. *Ibid.*, p. 164. The university town of Strasbourg would change hands following the Franco-Prussian War.
13. Thomas Neville Bonner, *American Doctors and German Universities* (Lincoln: University of Nebraska Press, 1963), p. 18.
14. Bonner, *American Doctors*, p. 253.
15. *Ibid.*
16. *Ibid.*, p. 254.

Chapter 1

1. Owsei Temkin, "The European Background of the Young Dr. Welch," *Bulletin of the History of Medicine* 24, no. 4 (1950): 316–317. Cited by Bonner, *American Doctors*.
2. Thomas Brock, *Robert Koch: A Life in Medicine and Bacteriology* (Washington, D.C.: American Society for Microbiology, 1999), p. 11.
3. *Ibid.*
4. *Ibid.*, p. 12; William Ford, "The Life and Work of Robert Koch," *Bulletin of the Johns Hopkins Hospital* 22, no. 250 (December 1911): 415–425.
5. Christoph Gradmann, *Laboratory Disease: Robert Koch's Medical Bacteriology* (Baltimore, MD: Johns Hopkins University Press, 2009), p. 25.

6. Ford, p. 416.
7. Brock, *Robert Koch*, p. 19.
8. *Ibid.*, pp. 19–20.
9. Edwin Klebs, *Beiträge zur Pathologischen Anatomie der Schusswunden* [Contributions to the Pathologic Anatomy of Battle Wounds] (Leipzig: Vogel, 1872), p. 106. Cited by Gradmann, *Laboratory Disease*, p. 42.
10. K. Codell Carter, "Koch's Postulates in Relation to the Work of Jacob Henle and Edwin Klebs," *Medical History* 29 (1985) 353–375. Cited by Gradmann, p. 42.
11. John Dirckx, "Virgil on Anthrax," *American Journal of Dermatopathology* 3, no. 2 (Summer 1981): 191–195. Virgil's poem, *Georgics*, consists of four books, each dealing with aspects of agriculture, including animal husbandry.
12. Brock, *Robert Koch*, p. 23.
13. Martin Kirchner, "Kreisphysikus in Wollstein," *Robert Koch* (Berlin: Julius Springer, 1924).
14. Brock, *Robert Koch*, pp. 27–28.
15. Kenneth Alibeck, Catherine Lobanova and Serguei Popov, "Anthrax: A Disease and a Weapon," in *Bioterrorism and Infectious Agents* (New York: Springer Science+Business Media), 2005, p. 2.
16. Brock, *Robert Koch*, p. 34.
17. *Ibid*.
18. *Ibid.*, p. 35. Once Koch had completed his studies of anthrax, he was able to obtain a supply of white mice for future investigations. Brock described the source of those animals. "An assistant of Ferdinand Cohn, Eduard Eidam, studied with Koch in Wollstein in 1876. Eidam was accompanied by his foster father, a kindly old gentleman who loved children and who made friends during his stay with Koch's daughter Gertrud. Upon returning to Berlin, the old gentleman sent the daughter some pet white mice in a special 'mouse house' (a cage in the form of a little house, with floors, tiny rooms, stairways and windows). The mice multiplied rapidly and Koch began to use the 'excess' mice for his experiments" (321).
19. Robert Koch, "Die Ätiologie der Milzbrandkrankheit, Begründet auf die Entwicklungs Geschichte des Bacillus Anthracis," *Beiträge zur Biologie der Pflanzen* [The Etiology of Anthrax ... Contributions to the Biology of Plants] 2 (July 1876): 277–310. Cited by Brock, *Robert Koch*, p. 35.
20. *Ibid.*, cited by Brock, *Robert Koch*, p. 36.
21. Bruno Heymann, *Robert Koch. I. Teil. 1843–1882* (Leipzig, Germany: Akademische Verlagsgesellschaft, 1932), p. 147, cited by Brock, *Robert Koch*, pp. 36–37.

22. Heymann, p. 178, cited by Brock, *Robert Koch*, p. 44.
23. Ford, p. 419.
24. Heymann, p. 345, cited by Gradmann, p. 51.
25. Brock, *Robert Koch*, p. 45. Cohnheim developed a technique for introduction of tubercle material into the anterior chamber of the eye of a rabbit. The procedure was later applied by Koch in demonstrating the etiological agent of tuberculosis.
26. Ford, p. 419.
27. Brock, *Robert Koch*, p. 71. As noted in Chapter 4, Burdon-Sanderson also demonstrated the anti-bacterial properties associated with the mold *Penicillium*.
28. *Ibid., Robert Koch*, p. 65.
29. *Ibid., Robert Koch*, p. 74.
30. P.L. Panum, "Bidrag Til Laeren Om Den Sakaldte Putride Eller Septiske Infektion" [Experimental Contribution to the Theory of the So-Called Putrid or Septic Infection], *Bibliotek Laeger* 4, no. 8 (1856): 253–285. Panum is better remembered for his study of an outbreak of measles among the natives of the Faroe Islands during the summer of 1846.
31. P.L. Panum, "Das Putride Gift, Die Bakterien, Die Putride Infektion, Oder Intoxication Und Die Septekämie [The Putrid Poison, the Bacteria, the Putrid Infection or Intoxication and Septicaemia]," *Arch Path Anat Physiol Klin Med* [Virchow's Archives] 60 (1874): 301–352; Hans Kolmos, "Panum's Studies on 'Putrid Poison' 1856," *Danish Medical Bulletin* 53 (2006): 450–452, cited by Gradmann, p. 55.
32. Robert Koch, *Untersuchungen uber die Aetiologie der Wundinfectionskrankheiten* [Studies on the Etiology of Wound Infectious Disease] (Leipzig: Vogel, 1878), p. 15. Gradmann has suggested the publication of Koch's small book by Vogel was due to support on the part of Cohnheim (n248).
33. *Ibid.*, in *Milestones in Microbiology*, ed. Thomas Brock (Washington, D.C.: American Society for Microbiology, 1975), p. 98.
34. Gradmann, p. 59.
35. Brock, *Milestones*, p. 98.
36. Gradmann.
37. Koch, *Untersuchungen*, p. 101, cited by Brock, *Milestones*.
38. Brock, *Robert Koch*, p. 80. It was Ernst Abbe (1840–1905), working as a consultant for the Carl Zeiss Microscope Company, who designed the oil-immersion lens (ca. 1873). A review of Abbe's contribution can be found in the Brock biography (pp. 67–78). The famous equation defining the limit of diffraction was devel-

oped and confirmed by German physicist Hermann von Helmholtz and John Ware Stephenson. (Xiang Hao, et al., "From Microscopy to Nanoscopy Via Visible Light," *Light: Science and Applications* 2, no. 10 (October 2013), http://www.nature.com/lsa/journal/v2/n10/full/lsa201364a.html.
  39. Brock, *Robert Koch*.
  40. *Ibid.*, p. 85.
  41. Ford, p. 420. Brock referred to the position as *Gerichtliche Stadtphysikus, Robert Koch*, p. 85.
  42. Brock, *Robert Koch*, pp. 86, 90.
  43. Ford, p. 421. Brock has suggested it was Cohn who intervened on Koch's behalf. It may very well have been both professors who supported Koch's nomination to the position.
  44. Heymann, pp. 289–290, cited by Brock, *Robert Koch*, pp. 87–88.
  45. Brock, *Robert Koch*. p. 90.
  46. Ford.
  47. Adler, *Cholera in Detroit*, pp. 183–190, Brock, *Robert Koch*, pp. 140–168.
  48. Norman Howard-Jones, *The Scientific Background of the International Sanitary Conferences, 1851–1938* (Geneva: WHO, 1975), p. 50, cited by Adler, *Cholera in Detroit*, p. 186.
  49. Not everyone was convinced. Dr. Max von Pettenkofer (1818–1901), among the most important historical figures in the science of hygiene—in 1878 Pettenkofer had founded an Institute of Hygiene at the University of Munich, the first such institute anywhere—and who was considered a foremost expert on the subject of cholera, so disagreed with Koch's analysis that he swallowed a beaker-full of the organism to support his argument. He suffered no significant ill effects. Nor was Koch the likely the first to identify the etiological agent of cholera. That "honor" arguably belongs to the Italian scientist Filippo Pacini, who in 1854 reported similar findings to those of Koch's.
  50. Brock, *Robert Koch*, p. 183.
  51. *Ibid.*, p. 184–185.
  52. *Ibid.*, p. 187.
  53. Christoph Gradmann, "Robert Koch and the Pressures of Scientific Research," *Medical History* 45 (February 2001): 1–32.

Chapter 2

  1. W.L. Schenck, "Septic Disease," Kansas State Medical Society, *Transactions* 1 (1877): 405–421, cited by Thomas Neville Bonner, *American Doctors and German Universities* (Lincoln: University of Nebraska Press, 1963). Dr. Washington Lafayette Schenck played a significant role in the advancement of medicine in Kansas in the years following the Civil War. Born in Ohio (1825), he was a graduate of Dartmouth Medical College (1848), following which he attended Jefferson Medical College in Philadelphia. Following brief service as a physician during the war, Schenck moved to Kansas about 1871. He was a member of the American Medical Association as well as serving as president of the Kansas State Medical Society. In that capacity he supported the establishment of the State Board of Health. Schenck died in 1910.
  2. Alfred Hershey and Martha Chase (1952), "Independent Functions of Viral Protein and Nucleic Acid in Growth of Bacteriophage," *Journal of General Physiology* 36, no. 1: 39–56.
  3. Oswald Avery, et al., "Studies on the Chemical Nature of the Substance Inducing Transformation of Pneumococcal Types: Induction of Transformation by a Desoxyribonucleic Acid Fraction Isolated from Pneumococcus Type III," *Journal of Experimental Medicine* 79, no. 2 (1944): 137–58.
  4. Hubert Lechevalier and Morris Solotorovsky, *Three Centuries of Microbiology* (New York: Dover, 1974), p. 3. Given van Leeuwenhoek's belief that masturbation was sinful, one wonders how he obtained his source of sperm. Nor was van Leeuwenhoek the first to apply this technology to observe the very small. In the 1620s Galileo Galilei, usually associated with observing the very distant, assembled a crude compound microscope of his own.
  5. William Bulloch, *The History of Bacteriology* (New York: Dover, 1979), p. 46–47. The word "yeast" is derived from the Old English referring to a bubble.
  6. *Ibid.*, pp. 49–51. Schwann referred to the organisms as "Zuckerpilz" ("sugar fungus"), from which the genus name *Saccharomyces* was derived. Despite its similarity, the name of Pilsner beer was not from the same designation. Pilsner was named for the Bohemian town in which it was first brewed; the term itself is from the Czech "damp."
  7. Gerald Geison, *The Private Science of Louis Pasteur* (Princeton, NJ: Princeton University Press, 1996).
  8. Bulloch, pp. 163–165; Brock, *Milestones*, pp. 76–79.
  9. Brock, *Milestones*, p. 78.
  10. Bulloch.
  11. Brock, *Milestones*, p. 76.
  12. *Ibid.*, p. 77. Henle considered miasmatic-contagious diseases to be those in which the contagium exits the body and is transmitted to

the susceptible individual either through an airborne mechanism, or through direct contact. Examples included cholera, plague and influenza.

13. *Ibid.*, p. 78.

14. J.A. Villemin, *Études sur la Tuberculose, Preuves Rationnelles et Expérimentales de sa Spécificité et de Son Inoculabilité* (Paris: J.B. Baillière et Fils, 1868), cited by Lechevalier, p. 121.

15. Joseph Lister, "On a New Method of Treating Compound Fracture, Abscess, and So Forth; with Observations on the Conditions of Suppuration," *Lancet* 1 (1867): 364–373, 418–420, cited in Brock, *Milestones*, pp. 83–85.

16. *Ibid.*

17. Lechevalier, p. 47.

18. Brock, *Milestones*, p. 79.

19. Jean Théodoridès, "Casimir Davaine: A Precursor of Pasteur," *Medical History* 10, no. 2 (April 1966): 155–165. The statement likely originated with Davaine, who sent it to Rayer, well-known among physicians in Paris, for publication (Bulloch, *Milestones*, p. 179) Davaine was born in the town of St. Amand-les-Eaux, the sixth of nine children, to a distiller. In 1835, he became an externe member of the Hôpital de la Charité, where he was first associated with Rayer. He received his medical degree two years later. Davaine carried out his research on anthrax independently while working in Rayer's department.

20. *Ibid.*, p. 159.

21. *Ibid.*, p. 160.

22. *Ibid.*, pp. 161–162. Spores would have survived that temperature. It is possible that growth conditions resulted in a lack of spore formation. Alternatively, it is now known that the genetic information for virulence of the organism resides on plasmids within the cell. Heating at that temperature may cause loss of the plasmids, resulting in the loss of virulence as well.

23. *Ibid.*, p. 162.

24. *Ibid.*

25. *Ibid.*

26. *Ibid.*, p. 164.

27. K. Codell Carter, "Koch's Postulates in Relation to the Work of Jacob Henle and Edwin Klebs," *Medical History* 29 (1985): 353–374.

28. *Ibid.*, p. 365.

29. *Ibid.*

30. *Ibid.*, p. 366.

31. Brock, *Milestones*, p. 95.

32. Brock, *Robert Koch*, p. 31.

33. Robert Koch, "Untersuchungen uber Bakterien V. die Aetiologie der Milzbrand-Krankheit, Begründet auf die Entwicklungsgeschichte des Bacillus Anthracis," *Beiträge zur Biologie der Pflanzen* [Investigations about Bacteria V: The Etiology of Anthrax Disease, Based on the Development History of *Bacillus Anthracis*," Contributions to the Biology of Plants] 2, no. 2 (1877): 277–310. Cited by Brock, *Milestones*, p. 90. Cohn also established the journal *Beiträge zur Biologie der Pflanzen* in 1870 as a means to publish much of the work with which they were involved.

34. Brock, *Milestones*, pp. 94–95.

35. Robert Koch, "Zur Untersuchung von Pathogenen Organismen" [Methods for the study of pathogenic organisms] *Mittheilungen aus dem Kaiserlichen Gesundheitsamte* 1 (1881): 1–48; Brock, *Milestones*, p. 101–108.

36. Brock, *Milestones*, p. 107. Gelatin as a hardening agent had certain disadvantages. For one, it could liquefy when incubated at 37 degrees C. Second, some bacteria produce a protease which hydrolyzes gelatin. It was subsequently superseded by agar as the hardening agent.

37. Brock, *Robert Koch*, p. 46.

38. *Ibid.*, p. 80.

39. Robert Koch, "Die Atiologie der Tuberkulose" [The Etiology of Tuberculosis], *Berliner Klinischen Wochenschrift* 15 (April 10, 1882): 221–230, cited by Brock, *Milestones*, p. 109. "Tappeiner, in a series of experiments which lasted from 1877 to 1888, demonstrated beyond doubt the infectiousness of phthisical sputum by inhalation experiments ... Tappeiner, in 1880, had failed to infect rabbits by exposing them to the breath of coughing consumptives, and concluded that the infection must be conveyed, if at all, by dried sputum arising as dust, and not by the breath of the patient. The danger of this mode of infection received practical confirmation when his servant, whom he had warned to protect himself from inhaling the dust of the room in which the animals were confined, developed pulmonary tuberculosis and died of it" (E.L. Trudeau, *Animal Experimentation and Tuberculosis* [Chicago: Press of American Medical Association, 1913], p. 5). Nor were these the first to propose the infectious nature of the disease. As noted by Koch in his report, Jean Antoine Villemin had proposed the same in 1865. Even earlier, in 1843, Philipp Friedrich Hermann Klenke had suggested that the disease was infectious.

40. Koch, "Die Atiologie der Tuberkulose," p. 110. The similarity to the leprosy bacillus is not a coincidence. The etiological agent of leprosy, also known as Hansen's Disease, was identified in 1880 by Gerhard Hansen. Both the tuberculosis agent and the leprosy agent are today classified in the same genus, *Mycobacterium*.

41. *Ibid.*, p. 111.

42. *Ibid.*
43. Christoph Gradmann, "Robert Koch and the Pressures of Scientific Research," *Medical History* 45 (February 2001): 1–32.
44. Koch, "Die Atiologie der Tuberkulose," pp. 112–113.
45. Koch, "Die Atiologie der Tuberkulose," p. 114.
46. Robert Koch, "Die Atiologie der Tuberkulose" [The Etiology of Tuberculosis], *Mittheilungen aus dem Kaiserlichen Gesundheitsamte* 2 (1884): 1–88, cited by Brock, *Milestones*, pp. 116–117.
47. Lechevalier, p. 123; Brock, *Robert Koch*, p. 180.

Chapter 3

1. Schenck, p. 412.
2. Joseph McFarland, "The Beginning of Bacteriology in Philadelphia," *Bulletin of the History of Medicine* 5 (1937): 149–198.
3. "Rabies Past and Present," http://www.preciousorganics.com.au/pages/rabies-past-and-present.
4. McFarland, p. 151. Edward Emanuel Klein (1844–1925) was born in Ersek, then part of Austria-Hungary, and studied medicine in Vienna. In 1869 he came to England. As a member of the faculty at St. Bartholomew's Hospital Medical School in London, he was the author of numerous texts on the subjects of histology and bacteriology. Among his students was Dr. Ronald Ross, later a Nobel laureate for his discovery of the method of transmission of the malarial parasite.
5. "The Early History of Bacteriology in the United States," *Journal of the American Medical Association* 70, no. 25 (June 22, 1918): 1946–1947; David Bergey, "Early Instructors in Bacteriology in the United States," *Journal of Bacteriology* 2, no. 6 (1917): 595–601.
6. McFarland.
7. "Tyndall on Koch's Work," *The New York Times*, May 3, 1882, p. 2.
8. *Ibid.*; John Keating, "The Presence of the Micrococcus in the Blood of Malignant Measles: Its Importance in Treatment," *Boston Medical and Surgical Journal* 107(5): (August 3, 1882): 101–105. Formad was associated with Dr. Horatio Wood in his study of diphtheria. Wood was an advocate of an unusual medicine for treatment of the sick: tomato juice mixed with flour and milk.
9. H.C. Wood, "On the Nature of the Diphtheritic Contagium," *Science* 2, no. 74 (November 26, 1881): 560–562.

10. "Fresh Researches on the Tubercle-Bacillus," *Medical Times and Gazette* 1 (April 21, 1883): 437.
11. Bergey, pp. 596–597.
12. Erwin F. Smith, "In Memoriam: Thomas Jonathon Burrill," *Journal of Bacteriology* 1, no. 3 (May 1916): 269–271.
13. Bergey, p. 597.
14. E.G. Hastings and C.B. Morrey, "Early Instructors in Bacteriology in the United States," *Journal of Bacteriology* 3, no. 3 (May 1918): 307–308.
15. *Ibid.*
16. "Russell, Harry Luman," http://www.asm.org/index.php/choma3/71-membership/archives/852-russell-harry-luman.
17. "Behind the Frieze—Hermann Michael Biggs," http://www.lshtm.ac.uk/library/archives/history/frieze/biggs.html.
18. "T. Mitchel Prudden and the First American Use of Vaccine," http://pathology.columbia.edu/mitchellprudden.html.
19. Gregg Cima, "Legends: Teacher, Researcher and Inventor: Heinrich J. Detmers," *Journal of American Medical Veterinary Association* 242, no. 11 (June 1, 2013), https://www.avma.org/News/JAVMANews/Pages/130601g.aspx.
20. Hastings, p. 308; "Transformation and Tradition," vet.osu.edu/assets/pdf/about/125Anniversary.pdf, p.10.
21. Bergey, p. 600.
22. C.-E.A. Winslow, "William Thompson Sedgwick," *Journal of Bacteriology* 6, no. 3 (May 1921): 255–262.
23. Bergey, pp. 600–601.
24. Barnett Cohen, *Chronicles of the Society of American Bacteriologists: 1899–1950*, Baltimore: Waverly, 1950, p. 2.
25. *Ibid.*
26. *Ibid.*, pp. 4–15.

Chapter 4

1. Groucho Marx.
2. "The Dean's Lecture Series: The Cartwright Lecture," http://www.cumc.columbia.edu/events/deanlectures/cartwright.html. Osborn, a geologist well-known for his theories of human evolution, was the long-time president of the American Museum of Natural History in New York. During the John Scopes "Monkey Trial" in 1925, he was requested to appear as a defense witness, but declined.
3. William F. Belfield, "Relations of Micro-Organisms to Disease," The Cartwright Lectures.

Delivered before the alumni association of the College of Physicians and Surgeons, New York, February 19, 21, 24 and 27, 1883. *The Medical Record* (February-March, 1883) (Chicago: W.T. Kleener, 1883), pp. 3-142.

4. *Ibid.*, pp. 8-9.
5. *Ibid.*, p. 5.
6. *Ibid.*, pp. 18-19. Cohn was actually correct. Morphologically, *Bacillus subtilis*, the hay bacillus, and *Bacillus anthracis*, the etiological agent of anthrax, are both spore-forming bacilli. The primary differences are the plasmid-encoded virulence factors produced by the anthrax organism.
7. *Ibid.*, pp. 21-24.
8. *Ibid.*, pp. 30-31.
9. *Ibid.*, pp. 35-36.
10. *Ibid.*, pp. 60-61.
11. *Ibid.*, pp. 62. Pasteur and Sternberg may have observed a different organism. One possibility would be *Proteus*, a urease-positive organism which might have been present in the urine. However, *Proteus* is a bacillus, and while Pasteur may have misidentified the morphology, it is unlikely Sternberg would make the same error. More likely, each had observed a different micrococcus, albeit one which today would be considered gram-positive. The procedure for the gram stain was published in 1884, and would not have been known to Sternberg at the time. It should also be pointed out that each of the successful examples referred to by Belfield were either Koch's students or associates.
12. *Ibid.*, pp. 62-63.
13. *Ibid.*, pp. 77-78. The phrase "survival of the fittest," often ascribed to Darwin, was originally coined by philosopher Herbert Spencer. Darwin adopted the phrase in *The Variation of Animals and Plants Under Domestication* (1868). It later appeared in the fifth edition of *On the Origin of Species* (1869).
14. "History of Medical Practice in Illinois," https://archive.org/details/historyofmedical02illi.
15. William Hunt, "Esmarch, Antisepsis and Bacillus," *The Medical News* 42, no. 4 (January 27, 1883): 93.
16. *Ibid.*
17. Belfield, p. 79.
18. Hunt, p. 94.
19. Belfield, p. 79, *n*1.
20. *Ibid.*, p. 80.
21. *Ibid.*, pp. 81-83.
22. *Ibid.*, pp. 85-86.
23. Hunt, p. 93.
24. Belfield, p. 86-87.
25. H.F. Formad, "The Bacillus Tuberculosis," *Philadelphia Medical Times* (November 18, 1882): pp. 1-2.
26. It is of course possible the animals contracted and died from tuberculosis, a respiratory infection. But it is also possible the animals contracted an illness now called "Snuffles," a highly contagious, and often fatal, respiratory illness common among confined animals such as rabbits and guinea pigs. The etiological agent is a bacterium, *Pasteurella multocida*. If so, Dr. Formad may not have recognized, or even ignored, the difference.
27. Burdon-Sanderson (1828-1905), a British physiologist, also observed the antibacterial effects of the mold *Penicillium* some fifty-five years before being "rediscovered" by Alexander Fleming.
28. Belfield, pp. 87-89. In a note, Belfield noted a paradox in Formad's reasoning: "Tubercle tissue is always infested by bacilli," yet "true tuberculosis may be produced without" them. *Ibid.*, *n*2, p. 89.
29. *Chicago Daily Tribune*, March 29, 1884, p. 4.
30. H.F. Formad, "The Bacillus Tuberculosis and the Etiology of Tuberculosis—Is Consumption Contagious?" *Journal of the American Medical Association* 2, no. 17 (April 26, 1884): 449-463. In a note, Formad conceded the bacterial nature of Koch's observations "The statements made by Beneke, Klebs and Schmidt, that the bacilli are crystalline bodies, have been withdrawn; while views to the effect that 'bacilli' are to be identified with blood-fibrin, etc, were at no time taken into serious consideration by microscopists." Formad had conceded this portion of Belfield's argument. *Ibid.*, *n*449.
31. *Ibid.*, p. 451.
32. *Ibid.*, pp. 451-452.
33. *Ibid.*, p. 453.
34. *Ibid.*, pp. 454-455.
35. *Ibid.*, p. 455.
36. *Ibid.*, pp. 457-458.
37. *Ibid.*, p. 458.
38. *Ibid.*, p. 459.
39. *Ibid.*, pp. 459-460.
40. *Ibid.*, pp. 460-462.
41. *Ibid.*, p. 463.
42. "Koch's Work Upon Tuberculosis, and the Present Condition of the Question," *Science* 4, no. 76 (July 18, 1884): 59-61.

Chapter 5

1. George W. Lewis, "Ten Days in the Laboratory with Dr. Robert Koch," *The Buffalo Med-*

ical and Surgical Journal 24 (August 1884-July 1885): 343–355.
  2. Ibid., p. 347.
  3. Ibid., p. 352.
  4. Brock, Robert Koch, p. 101; http://www.labnews.co.uk/features/history-of-the-agar-plate-01-11-2005/.
  5. Lewis, p. 352.
  6. Ibid., pp. 353–355.
  7. T. Mitchell Prudden, "On Koch's Methods of Studying the Bacteria, Particularly Those Causing Asiatic Cholera," Eighth Annual Report of the State Board of Connecticut for the Year Ending November 1, 1885 (New Haven, 1886), pp. 213–230, also cited by Brock, Robert Koch, pp. 188–189.
  8. Prudden, pp. 215–217.
  9. Ibid., pp. 217–226.
  10. Frederick G. Novy, "The Hygienic Institute at Berlin," The Pharmaceutical Era 2 (November 1888): 426–427. This author remembers when smoking in the laboratory, while not encouraged, was still common in the 1970s. When working on a research fellowship in an unidentified laboratory, I was advised to never let the director actually help me with setting up an experiment. I soon discovered why. While the two of us were working with cell cultures in the laminar-flow hood, ashes from his ever-present cigar had fallen on the mat, creating a fire of which he was completely unaware.
  11. Ibid.
  12. Harry Russell, Diary, book 10, University of Wisconsin Archives, pp. 63–64, cited by Brock, Robert Koch, pp. 189–190. A brief description of Russell's professional career is also found in Chapter 3.
  13. Bonner, American Doctors and German Universities, p. 116.

Chapter 6

  1. T. Mitchell Prudden, "Pathology and the Department of Pathology," Columbia University Bulletin 19 (1898): 103–119, cited by Ludvig Hektoen, "Biographical Memoir of Theophil Mitchell Prudden (1849–1924)," National Academy of Sciences XII-Third Memoir (1925): 71–98.
  2. Lillian Prudden, Biographical Sketches and Letters of T. Mitchell Prudden (New Haven, CT: Yale University Press, 1927), p. 12.
  3. For the baseball enthusiast, among the alumni was Thomas Yawkey, longtime owner of the Boston Red Sox.
  4. Hektoen, p. 75. Russell would in time become professor of surgery at Yale Medical School. Russell's father, Major-General William Huntington Russell, a military appointment conferred by the governor of Connecticut for his service in recruiting soldiers during the Civil War, was among the figures credited with establishment of the Republican Party in 1854. The elder Russell was also a Yale alumnus, graduating as valedictorian in 1833.
  5. Ibid., p. 76.
  6. Lillian Prudden, p. 16.
  7. Ibid., p. 17.
  8. Ibid.
  9. Ibid., p. 25. In 1901, Delafield would be the attending physician at the bedside of the mortally wounded President William Mckinley.
  10. Ibid., p. 26.
  11. T.M. Prudden, "Progress and Drift in Pathology," Medical Record 57 (1900): 397–405, cited by Hektoen, p. 78.
  12. Hektoen, Ibid.
  13. A specialist in abdominal disorders, Fitz had coined the term appendicitis.
  14. Lillian Prudden, p. 33.
  15. Hektoen, p. 80.
  16. Lillian Prudden, pp. 34–35.
  17. Ibid., p. 36.
  18. Ibid.
  19. T. Mitchell Prudden, "Pathology," cited by Hektoen, p. 81.
  20. Lillian Prudden, p. 38.
  21. Ibid., p. 59. Cited also by Hektoen, p. 82. It may be noted that much of the material presented by Hektoen in the "Biographical Memoir" was obtained verbatim from the biography written by Lillian Prudden, T. Mitchell's niece.
  22. T. Mitchell Prudden, "Occurrence of the Bacillus Tuberculosis in Tuberculous Lesions," Medical Record 23 (1883): 397–400.
  23. T. Mitchell Prudden, "On the Occurrence of Tubercles in Which the Bacillus Tuberculosis Is Not Demonstrable by the Ordinary Method of Staining," Medical Record 23 (1883): 645–648.
  24. Hektoen, p. 84.
  25. T. Mitchell Prudden, "On Koch's Methods of Studying the Bacteria, Particularly Those Causing Asiatic Cholera," Eighth Annual Report of the State Board of Connecticut for the Year Ending November 1, 1885 (New Haven, 1886), pp. 213–230.
  26. Ibid.
  27. Ibid.
  28. C.J. Foote, "Early Years of Bacteriology in the Yale Medical School and in the City of New Haven," The Yale Journal of Biology and Medicine 13, no. 3 (1941): 309–314. Yale College became Yale University in 1887, among Dwight's achievements.

29. Paul F. Clark, "The Great Metropolis and New York State," in *Pioneer Microbiologists of America*, (Madison: University of Wisconsin Press, 1961), pp. 154–189.
30. Lillian Prudden, p. 63.
31. N. Paul Hudson, "Edwin Oakes Jordan, 1866–1936," *Journal of Bacteriology* 33, no. 3 (March 1937): i2, 243–248.
32. Daniel M. Fox, "Social Policy and City Politics: Tuberculosis Reporting in New York, 1889–1900," in *Sickness and Health in America*, edited by Judith Walzer Leavitt and Ronald L. Numbers (Madison: University of Wisconsin Press, 1978), pp. 415–431. In 1893, Bryant would be the primary surgeon in an operation, carried out in secret, in which a malignant tumor of the jaw was removed from President Grover Cleveland. The operation was carried out aboard the yacht *Oneida* sailing on the East River. The actual tumor is now on display in the Mütter Museum in Philadelphia (Matthew Algeo, *The President Is a Sick Man* [Chicago: Chicago Review, 2011]).
33. H.M. Biggs, "A Brief History of the Campaign Against Tuberculosis in New York City" (New York: New York City Department of Health, 1908).
34. Thomas Frieden, et al., "Tuberculosis in New York City—Turning the Tide," *The New England Journal of Medicine* 333 (July 27, 1995): 229–233.
35. Biggs.

Chapter 7

1. Simon Flexner and James Thomas Flexner, *William Henry Welch and the Heroic Age of American Medicine* (Baltimore: The Johns Hopkins University Press, 1993), pp. 148–149. Prudden's account of the incident, as Flexner described it some thirty-five years later, was less dramatic. As Simon Flexner pointed out, Welch was known for embellishing a good story. N3, p. 481.
2. *Ibid.*, p. 23; W.H. Welch, "Remarks at the Unveiling of a Tablet in Memory of Miss Isabella Eldridge in the Congregational Church, Norfolk, Conn.," *Litchfield County Leader*, July 1, 1921, cited by Barry Silverman, "William Henry Welch (1850–1934): The Road to Johns Hopkins," *Proceedings Baylor University Medical Center* 24, no. 3 (2011): 236–242.
3. Silverman, p. 238.
4. Flexner and Flexner, p. 25.
5. *Ibid.*, pp. 62–63.
6. *Ibid.*
7. *Ibid.*, pp. 70–71.
8. *Ibid.*, p. 78.
9. *Ibid.*, p. 79.
10. Among Hoppe-Seyler's students was Friedrich Miescher, who discovered DNA in cell nuclei during the 1860s. A common misconception, even among some beginning biology students, is that DNA was discovered by James Watson and Francis Crick. In fact, they, along with Maurice Wilkins and Rosalind Franklin, determined its structure, not its existence.
11. Flexner and Flexner, pp. 82–83.
12. *Ibid.*, p. 85. The "new and improved methods" to which Welch referred had been developed by Julius Cohnheim, and involved "impregnating" nerve fibers with gold chloride (p. 86).
13. Silverman, p. 240.
14. Flexner and Flexner, p. 83.
15. *Ibid.*, pp. 94–95.
16. W. Welch, "Zur Pathologie Des Lungenödems," *Virchows Archiv* 72 (1878): 375–413.
17. Owsei Temkin, "The European Background of the Young Dr. Welch," *Bulletin of the History of Medicine* 24 (January 1, 1950): 308–318.
18. Flexner and Flexner, p. 104.
19. Silverman, p. 240.
20. Donald Fleming, *William H. Welch and the Rise of Modern Medicine* (Boston: Little, Brown, 1954), p. 56.
21. Flexner and Flexner, p. 109.
22. Carl Weigert, *Gesammelte Abhandlungen*, vol. 2 (Berlin: Springer, 1906), p. 426, cited by Temkin, p. 316.
23. Julius Cohnheim, *Gesammelte Abhandlungen* (Berlin: Springer, 1885), p. 615, cited by Temkin, p. 316.
24. Flexner and Flexner, p. 112.
25. Goldthwaite (1842–1895) had been born in Mobile, Alabama. An 1860 graduate of Princeton, he served with the Confederacy during the Civil War, rising to the rank of major. Eschewing a career in business after the war, he entered the field of medicine, graduating from Bellevue Hospital Medical College in 1876.
26. Fleming, p. 65.
27. *Ibid.*; Flexner and Flexner, p. 120; S.J. Meltzer and W. Welch, "The Behavior of the Red Blood-Corpuscles When Shaken with Indifferent Substances," *Journal of Physiology (London)* 5 (1884): 255–260.
28. Silverman, p. 242; Flexner and Flexner, p. 128. Ponfick was well known for his study of the role played by the bacterium *Actinomyces* as the agent of actinomycosis, an infection of the face, lungs or gastrointestinal tract.
29. Fleming, pp. 66–67. Remsen (1846–1927)

and his associate Constantin Fahlberg discovered the artificial sweetener saccharin in 1879 when the coal tar derivative happened to contaminate food they were eating. Martin, a British physiologist, was the first professor of physiology at Johns Hopkins.

30. Ibid.
31. Flexner and Flexner, p. 130.
32. Ibid., p. 131.
33. Ibid.
34. Fleming, p. 71-72. In Flint's *A Treatise on the Principles and Practice of Medicine*, 6th ed. (1886), a text for which Welch played a significant part in revising, the section on bacteriology "may be regarded as the first complete treatise on [this] subject to reach the rank and file of the medical profession" (Flexner, p. 478f).
35. Fleming, p. 72. Because of the unusual nature of the mycolic acid lipid layer on the surface of the tubercle bacillus, the standard method of staining uses hot carbol fuchsin (red), followed by a counterstain of a different color such as methylene blue. The method usually goes by the designation of acid-fast stain. The answer to the question of which city established the first municipal public health department, is muddled. A city board of health was established in New York in 1866, shortly after the end of the Civil War, in response to the poor sanitation facilities and spread of disease, the solution to which was previously helped in no part by the corruption inherent in the political climate run by Tammany Hall. In 1888, a public health laboratory was established in Providence, Rhode Island. Since biologists from the Massachusetts Institute of Technology worked with the laboratory in applying bacteriology to the sanitation problem, some consider that to be the first such municipal program (Patricia Gossel, "Pasteur, Koch and American Bacteriology," *History and Philosophy of the Life Sciences* 22 [2000]: 81-100).
36. Flexner and Flexner, p. 138. On Formad, see Chapter 4.
37. Ibid., p. 139. Among Frobenius' students was Theodor Escherich, one of the first pediatric infectious disease physicians, and the scientist given credit for identification of the eponymous colon bacillus, *Escherichia coli*.
38. Ibid., pp. 142-143.
39. Ibid., p. 145. Prince Albert's father, Albert Edward, Prince of Wales, would succeed Victoria upon her death in 1901. Tragically, Albert Victor had died during the influenza epidemic in 1892.
40. Ibid., p. 147.
41. Ibid.
42. Ibid., p. 482n2.

43. Ibid., p. 153; Simon Flexner, "Biographical Memoir of William Henry Welch," presented to the Academy at the Autumn Meeting, *National Academy of Sciences* 22 (1942): 213-231.
44. W. Welch and G.H.F. Nuttall, "A Gas-Producing Bacillus (*Bacillus Aerogenes Capsulatus* Nov. Spec.), Capable of Rapid Development in the Blood-Vessels After Death," *Johns Hopkins Hospital Bulletin* 3 (1892): 81-91.
45. William Welch and Simon Flexner, "Observations Concerning the *Bacillus Aerogenes Capsulatus*," *Journal of Experimental Medicine* 1 (January 1896): 5-45. Welch was the first editor of the *JEM*.
46. Brendan Lucey and Grover Hutchins, "William H. Welch, MD, and the Discovery of *Bacillus Welchii*," *Archives of Pathology & Laboratory Medicine* 128, no. 10 (October 2004): 1193-1195. Welch, along with Osler, Halsted and Kelly, were known as the "Big Four," the four founding physicians of the hospital. In 1905, they sat for a famous portrait by the artist John Singer Sargent; the painting now hangs in the Welch Medical Library at the university.

Chapter 8

1. Edward Oram Shakespeare, Obituary, *The New York Times*, June 2, 1900, p. 9.
2. Edward Shakespeare, "A New Ophthalmoscope and Ophthalmometer Devised for Clinical Use and for Physiological and Therapeutical Investigation on Men and Animals," *The American Journal of Medical Sciences* 71 (January 1876): 45-61.
3. H.R.M. Landis, "The Reception of Koch's Discovery in the United States," *Annals of Medical History* 4 (September 1932): 531-537.
4. Ibid., p. 534.
5. *The Medical Annals, Medical Society of the County of Albany* V (April 1884), pp. 113-114. As noted by the (anonymous) editor of the journal, Formad's understanding of predisposition meant "not merely a peculiar soil suited to the bacillus, but a condition of embryonic tissue development, and that in an animal whose tissues are of an embryonic character tuberculosis is set up by any irritant" (p. 114).
6. *The Medical Annals, Medical Society of the County of Albany* V (July 1884), p. 210.
7. H.F. Formad, "The Philadelphia Debate on the Tubercle Bacillus," *The New York Medical Journal* 39 (June 28, 1884): 723-724. The difficulty in staining the tubercle bacilli was the result of the layer of mycolic acids on their surface, requiring the use of what subsequently became

known as the Ziehl-Neelson, or acid-fast stain. An earlier version of the procedure was developed by Koch's colleague, Dr. Paul Ehrlich.

8. Edward O. Shakespeare, "A Criticism of Dr. Formad's Printed Statements and Conclusions Concerning the Etiology of Tuberculosis," *The New York Medical Journal* 40 (August 9, 1884): 141–146.

9. *Ibid.*

10. C.E.A. Winslow, *The Life of Hermann Biggs* (Philadelphia: Lea & Febiger, 1929), pp. 65–66. According to Dr. Hermann Biggs, who had been requested by the Carnegie Foundation in New York to also investigate the outbreak, a member of the Davis family which owned the farm suffered from typhoid. Feces from the patient was thrown into the snow near the stream (*Commonwealth of Pennsylvania, State Board of Health*, July 3 and November 11, 1885, p. 25).

11. Morris Stroud French, *Report Upon the Epidemic of Typhoid Fever at Plymouth, Luzerne County, Pennsylvania* (Philadelphia: Ledger Job Print, 1885); *The Lancet* 121 (August 8, 1885): 256.

12. M.S. French and E.O. Shakespeare, "The Lesson Taught by the Epidemic at Plymouth Concerning Typhoid Fever," *New York Medical Journal* 41 (June 13, 1885): 666–667.

13. George A. Johnson, *The Purification of Public Water Supplies* (Washington, D.C.: Government Printing Office, 1913).

14. Actually Koch had "rediscovered" the organism, the role of which in cholera had previously been reported by the Italian physician Filippo Pacini (1812–1883) in 1854.

15. Edward O. Shakespeare, *Report on Cholera in Europe and India* (Washington, D.C.: Government Printing Office, 1890), p. iii.

16. *Ibid.*, p. v.

17. *Ibid.*, pp. 625–630. The Spanish physician Jaime Ferrán y Clua (1851–1929) had observed during the cholera epidemic in Spain in 1884 that when he immunized guinea pigs with the cholera bacillus, the survivors were immune to further infection. He tested an inactive form of the bacillus on himself, then arranged for the immunization of volunteers who paid for the "privilege." While he published the work, information such as the source of the inoculum, or the number of volunteers who subsequently developed cholera, remained a mystery. Most authorities discounted his work (Richard Adler, *Cholera in Detroit: A History* [Jefferson, NC: McFarland, 2013], pp. 193–194).

18. Klein was born and educated in central Europe, but spent much of his professional career in England. He is considered by some as the father of bacteriology in England. Klein acknowledged finding the comma bacillus in the water supply, and though accepting the contagious nature of cholera, was not convinced it was the actual etiological agent. Gibbes subsequently joined the faculty at the University of Michigan, where he opposed the ideas of germ theory expressed by Victor Vaughan and Frederick Novy. (See Chapter 9.)

19. Max von Pettenkofer, "On Cholera, with Reference to the Recent Epidemic at Hamburg," *The Lancet* (November 19, 1892): 1182–1185.

20. E. Klein and Henneage Gibbes, "An Inquiry into the Etiology of Asiatic Cholera," in Shakespeare, *Report*, pp. 477–481. Pettenkofer would later acknowledge the importance of the presence of the organism in development of cholera. However, in order to support his argument that its presence was not in itself sufficient, Pettenkofer swallowed a solution of the bacillus, with little noticeable effect.

21. S.N. De, "Enterotoxicity of Bacteria-Free Culture Filtrate of *Vibrio cholerae*," *Nature* 183 (May 30, 1959): 1533–1534.

22. Shakespeare, *Report*, pp. 885–886.

23. *Ibid.*, pp. 848–850.

24. Walter Wyman, "Government Aids to Public Health," *Journal of the American Medical Association* 15, no. 1 (July 5, 1890): 1 and 19, no. (1) (July 2, 1892): 4.

25. Edward T. Morman, "Guarding Against Alien Impurities: The Philadelphia Lazaretto, 1854–1893," *The Pennsylvania Magazine of History and Biography* 108, no. 2 (April 1984): 131–150.

26. *Journal of the American Medical Association* 19, no. 18 (October 29, 1892): 533.

27. Walter Reed, Victor Clarence Vaughan and Edward Oram Shakespeare, *Report on the Origin and Spread of Typhoid Fever in United States Military Camps During the Spanish War of 1898* (Washington, D.C.: Government Printing Office, 1904), p. xv. Henry Clark Corbin had previously been cited for "gallant and meritorious service" during the Civil War. He had been at the side of President James Garfield when the latter was shot by the assassin Charles Guiteau at the Baltimore and Potomac Railroad Station in Washington in 1881.

28. Bobby Wintermute, *Public Health and the U.S. Military: A History of the Army Medical Department, 1818–1917* (New York: Routledge, 2011); Reed, et al., *Report*.

Chapter 9

1. S.B. Wolbach, "Harold Clarence Ernst," *Proceedings of the American Academy of Arts*

and Sciences 60, no. 14 (December 1925): 621–624.
2. http://bestblog.mlblogs.com/2006/02/16/the-invention-of-the-catchers-mask/.
3. Peter Morris, *Catcher* (Chicago: Ivan R. Dee, 2009), pp. 120–121.
4. *The Medical Times and Gazette* 2 (October 13, 1883): 443; H.C. Ernst, "A Contribution to the Study of the Tubercle-Bacillus," *The Boston Medical and Surgical Journal* 109, no. 5 (August 2, 1883): 100–104, and 109, no. (August 9, 1883): 121–125.
5. H.C. Ernst, "Koch's Treatment of Tuberculosis," *The Boston Medical and Surgical Journal* 124, no. 4 (January 22, 1891): 77–79.
6. *Ibid.*
7. *Ibid.*
8. *Ibid.*
9. H.C. Ernst, "Koch's Treatment of Tuberculosis." *The Boston Medical and Surgical Journal* 124, no. 5 (January 29, 1891): 105–108.
10. W. Gilman Thompson, *Practical Dietetics, with Special Reference to Diet in Disease* (New York: Appleton, 1903), p. 386.
11. Henry Shumway, *A Hand-Book on Tuberculosis Among Cattle* (Boston: Roberts Brothers, 1895), p. 67.; H.C. Ernst, *Infectiousness of Milk: Result of Investigations Made for the Trustees of the Massachusetts Society for Promoting Agriculture* (Cambridge, UK: The Riverside Press, 1895).
12. S.B. Wolbach, *Harvard Alumni Bulletin* 25, no. 1 (September 22, 1922): 1006–1011.

Chapter 10

1. W.J. Nungester, "Frederick George Novy (1864–1957)," *Journal of Bacteriology* 74, no. 5 (November 1957): 545–547. The professor of pathology was likely Dr. Heneage Gibbes (1837–1912). Gibbes was a British-born pathologist who came to the University of Michigan in 1887. His ideas related to the basis of disease were controversial, even for that period. While acknowledging the presence of bacteria in tissues, Gibbes remained skeptical of the germ theory, arguing no causal relationship had been proven. In 1895, Gibbes moved to the Detroit College of Medicine in Detroit—now Wayne State University College of Medicine—as professor of theory and practice of medicine and of pathology.
2. Emily Chenault Runyon, "Remembering Victor C. Vaughan." Notes from Dr. Emily C. Runyon concerning her medical student days at Ann Arbor. http://www.vaughan.org/bios/vcv/images/winfreyLetter.jpg.

3. Victor Vaughan, *A Doctor's Memories* (Indianapolis: Bobbs-Merrill, 1926), pp.14, 21.
4. *Ibid.*, p. 9. William Dameron, Victor Vaughan's grandfather, had fought in the 1832 Black Hawk War, rising to the rank of colonel. He died in 1839 at the age of forty.
5. *Ibid.*, p. 50. The massacre took place September 27, 1864. Vaughan was mistaken in associating the Centralia massacre with Quantrill. The Centralia massacre, the murder of some 150 unarmed Union soldiers, was carried out by "Bloody Bill" Anderson. Either Vaughan mistook one Southern guerilla fighter for another, or he had the date incorrect. Quantrill, of course, was associated with the massacre at Lawrence, Kansas, a year earlier.
6. *Ibid.*, p. 77. In 1882, a fire burned destroyed most of the buildings, and the college was forced to close.
7. *Ibid.*, p. 96. After leaving Ann Arbor in 1876, Mark Walrod Harrington (1848–1926) spent much of the next two decades traveling. His path included studies at the University of Leipzig in Germany, serving as a professor of mathematics at the University of Peking in China, and, in 1891, appointed as the first civilian chief of the Weather Bureau in Washington, D.C. Fired from that position by President Grover Cleveland in 1895, he was appointed president of the University of Washington. Harrington mysteriously disappeared in 1899, leaving for a dinner appointment and never returning. Harrington reappeared nine years later as an inmate in the New Jersey State Hospital in Morristown, New Jersey. According to his wife, Rose, Harrington's condition was the result of having been struck by lightning while studying the atmosphere while at the University of Washington. Rose and Mark's son, Mark Raymond Harrington, became a field archaeologist, serving as curator at the Southwest Museum of the American Indian in Los Angeles, California, for thirty-six years.
8. *Ibid.*, p. 98. Hilgard (1833–1916) remained at the University of California, Berkeley, until 1904, retiring as professor of agricultural chemistry. His book, *Soils: Their Formation, Properties, Composition, and Relations to Climate and Plant Growth in the Humid and Arid Regions* (1906), is considered a classic in associating climate with soil formation.
9. *Ibid.*, p. 99–100. The Ph.D. program at the university had only recently been established. Prior to this, the degree was merely honorary. If a student wished to be awarded a doctorate, it was routine to travel to Germany, where, following two years of study, he would receive that degree.

10. Silas Hamilton Douglas, et al., University of Michigan Board of Regents, *The Regents of the University of Michigan Vs. Preston B. Rose, Silas H. Douglas, Appellant,* State of Michigan, Supreme Court, in Chancery, 1881, p. 2.

11. University of Michigan, Board of Regents. *Proceedings of the Board of Regents (1876–1881)* (June 26, 1877), p. 136.

12. "Department of Bacteriology and Serology and the Hygienic Laboratory," www.umhistory.dc.umich.edu/history/Faculty_History/Medical_Depertment_History/Department_of_Bacteriology.html.

13. "A Brief History of Public Health." www.muskegonhealth.net/aboutus/documents/history.pdf; *First Annual Report of the Secretary of the State of Michigan* (Lansing, 1873).

14. The Battle Creek Sanitarium had been founded in 1866 as the Western Health Reform Institute. In 1876, Kellogg (1852–1943) became superintendent. As the medical officer as well for the institution, Kellogg was a strong advocate of vegetarianism and holistic medicine, focusing on nutrition, enemas and exercise as a means to prevent or treat disease. Kellogg is best remembered for his development of the breakfast cereal corn flakes in 1878. His brother, Will Kellogg (1860–1951), founded the Battle Creek Toasted Corn Fake Company in 1906, the result of a dispute with his brother about Will's idea of adding sugar to the cereal. The company is recognized today simply as Kellogg Company.

15. *Twelfth Annual Report of the Secretary of the State Board of Health of the State of Michigan for the Fiscal Year Ending September 30, 1884* (Lansing: W.S. George, 1885), January 8, 1884, p. xxxvii.

16. *Ibid.,* "Poisonous Cheese." p. 122–123.

17. *Thirteenth Annual Report of the Secretary of the State Board of Health of the State of Michigan for the Fiscal Year Ending September 30, 1885* (Lansing: W.S. George, 1886), pp. 221–226.

18. *Ibid.* The word ptomaine (Gr. *corpse*) has long been a generic term referring to any bacterial toxin. Vaughan, and Frederick Novy as well, believed two classes of such toxins could be observed as a result of putrefaction: ptomaines and leucomaines. Ptomaines were believed to arise from decomposition of tissue, while leucomaines were a product of tissue metabolism.

19. Victor C. Vaughan, "Preliminary Note on the Chemistry of Tyrotoxicon." *The Medical News* 50 (April 2, 1887): 369–370. The increasingly common illness associated with milk products such as ice cream became so common, that a name was given to the disorder: "ice cream poisoning." It was often attributed to toxic vanilla, galvanism (electric currents) in ice cream freezers, and even simple indigestion. Edward Geist, "When Ice Cream Was Poisonous: Adulteration, Ptomaines, and Bacteriology in the United States, 1850–1910," *Bulletin of the History of Medicine* 86, no. 3 (Fall 2012): 333–360; Victor Clarence Vaughan and Frederick George Novy, *Ptomaines and Leucomaines: Or the Putrefactive and Physiological Alkaloids* (Philadelphia: Lea Brothers & Co., 1888).

20. *Fifteenth Annual Report of the Secretary of the State Board of Health of the State of Michigan for the Fiscal Year Ending June 30, 1887* (Lansing: Thorp and Godfrey, 1887), pp. xliv–xlv.

21. *Ibid.,* p. xlv.

22. *Ibid.,* p. 259, cited by Powel Kazanjian, "The Beginnings of Bacteriology in American Medicine: Works of Frederick Novy, 1888–1933," Dissertation Submitted for Degree of Doctor of Philosophy (Ann Arbor: University of Michigan, 2012).

23. *Journal of the Senate of the State of Michigan, 1887,* vol. 2 (Lansing: Thorp and Godfrey, 1887), p. 1659.

24. University of Michigan, Board of Regents, *Proceedings of the Board of Regents* (July 8, 1887), pp. 143–144.

25. *Ibid.,* pp. 138–139.

26. *Ibid.,* p. 144.

27. Esmond R. Long, "Frederick George Novy (1864–1957)," *A Biographical Memoir* (Washington, D.C.: National Academy of Sciences, 1959): 325–350.

28. http://encyclopedia.chicagohistory.org/pages/878html.

29. S.E. Gould, "Frederick George Novy, Microbiologist, 1864–1957," *American Journal of Clinical Pathology* 29, no. 4 (April 1958): 297–309.

30. *Ibid.* De la Fontaine (1837–1911) was credited in these sources as having discovered element number 62, salarium, though credit for that isolation is generally given to the French chemist Paul Lecoq de Boisbaudran. De la Fontaine is correctly credited as co-discoverer of element 67, holmium, in 1878. His research laboratory in Chicago had been destroyed during the Great Fire, as a result of which he taught high school chemistry (Mary Elvira Weeks, "The Discovery of the Elements, XVI: The Rare Earth Elements," *Journal of Chemical Education* 9, no. 10 [October 1932]: 1751–1773).

31. Gould, "Frederick George Novy." The London company was founded by brothers Richard Beck and James Smith during the 1830s, later joined by Beck's brother Joseph. The company also manufactured early cameras.

32. Gould, "Frederick George Novy." The Chicago Microscopical Club was founded in December 1868. Many of the founders were also members of the Chicago Academy of Sciences. Dr. Walter Allport, a Chicago dentist, was elected first president. www.smsi.org/history.html.

33. Gould, "Frederick George Novy." During the latter decades of the 19th century, hog cholera was a devastating disease of pigs. A bacillus, a member of the genus *Salmonella*, and thought to be the etiological agent, had been isolated by Theobald Smith in 1881, and incorrectly identified. The etiological agent was later correctly identified as a virus (Richard Adler and Elise Mara, *Typhoid Fever: A History* [Jefferson, NC: McFarland, 2016]).

34. Frederick Novy, "University of Michigan Student Notebooks." Independent Study in Chemistry (1885), Frederick Novy Papers, Bentley Historical Library (BHL), Ann Arbor: University of Michigan. Cited by Kazanjian, pp. 59–60.

35. Albert B. Prescott, "Recommendation Letter" (1886). Frederick Novy Papers. BHL, Ann Arbor: University of Michigan. Cited by Kazanjian, p. 61.

36. "Albert Benjamin Presott," Memorial Service. Ann Arbor, MI: Private printing, 1906.

37. Proceedings of the Board of Regents (1886–1891), University of Michigan. The other two graduates in the chemistry program were equally successful in their respective fields. Louis Munroe Dennis (1863–1936) became a pioneer in the subject of industrial chemistry at Cornell University, where he taught from 1887 to 1930; Edward Demill Campbell (1863–1925), after four years as a chemist working in industry, returned to the University of Michigan in 1890 as an assistant professor of metallurgy. In 1905, he was appointed director of the Chemical Laboratory, remaining at the university until his death.

38. Ruth Good, "Dr. Frederick G. Novy: Biographic Sketch," *University of Michigan Medical Bulletin* 16 (1950): 257–268.

39. Frederick Novy, "The Hygienic Institute at Berlin," *The Pharmaceutical Era* 2 (November 1888): 426–427.

40. Ibid.

41. Vaughan, *A Doctor's Memories*.

42. F.G. Novy, "The Hygienic Laboratory," *The Michigan Alumnus* 6 (1900): 242–244.

43. Ibid.

44. Ibid.

45. Victor Vaughan, "First Quarterly Report, Michigan State Laboratory of Hygiene," *Report of the Michigan State Board of Health* 15 (1887): 2–23.

46. Good, p. 261.

47. Vaughan, *A Doctor's Memories*; Richard Adler, *Victor Vaughan: A Biography of the Pioneering Bacteriologist, 1851–1929* (Jefferson, NC: McFarland, 2015).

48. Frederick G. Novy, *Directions for Laboratory Work in Bacteriology* (Ann Arbor: George Wahr, 1894).

49. Frederick Novy Papers, BHL.

50. Long, pp. 329–330.

51. Ibid.

52. Howard Markel, "Prescribing *Arrowsmith*," September 28, 2000, www.nytimes.com/books/00/09/24/bookend/bookend.html.

53. F.G. Novy, W.A. Perkins, R. Chambers and P.H. DeKruif, "The Rat Virus," *Journal of Infectious Diseases* 93, no. 2 (September-October 1953): 111–123. The story of the re-discovery of the rat virus provides an interesting scientific story. While studying trypanosome infections in rats during the first decades of the 20th century, Novy observed that infection with an unknown "filterable agent" was killing the animals. In 1935, samples of blood from infected animals were placed in storage, initially in a refrigerator, but later removed to a storage shelf, where they were forgotten. In 1951, the samples were discovered, and used to infect laboratory rats. What was by then recognized as a (Kilham) rat virus was still viable.

Chapter 11

1. The caveat here was that while education for middle-class Jews was stressed, most of the Jewish population was orthodox and literally dirt-poor. Education, such as it was, was primarily religious and generally provided for only the males. Think *Fiddler on the Roof* without the singing.

2. Harriet Pass Freidenreich, *Female, Jewish and Educated: The Lives of Central European University Women* (Bloomington: Indiana University Press, 2002), p. 7–8.

3. "Kovno," http://www.jewishencyclopedia.com/articles/9490-kovno.

4. Freidenreich, p. 8.

5. Mary R.S. Creese, *Ladies in the Laboratory II: West European Women in Science, 1800–1900* (Lanham, MD: Scarecrow, 2004, p. 130). Augsburg (1857–1943) was a member of the Association of Progressive Women's Organizations, arguing for "radical" ideas such as free rather than state-approved marriages and women's suffrage. She was also a member of the

Independent Social Democrats and a member of the pacifist movement between the world wars. Her stand against the Nazis, and Adolf Hitler in particular, forced her in exile in Switzerland. Luxemburg (1864–1919), socialist, and founder of the Spartacus League, forerunner of the German Communist Party, was a participant in the Marxist uprising which followed the war. During the rioting she was arrested and subsequently murdered.

6. Ibid., p. 255.
7. Ibid., pp. 130–131, 255.
8. Joseph Longshore, "An Introductory Lecture at the Opening of the Female Medical College of Pennsylvania," http://doctordoctress.org/islandora/object/islandora%3A1496.
9. *Laws of the General Assembly of the Commonwealth of Pennsylvania Passed at the Session of 1850*, Act 148: 171, "Laws of the General Assembly," http://archive.org/stream/lawsofgeneralas1850penn/lawsofgeneralas1850penn_djvu.txt, cited by Steven Peitzman, *A New and Untried Course: Woman's Medical College and Medical College of Pennsylvania, 1850–1998* (New Brunswick, NJ: Rutgers University Press, 2000), p. 11.
10. "An Inventory of the Lewis-Fussell Family Papers," http://www.swarthmore.edu/library/friends/ead/5087lefu.xml; "Graceanna Lewis in the Delaware Valley," http://www.dvoc.org/DelValOrniHistory/LewisGraceanna/LewisGraceanna.htm; Lewis would become among the most important ornithologists in the region.
11. "Graceanna Lewis."
12. "Longshore Family Papers," http://dla.library.upenn.edu/dla/pacscl/ead.html?id=PACSCL_DUCOM_WMSC075. Also cited by Peitzman, p. 10.
13. Elizabeth Fee and Theodore Brown, "An Eventful Epoch in the History of Your Lives," *American Journal of Public Health* 94, no. 3 (March 2004): 367.
14. "William James Mullin," http://www.findagrave.com/cgi-bin/fg.cgi?page=gr&GRid=14434523.
15. "Changing the Face of Medicine: Dr. Ann Preston," https://www.nlm.nih.gov/changingthefaceofmedicine/physicians/biography_256.html.
16. Marilyn Ogilvie, Joy Harvey and Margaret Rossite, eds., *The Biographical Dictionary of Women in Science* (New York: Routledge, 2000), "Hannah Myers Longshore," pp. 802–803.
17. *Eighteenth Annual Announcement of the Woman's Medical College of Pennsylvania, for the Session of 1867–1868* (Philadelphia: Jas. B. Rodgers, 1867), p. 5–6. Cited by Peitzman, p. 28.
18. Peitzman. Hale was also the composer of the nursery rhyme "Mary Had a Little Lamb."

19. *Ibid.*, and Alice Felt Tyler, *Freedom's Ferment: Phases of American Social History to 1860* (Minneapolis: Lund, 1944), p. 438. The context of the term "female" during the 1860s is important in understanding the opposition of Hale, and indeed other women, many of whom were associated with the abolitionist movement. The British naturalist Charles Darwin had recently published his work *On the Origin of Species*, in which the term "female" was liberally applied in describing the sexual reproduction of animals. In what may appear quaint (or perhaps not) in the 21st century, the equation of humans and less evolved animals appeared offensive to a portion of the population (Renee Bergland, *Maria Mitchell and the Sexing of Science* [Boston, MA: Beacon, 2008], p. 173).
20. Lori Walsh and James Poupard, "Lydia Rabinowitsch, Ph.D., and the Emergence of Clinical Pathology in Late 19th-Century America," *Archives of Pathology and Laboratory Medicine* 113, no. 11 (November 1989): 1303–1308.
21. Creese, p. 131.
22. *Report of the Provost of the University of Pennsylvania for the Three Years Ending October 31, 1892* (Philadelphia: University of Pennsylvania Press, 1893),p. 90. Also cited by Walsh, p. 1304. Joseph McFarland, "The Beginning of Bacteriology in Philadelphia," *Bulletin of the History of Medicine* 5 (1937): 149–198. The Class of 1893–1894 included David Hendricks Bergey. Bergey would be appointed as Thomas A. Scott Fellow at the University of Pennsylvania a year later. Bergey would become known to future microbiologists as a result of serving several decades later as chair of a committee within the Society of American Bacteriologists—now known as the American Society for Microbiology—which produced the first edition of *Bergey's Manual of Determinative Bacteriology* (1925).
23. Richard Adler, *Victor Vaughan: A Biography of the Pioneering Bacteriologist* (Jefferson, NC: McFarland, 2014).
24. Cited by Walsh.
25. Walsh, p. 1305. Henry (1844–1919) attended Princeton University in the 1860s, though he did not graduate. In 1863, as a pitcher for the Princeton Nassaus, Henry allegedly became the first player to develop a curve ball (Donald Grant Herring, "The Pioneer of Curved Pitching Coming Back," *Princeton Alumni Weekly* 16, no. 34 (May 31, 1916): 798. Henry received his medical degree from the College of Physicians and Surgeons in New York in 1868.
26. Walsh; "Helen L. Betts," *Viennapedia*, http://viennapedia.viennahistory.org/people/betts-helen-l.

27. Woman's Medical College of Pennsylvania, *Faculty Minutes* (October 5, 1895): 358–359, cited by Walsh.

28. Woman's Medical College of Pennsylvania, *Faculty Minutes* (October 19, 1895): 363–364, cited by Walsh. The presence of yeast in some tumors gave rise to a popular theory during that period that yeast was the etiological agent of cancers. Some believed that yeast was the agent of rabies as well.

29. Woman's Medical College of Pennsylvania, *Faculty Minutes* (May 16, 1896): 434–435, cited by Walsh, p. 1305.

30. Walsh.

31. Walsh.

32. Peitzman, p. 77.

33. Walsh, pp. 1305–1306.

34. Catherine Macfarlane, unpublished autobiography, p. 21; Archives and Special Collections on Women in Medicine, Medical College of Pennsylvania Hahnemann University (now Drexel University College of Medicine), cited by Peitzman, p. 77. Dr. Macfarlane (1877–1969) was a student at WCM from 1895 to 1898, later becoming a member of the faculty. She was a well-known gynecologist and cancer researcher, honored in 1951 with the Lasker Clinical Medical Research Award for establishment of treatment centers for women.

35. Creese, p. 131.

36. B. Orland, "Cow's Milk and Human Disease: Bovine Tuberculosis and the Difficulties Involved in Combating Animal Diseases," *Food and History* 1 (2003):179–202.

37. Sandra Chaff, et al., eds., *Women in Medicine: A Bibliography of the Literature on Women Physicians* (Metuchen, NJ: Scarecrow, 1977), p. 942.

38. Walsh, p. 1306.

39. WMC *Faculty Minutes* (February 19, 1898): 105, cited by Walsh, p. 1306.

40. WMC *Faculty Minutes* (March 19, 1898): 111, cited by Walsh.

41. WMC *Faculty Minutes* (April 16, 1898): 122, cited by Walsh.

42. Adelaide Ward Peckham, "The Influence of Environment Upon the Biological Processes of the Various Members of the Colon Group of Bacilli: An Experimental Study," *Science* 5, no. 130 (June 25, 1897): 981–985.

43. Creese, p. 134.

44. *Ibid.*, p. 131.

Chapter 12

1. Simon Flexner and James Thomas Flexner, *William Henry Welch and the Heroic Age of American Medicine* (Baltimore, MD: The Johns Hopkins University Press, 1941), p. 138.

2. J. Howard Brown, "Theobald Smith, 1859–1934," *Journal of Bacteriology* 30,, no. 1 (July 1935): 1–3.

3. Theobald Smith, "The Diagnostic and Prognostic Value of the Bacillus Tuberculosis in the Sputum of Pulmonary Diseases," *Albany Medical Annals* 5, no. 7 (July 1884): 193–198, and *Albany Medical Annals* 5, no. 8 (August 1884): 233–236. William Welch had by this time also published an account of Koch's bacteriological procedures. So whether Smith was the first to introduce these to American researchers, or was one of several, falls into the permanently unresolved category of scientific priority.

4. Hans Zinsser, "Biographical Memoir of Theobald Smith," *National Academy of Sciences of the United States of America* 17 (1936): 259–303; Theobald Smith, "Relation Between Bovine and Human Tuberculosis," *Medical News* 80, no. 8 (February 22, 1902): 343–346.

5. Smith, "Relation," and Theobald Smith, "Preliminary Observations on the Microorganism of Texas Fever," *Medical News* 55 (1889): 689–693.

6. Flexner and Flexner, p. 163.

7. "William Hallock Park," *American Journal of Public Health* 29, no. 5 (May 1939): 530–531.

8. *Ibid.*

9. Thomas Neville Bonner, *American Doctors and German Universities* (Lincoln: University of Nebraska Press, 1963), p. 116.

10. "Rufus Cole," www.nap.edu/catalog/573/biographical-memoirs-v50, (1979), pp. 118–129.

Bibliography

Books

Adler, Richard. *Cholera in Detroit: A History.* Jefferson, NC: McFarland, 2013.

Adler, Richard. *Victor Vaughan: A Biography of the Pioneering Bacteriologist, 1851–1929.* Jefferson, NC: McFarland, 2015.

Adler, Richard, and Elise Mara. *Typhoid Fever: A History.* Jefferson, NC: McFarland, 2016.

Algeo, Matthew. *The President Is a Sick Man.* Chicago: Chicago Review, 2011.

Alibeck, Kenneth, Catherine Lobanova and Serguei Popov. *Bioterrorism and Infectious Agents.* New York: Springer Science+Business Media, 2005.

Bergland, Renee. *Maria Mitchell and the Sexing of Science.* Boston: Beacon, 2008.

Biggs, H.M. *A Brief History of the Campaign Against Tuberculosis in New York City.* New York: New York City Department of Health, 1908.

Bonner, Thomas Neville. *American Doctors and German Universities.* Lincoln: University of Nebraska Press, 1963.

Bonner, Thomas Neville. *Becoming a Physician: Medical Education in Great Brirain, France, Germany and the United States, 1750–1945.* New York: Oxford University Press, 1995.

Brock, Thomas. *Robert Koch: A Life in Medicine and Bacteriology.* Washington, D.C.: American Society for Microbiology, 1999.

Brock, Thomas, ed. *Milestones in Microbiology.* Washington, D.C.: American Society for Microbiology, 1975.

Bulloch, William. *The History of Bacteriology.* New York: Dover, 1979.

Chaff, Sandra, et al., eds. *Women in Medicine: A Bibliography of the Literature on Women Physicians.* Metuchen, NJ: Scarecrow, 1977.

Clark, Paul F. *Pioneer Microbiologists of America.* Madison: University of Wisconsin Press, 1961.

Cohen, Barnett. *Chronicles of the Society of American Bacteriologists: 1899–1950.* Baltimore: Waverly, 1950.

Creese, Mary R.S. *Ladies in the Laboratory II: West European Women in Science, 1800–1900.* Lanham, MD: Scarecrow, 2004.

Ernst, H.C. *Infectiousness of Milk: Result of Investigations Made for the Trustees of the Massachusetts Society for Promoting Agriculture.* Cambridge, UK: The Riverside, 1895.

Fleming, Donald. *William H. Welch and the Rise of Modern Medicine.* Boston: Little, Brown, 1954.

Flexner, Simon, and James Thomas Flexner. *William Henry Welch and the Heroic Age of American Medicine.* Baltimore: Johns Hopkins University Press, 1993.

Freidenreich, Harriet Pass. *Female, Jewish and Educated: The Lives of Central European University Women.* Bloomington: Indiana University Press, 2002.

Geison, Gerald. *The Private Science of Louis Pasteur.* Princeton, NJ: Princeton University Press, 1996.

Gradmann, Christoph. *Laboratory Disease: Robert Koch's Medical Bacteriology.* Baltimore: Johns Hopkins University Press, 2009.

Heymann, Bruno. *Robert Koch. I. Teil. 1843–1882.* Leipzig, Germany: Akademische Verlagsgesellschaft, 1932.

Hubbard, William M., and Nicholas H. Steneck. *The Origins of Michigan's Leadership in the Health Sciences.* Ann Arbor, MI: Historical Center for the Health Sciences, 1995.

Johnson, George A. *The Purification of Public Water Supplies*. Washington: Government Printing Office, 1913.

Kazanjian, Powel. "The Beginnings of Bacteriology in American Medicine: Works of Frederick Novy, 1888-1933." Dissertation Submitted for Degree of Doctor of Philosophy. Ann Arbor: University of Michigan, 2012.

Kirchner, Martin. "Kreisphysikus in Wollstein." *Robert Koch*. Berlin: Verlag Julius Springer, 1924.

Klebs, Edwin. *Beiträge Zur Pathologischen Anatomie Der Schusswunden* [Contributions to the Pathologic Anatomy of Battle Wounds]. Leipzif: Vogel, 1872.

Koch, Robert. *Untersuchungen Uber Die Aetiologie Der Wundinfectionskrankheiten* [Studies on the Etiology of Wound Infectious Disease]. Leipzig: Vogel, 1878.

Leavitt, Judith Walzer, and Ronald L. Numbers, eds. *Sickness and Health in America*. Madison: University of Wisconsin Press, 1978.

Lechevalier, Hubert, and Morris Solotorovsky. *Three Centuries of Microbiology*. New York: Dover, 1974.

Manley, James R. *Letters Addressed to the Board of Health and to Richard Riker, Recorder of the City of New-York*. New York: Peter van Pelt, 1832.

Morris, Peter. *Catcher*. Chicago: Ivan R. Dee, 2009.

Novy, Frederick. "University of Michigan Student Notebooks." Independent Study in Chemistry (1885). Frederick Novy Papers. Bentley Historical Library (BHL), Ann Arbor: University of Michigan.

Novy, Frederick G. *Directions for Laboratory Work in Bacteriology*. Ann Arbor: George Wahr, 1894.

Ogilvie, Marilyn, Joy Harvey and Margaret Rossiter, eds. *The Biographical Dictionary of Women in Science*. New York: Routledge, 2000.

Peitzman, Steven. *A New and Untried Course: Woman's Medical College and Medical College of Pennsylvania, 1850-1998*. New Brunswick, NJ: Rutgers University Press, 2000.

Prudden, Lillian. *Biographical Sketches and Letters of T. Mitchell Prudden*. New Haven, CT: Yale University Press, 1927.

Reed, Walter, Victor Clarence Vaughan and Edward Oram Shakespeare. *Report on the Origin and Spread of Typhoid Fever in United States Military Camps During the Spanish War of 1898*. Washington, D.C.: Government Printing Office, 1904.

Shah, Sonia. *Pandemic*. New York: Farrar, Straus and Giroux, 2016.

Shakespeare, Edward O. *Report on Cholera in Europe and India*. Washington, D.C.: Government Printing Office, 1890.

Shumway, Henry. *A Hand-Book on Tuberculosis Among Cattle*. Boston: Roberts Brothers, 1895.

Thompson, W. Gilman. *Practical Dietetics, with Special Reference to Diet in Disease*. New York: Appleton, 1903.

Tyler, Alice Felt. *Freedom's Ferment: Phases of American Social History to 1860*. Minneapolis: Lund, 1944.

Vaughan, Victor. *A Doctor's Memories*. Indianapolis: Bobbs-Merrill, 1926.

Vaughan, Victor Clarence, and Frederick George Novy. *Ptomaines and Leucomaines: Or the Putrefactive and Physiological Alkaloids*. Philadelphia: Lea Brothers & Co., 1888.

Winslow, C.E.A. *The Life of Hermann Biggs*. Philadelphia: Lea & Febiger, 1929.

Wintermute, Bobby. *Public Health and the U.S. Military: A History of the Army Medical Department, 1818-1917*. New York: Routledge, 2011

Periodicals and Reports

Albany Medical Annals.
American Journal of Clinical Pathology.
American Journal of Dermatopathology.
American Journal of Medical Sciences.
American Journal of Public Health.
Annals of Medical History.
Arch Path Anat Physiol Klin Med [Virchow's Archives].
Archives of Pathology & Laboratory Medicine.
Beiträge Zur Biologie Der Pflanzen.
Berliner Klinischen Wochenschrift.
Bibliotek Laeger.
Boston Medical and Surgical Journal.
Buffalo Medical and Surgical Journal.
Bulletin of the History of Medicine.
Bulletin of the Johns Hopkins Hospital.
Columbia University Bulletin.
Commonwealth of Pennsylvania, State Board of Health.

Danish Medical Bulletin.
Eighteenth Annual Announcement of the Woman's Medical College of Pennsylvania, for the Session of 1867–1868.
Eighth Annual Report of the State Board of Connecticut for the Year Ending November 1, 1885.
Fifteenth Annual Report of the Secretary of the State Board of Health of the State of Michigan for the Fiscal Year Ending June 30, 1887.
First Annual Report of the Secretary of the State of Michigan.
Food and History.
Gesammelte Abhandlungen.
Harvard Alumni Bulletin.
History and Philosophy of the Life Sciences.
Johns Hopkins Hospital Bulletin.
Journal of American Medical Veterinary Association.
Journal of Bacteriology.
Journal of Chemical Education.
Journal of Experimental Medicine.
Journal of General Physiology.
Journal of Infectious Diseases.
Journal of Physiology [London].
Journal of the American Medical Association.
Journal of the Senate of the State of Michigan, 1887, Vol. 2.
Lancet.
Laws of the General Assembly of the Commonwealth of Pennsylvania Passed at the Session of 1850.
Light: Science and Applications.
Medical Annals, Medical Society of the County of Albany.
Medical History.
Medical News.
Medical Times and Gazette.
Michigan Alumnus.
Mittheilungen aus dem Kaiserlichen Gesundheitsamte.
National Academy of Sciences.
Nature.
New England Journal of Medicine.
New York Medical Journal.
Pennsylvania Magazine of History and Biography.
Pharmaceutical Era.
Philadelphia Medical Times.
Princeton Alumni Weekly.
Proceedings of the American Academy of Arts and Sciences.
Proceedings (Baylor University Medical Center).
Regents of the University of Michigan vs. Preston B. Rose, Silas H. Douglas, Appellant, State of Michigan, Supreme Court, in Chancery, 1881.
Report of the Michigan State Board of Health (1887).
Report of the Provost of the University of Pennsylvania for the Three Years Ending October 31, 1892.
Science.
Thirteenth Annual Report of the Secretary of the State Board of Health of the State of Michigan for the Fiscal Year Ending September 30, 1885.
Transactions.
Twelfth Annual Report of the Secretary of the State Board of Health of the State of Michigan for the Fiscal Year Ending September 30, 1884.
University of Michigan, Board of Regents. *Proceedings of the Board of Regents (1876–1881.)*
University of Michigan Medical Bulletin.
Woman's Medical College of Pennsylvania. *Faculty Minutes.*
Yale Journal of Biology and Medicine

Newspapers

Litchfield County Leader.
New York Times.

Websites

"Behind the Frieze—Hermann Michael Biggs." http://www.lshtm.ac.uk/library/archives/history/frieze/biggs.html.
"A Brief History of Public Health." www.muskegonhealth.net/aboutus/documents/history.pdf.
"Changing the Face of Medicine: Dr. Ann Preston." https://www.nlm.nih.gov/changingthefaceofmedicine/physicians/biography_256.html.
"Chicago." http://encyclopedia.chicagohistory.org/pages/878html.
Cima, Gregg. "Legends: Teacher, Researcher and Inventor: Heinrich J. Detmers." https://www.avma.org/News/JAVMANews/Pages/130601g.aspx.
"The Dean's Lecture Series: The Cartwright Lecture." http://www.cumc.columbia.edu/events/deanlectures/cartwright.html.

"Department of Bacteriology and Serology and the Hygienic Laboratory." www.umhistory.dc.umich.edu/history/Faculty_History/Medical_Depertment_History/Department_of_Bacteriology.html.

"Graceanna Lewis in the Delaware Valley." http://www.dvoc.org/DelValOrniHistory/LewisGraceanna/LewisGraceanna.htm.

"Helen L. Betts." *Viennapedia*, http://viennapedia.viennahistory.org/people/betts-helen-l.

"History of Medical Practice in Illinois." https://archive.org/details/historyofmedical02illi.

"History of the Agar Plate." http://www.labnews.co.uk/features/history-of-the-agar-plate-01-11-2005/.

"History, State Microscopical Society of Illinois." www.smsi.org/history.html.

"Invention of the Catcher's Mask." http://bestblog.mlblogs.com/2006/02/16/the-invention-of-the-catchers-mask/.

"An Inventory of the Lewis-Fussell Family Papers." http://www.swarthmore.edu/library/friends/ead/5087lefu.xml.

"Kovno." http://www.jewishencyclopedia.com/articles/9490-kovno.

Longshore, Joseph. "An Introductory Lecture at the Opening of the Female Medical College of Pennsylvania." http://doctordoctress.org/islandora/object/islandora%3A1496.

"Longshore Family Papers." http://dla.library.upenn.edu/dla/pacscl/ead.html?id=PACSCL_DUCOM_WMSC075.

Markel, Howard. "Prescribing *Arrowsmith*." www.nytimes.com/books/00/09/24/bookend/bookend.html.

"Rabies Past and Present." http://www.preciousorganics.com.au/pages/rabies-past-and-present.

"Rufus Cole." www.nap.edu/catalog/573/biographical-memoirs-v50.

Runyon, Emily Chenault. "Remembering Victor C. Vaughan." Notes from Dr. Emily C. Runyon concerning her medical student days at Ann Arbor. http://www.vaughan.org/bios/vcv/images/winfreyLetter.jpg.

Russell, Harry Luman." http://www.asm.org/index.php/choma3/71-membership/archives/852-russell-harry-luman.

"Stanford Medicine." http://elane.stanford.edu/wilson/html/chap22/chap22-sect3.html.

"T. Mitchel Prudden and the First American Use of Vaccine." http://pathology.columbia.edu/mitchellprudden.html.

"Transformation and Tradition." vet.osu.edu/assets/pdf/about/125Anniversary.pdf.

"William James Mullin." http://www.findagrave.com/cgi-bin/fg.cgi?page=gr&GRid=14434523.

Index

Numbers in ***bold italics*** refer to pages with photographs.

Abbe, Ernst 222*n*38
Abbott, Alexander Crever 61, ***61***, 68, 69, 150, 217, 220
Abbott, William Osler 61, 62
Abel, John 8
Allport, Walter 233*n*32
American Medical Association, reform in medical education 7
Anderson, Thomas 40
anthrax 17–23, ***20***, 44, 45, 50
Arnold, Julius 109, 117
Arrowsmith 197, 198
Audouin, Jean Victor 40
Aufrecht, Emanuel 74
Augsberg, Anita 202, 233*n*5
Avery, Charles 168, 220
Avery, Oswald 33

Bacon, Francis 108
Baker, Henry 180, 181
Ball, Michael Valentine 208
Bartholow, Robert 69
Belfield, William 11, 70, 71, 226*n*10; addressing Koch's critics 78–80; demonstration of Koch's postulates 72–74
Bellevue Medical College 59, 63, 110, 111, 129, 131, 137, 139, 141
Bergey, David 61, 234*n*22
Betts, Helen 207, 208
Bigelow, Henry Jacob 129
Biggs, Hermann Michael 63, 64, 124, ***124***, 125, 145, 218, 219
Billings, John Shaw ***141***, 142
Billroth, Theodor 10, 27, 77
Birge, Edward Ashael 62, 64
Bollinger, Otto 146
Bottini, Enrico 40
Bowditch, Henry 5, 170
Bretonneau, Pierre 51
Broomall, Anna Elizabeth 211
Bryan, William Jennings 63
Bryant, Joseph 124, 228*n*32
Burdon-Sanderson, John 23, 81, 136, 222*n*27, 226*n*26
Burrill, Thomas Jonathan 59, 60, ***60***, 214

Cagniard-Latour, Baron Charles 34, 35, 37
Campbell, Edward Demill 233*n*37
Cartwright Lecture 11; origin 70
Carver, George Washington 64
Chauveau, Auguste 75
Cheesman, Timothy Matlack 123
cholera 18; German Commission 29, ***159***
Clark, Alonzo 129
Cleveland, Pres. Grover 62, 160, 165, 228*n*32, 231*n*7
Cohn, Ferdinand 19, 22, 23, 26, 45, 60, 71, 83, 136, 222*n*18, 223*n*43, 224*n*33, 226*n*5
Cohnheim, Julius 10, 22, 23, 47, 48, 77, 81, 109, ***135***, 135–139, 142, 222*n*25, 228*n*12; death 146
Cole, Rufus 219, 220
Columbia University 59
Conn, Herbert William 61, 65, 68, 69
Corbin, Henry Clark 230*n*27
Councilman, William 65
Crookshank, Edgar 54

Darwin, Charles 76, 135, 226*n*12, 234*n*19
Davaine, Casimir 19, 24, 40–45, 224*n*19
Davis, Nathan 7
de Forest, Lee 106
de Kruif, Paul Henry 197, ***197***, 198
Delafield, Francis ***107***, 108, 110–113, 123, 130, 131, 137, 139, 140, 227*n*9
de la Fontaine, Marc 186, 188, 232*n*30
Dennis, Frederic 139, 144
Dennis, Louis Munroe 233*n*37
Detmers, Heinrich Janssen 64, 65
Douglas, Silas 177–179
Dulles, Charles Winslow 54

Ehrlich, Paul 74, 85, 103, 219, 229*n*7
Eidam, Eduard 22, 222*n*18
Eliot, Charles 173
Ernst, Harold 59, 69, 103, 104, ***169***, 216; death 173; education 168, 169; study with Koch 170
Escherich, Theodor 229*n*37

Farnam, George Bronson 108
Finkelnberg, Karl 28

Finlay, Carlos 55
Fischer, Bernhard 29
Fischer, Eduard 201, 202
Fishbein, Morris 197
Fisher, Henry Middleton 207
Fleming, Alexander 226n26
Flexner, Abraham 220
Flexner, Simon 69, 150, 151, 217, 220
Flint, Austin 140, 141, 144
Flügge, Carl 126, 147–149
Formad, Henry 3, 11, 57, 60, 76–78, 80–83, 145, 152, *155*, 156, 157, 214, 220, 225n8, 226n25, n29, 229n5; death 90; on lack of contagion 85–89; skepticism on bacillus as agent of tuberculosis 153, 154
Formad, Marie 61
Fracastoro, Girolamo 33
Fraenkel, Carl 67, 100, 101, 191–193
Franco-Prussian War 2, 16, 43, 44, 171, 221n12
French, Morris 157, 159
Frobenius, Wilhelm 145–148 229n37
Frosch, Paul 103

Gaffky, Georg 28, 29, 31, 74, 161
Garfield, Pres. James 230n27
Germ Theory of Disease 6, 68, 117, 139, 206; see also Henle, Jacob
Gibbes, Heneage 84, *161*, 162, 164, 192, 220, 230n18, 231n1
Gibbs, Josiah 106
Gilman, Daniel Coit 142, 143, 145, 147
Goldthwaite, Henry 140, 228n25
The Greater Journey: Americans in Paris 5

Hallier, Ernst 17
Halstead, William 150, 229n46
Hansen, Gerhard Henrik Armaur 52, 224n40
Harrington, Mark 178, 231n7
Harvard 8, 59, 69, 76, 103, 110, 168–170
Hasse, Karl Ewald 14
Hektoen, Ludvig 69, 109
Henle, Friedrich Gustav Jacob 14, 35, *35*, 36; role in Germ Theory 36–38, 40, 41, 43, 54, 115, 223n12
Henry, Frederick Porteous 207, 234n25
Hershey-Chase Experiment 32, 33
Hesse, Angelina Fannie 92
Hesse, Walther 28, 92
Heubner, Johann 133
Hilgard, Eugene 178, 179
Holmes, Bayard Taylor 65
Holmes, Oliver Wendell, Sr. 5, 38
Hoppe-Seyler, Felix 10, 228n10
Hueppe, Ferdinand 94, 117, 190
Hunt, William 76, 77, 80
Hygienic Laboratory, University of Michigan *193*, 194

Jackson, James, Jr. 5
Jackson, John Barnard Swett 110
Jacobi, Abraham 131

Janeway, Edward Gamaliel 110, 131
Johns Hopkins School of Medicine 8, 53, 59
Johnston, Wyatt 69
Jordan, Edwin Oakes 61, 68, 69, *69*, 123, 124, 196

Kellogg, John 181, 232n14
Kelly, Howard 150, 229n46
Klebs, Edwin 10, 16, 17, 24, 43, *43*, 44, 51, 73, 82, 104, 136
Klein, Edward 54
Klein, Emanual 162, 164, 225n4, 230n18
Knapp, Hermann 64
Koch, Heinrich Hermann Robert 10, 11; childhood 13; death 31; director Hygiene Laboratory 30, 91; early education 14, 15; early practice 15, 17, 18; laboratory course in bacteriology 91, *100*; laboratory director 26; marriage 15, *16*, 17; member of *Gesundheitsamt* 28, 30; military career 16, 17; Sleeping Sickness Commission 31; study of anthrax 19–23, 28; University of Berlin 30; see also anthrax; cholera; Koch's Postulates; tuberculosis
Koch's Postulates 17, 29, 43–52, 115
Krause, Wilhelm 14, 15
Kützing, Friedrich Traugott 34

Lang, Arnold 201
Langley, John 185, 188
Leukort, Rudolf 134, 135
Lewis, George 91–93, 95
Lewis, Sinclair 197, 198
Lister, Joseph 29, 38, 39, *39*, 40, 71, 73, 118, 192
Loeffler, Friedrich 28, 30, 31, 43, 51, *51*, 61, 92, 125, 217
Longshore, Joseph Skelton 203, 204, 210
Longworth, Landon Rives 132
Loomis, Alfred 124, 125, 218
Louis, Pierre-Charles-Alexandre 5, 129
Ludwig, Carl 10, 133, *133*, 134, 146
Luxemburg, Rosa 202

MacFarland, Joseph 67
Magnin, Antoine 55, 214
Mall, Franklin 8, 68
Manley, James 6
Marx, Groucho 69
McGill University 69
McKinley, Pres. William 227n9
Meissner, George 14
Meltzer, Samuel 141
Meynert, Theodor 138
Microbe Hunters 197
Miescher, Friedrich 228n10
Missouri Botanical Gardens 62
Mixter, William 107
Moseley, Nathaniel 204
Müller, Johannes 9

Nasse, Friedrich 9
Neisser, Albert 52, 74

Index 243

New York University School of Medicine 64
Nichols, William 66
Northrup, William 113
Novy, Frederick George 8, 65, 69, 100, 103, 114, 185, *187*, 197, 233*n*53; death 198; education 186, 187; member Michigan faculty 189; participant in Koch's course 191
Nuttall, George 150, 217

Ogston, Alexander 27
Osborn, Henry Fairfield 70, 225*n*1
Osler, Georgina 61
Osler, Sir William 61, 70, 150, 152, 229*n*46

Pacini, Filippo 223*n*49, 230*n*14
Pammel, Louis Hermann 64
Panum, Peter Ludwig 24, 25, 222*n*30
Park, William Hallock 67, 69, 218, 219
Parke, Davis & Company 189
Pasteur, Louis 3, 32, 33, *33*, 34, 35, 39, 41–43, 52, 53, 63, 70, 71, 74, 118, 191, 221*n*2, 226*n*10
Peabody, George Livingston 132
pébrine 35
Peckham, Adelaide Ward 207, 212
Pengra, Charles 182
Pfeiffer, Richard 31, 103
Polle, Adolf 14
Pollender, Aloys 19, 41
Prescott, Albert 177, 178, 185, 188, 189
Preston, Ann 204
Prudden, Theophil Mitchell 59, 64, 91, 94, 95, 98, 103, 126, 129, 141, 145, 148, 149, 169, 170, 216, 218, 228*n*1; death 125; education 105–107, *108*; training in pathology 110–112
puerperal fever 38, 54

Quantrill, William 176, 231*n*5

Rabinowitsch-Kempner, Lydia 11; death 231; education 200, 201, *201*, 207; faculty, Woman's Medical College 209–212; Koch's laboratory 202; *see also* Woman's Medical College
Ranvier, Louis-Antoine 134, 138
Rayer, Pierre Francois 41, 224*n*19
Reed, Walter 55, 166, 167, 175, 217
Roberts, John 211
Roosevelt Hospital 113
Roscoe, Henry 188
Rose, Preston 179, 180
Ross, Ronald 225*n*4
Rous, Peyton 218
Roux, Emile 63, 196, 197
Rush Medical College 10, 70
Russell, Harry Luman 63; description of Koch's course 102, 103
Russell, Thomas Hubbard 106, 108, 218

Salmon, Daniel 65, 215
Salomonsen, Carl 48, 137, 149

Sargent, John Singer 229*n*46
Schenck, Leopold 138
Schorlemmer, Carl 188
Schwann, Theodor 34–37, 223*n*6
Sedgwick, William Thompson 66, *66*, 69
Seguin, Edward 129, 131
Sell, Eugen 27
Semmelweis, Ignaz 38
Sewall, Henry 195
Shakespeare, Edward Oram 11, *154*, 207; death 167; education 152; investigation of Asiatic 160, 161; member, Typhoid Board 166, 175; Philadelphia debate 154–156; typhoid epidemic in Pennsylvania 157–159
Sheffield Scientific School 106, 107, 129
Shibasaburo, Kitasato 52
Smith, Theobald 69, 215, *215*, 216, 233*n*33, 235*n*3
Society of American Bacteriologists 60, 61, 65, 66; origin 68, 69, 151, 234*n*22
Spanish-American War 195, 217
Spencer, Herbert 226*n*12
Sternberg, George 52, 55, 61, *62*, 74, 84, 150, 214, 217, 226*n*10
Stevens, Arthur Albert 208, 211
Stricker, Salomon 109, 138
Struck, Heinrich 27, 28

Thayer, Frederick 169
Traube, Ludwig 10
Trelease, William 62, 64
Treskow, Hermann 29
tuberculin 31, 63, 103, 170, 172, 219
tuberculosis 29, 31; agent *75*; infectious nature 37, 47, 48, 56, 75, 114
Tuskegee Institute 64
tyrotoxicon 182, 183

University of Berlin 30
University of Bern 43
University of Breslau 22, 23, 26, 27, 47, 135
University of Chicago 61, 103, 124
University of Glasgow 38, 40
University of Göttingen 14, 30
University of Illinois 59, 60
University of Maryland 61
University of Michigan 8, 53, 65, 100, 103, 128, 129, 177; *see also* Hygienic Laboratory
University of Pennsylvania 54, 57, 61, 67, 155, 206
University of Vienna 67
University of Wisconsin 62–64, 103

van Leeuwenhoek, Antonie 33, 34, 70, 223*n*4
Vaughan, Victor Clarence 8, 65, 69, 100, 128, 166, *175*, 188, 190; Dean 195; education 174–177; faculty appointment 180; member, Michigan State Board of Health 181, 182; participant in Koch's course 191
Victor Vaughan, a Biography of the Pioneering Bacteriologist 1

Villemin, Jean Antoine 37, 38, *46*, 47, 48, 78, 224*n*39
Virchow, Rudolf 10, 15, 44, 47, 77, 132, 135, 138, 153, 208
Virgil 222*n*11
von Baumgarten, Paul Clemens 48
von Behring, Emil 31, 196, 208, 219
von Bismarck, Otto 16, 27
von Bollinger, Otto 21, 22
von Hebra, Ferdinand 138
von Leyden, Ernst 132
von Pettenkofer, Max 3, 18, 30, 53, 146, 162, 164, 192, 194, 220, 223*n*49, 230*n*20
von Recklinghausen, Friedrich Daniel 10, 132, 133, 138
von Waldeyer-Hartz, Heinrich Wilhelm 132
von Wassermann, August Paul 220

Wagner, Ernst 134, 135
Warthin, Alfred Scott 195
Washington University 62
Watson, James Craig 178
Weeks, John Elmer 64
Weigert, Carl 25, 77, 136, 139, 146
Welch, William 8, 23, 59, 61, 63, 69, 70, 103, 111, 126, 127, *128*, 169, 170, 196, 214, 216–218, 228*n*1, 229*n*46; death 151; early education 127–129; studying pathology in Germany 131–139; working in Koch's laboratory 145–149
Wesleyan University 61, 69
Whipple, George 218
Wilhelm, Kaiser I 30
Williams, Charles Theodore 85
Winchell, Alexander 178
Wisconsin Geological and Natural History Survey 62, 63
Wöhler, Friedrich 14
Wolffhügel, Gustav 27
Woman's Medical College 11, 61, 67, 198, 201, 202; bacteriology department 208; establishment 202–205
Wood, Horatio 57, 225*n*8
Wood, James 131

Yale College 105–107, 110, 111, 113, 122, 128, 168
Yawkey, Thomas 227*n*3
Yellow Fever Commission 55
Yersin, Alexandre 52, 196

www.ingramcontent.com/pod-product-compliance
Lightning Source LLC
Chambersburg PA
CBHW051219300426
44116CB00006B/631